Memory Distortion

Memory Distortion

How Minds, Brains, and Societies
Reconstruct the Past

Editor
Daniel L. Schacter

Contributing Editors
Joseph T. Coyle
Gerald D. Fischbach
Marek-Marsel Mesulam
Lawrence E. Sullivan

Harvard University Press

Cambridge, Massachusetts
London, England / 1995

Library of Congress Cataloging-in-Publication Data

Memory distortion : how minds, brains, and societies reconstruct the
past / Daniel L. Schacter, editor ; Joseph T. Coyle . . . [et al.],
contributing editors.
    p.   cm.
  Papers originally presented at the first conference sponsored by
the Harvard Center for the Study of Mind, Brain, and Behavior in
Cambridge, Mass., May 6–8, 1994.
  Includes bibliographical references and index.
  ISBN 0-674-56675-0 (alk. paper)
  1. Memory disorders—Congresses. I. Schacter, Daniel L.
II. Coyle, Joseph T. III. Harvard Center for the Study of Mind,
Brain, and Behavior.
BF376.M46 1995
153.1'2—dc20   95-30479

Contents

Part VI   Concluding Reflections

    Memory Distortion: A Neurologist's Perspective   379
       MAREK-MARSEL MESULAM

16 Memory Distortion and Anamnesis:
    A View from the Human Sciences   386
       LAWRENCE E. SULLIVAN

    Contributors   403
    Index   407

Preface

Memory is the scaffolding upon which all mental life is constructed. It is, therefore, a worthy subject for the first conference sponsored by the Harvard Center for the Study of Mind, Brain, and Behavior (MBB), whose mission, broadly stated, is to chart the human mind, integrating the perspectives of neuroscience, the social sciences, and the humanities. MBB is one of five university-wide programs initiated by President Neil Rudenstine as part of a search for common ground among the diverse faculties that constitute Harvard University.

The Center is currently composed of twenty-five faculty who gather every six weeks or so to debate issues raised during a formal presentation by one of the members. These stimulating discussions have lowered the intellectual barriers that isolate one discipline from another, and they have raised expectations so that new research collaborations now seem likely. We want to know what questions and theoretical constructs arise at the interface between disciplines that may lead to a more profound understanding of mental life. What is it that needs to be explained? Success in this exciting effort depends on the willingness of established investigators to ask questions that might seem naive within the confines of their native disciplines. The going is slow at times, but it is precisely this interplay across discipline boundaries that defines one of the most significant benefits of university life.

Small study groups emerge from the parent MBB fellowship from time to time in order to explore a particular subject in a more intense, sustained manner. Memory, in all forms from cells to institutions, is the focus of the subgroup (Coyle, Fischbach, Mesulam, Schacter, and Sullivan) that planned the conference on which this volume is based. The conference was held at the American Academy of Arts and Sciences in Cambridge, Massachusetts, May 6–8, 1994.

We decided to emphasize memory *distortion* because this phenomenon sits at a crucial interface between neurobiology and psychology. It also raises important issues regarding institutional and societal memory and how distortion at these levels relates to the function of individuals. We also wanted to begin a constructive, candid discussion of the relationship between recognized forms of memory distortion and the politically charged subject of repressed memories. The so-called "false memory syndrome" is currently the subject of intense discussion in the lay press. But the issues should not be ignored by academics. On the contrary, one important goal of MBB is to determine how scientists and scholars from different fields might come together to contribute constructively to this type of debate.

Memories are never exact replicas of external reality. Psychophysical studies and electrical recordings from the brain have shown that incoming sensory information is not received passively. Survival depends on rapid transformation and interpretation of sensory stimuli based on expectations about how the world works. We interpret patterns of light that fall on a two-dimensional array of receptors in the retina as three-dimensional, richly textured scenes. In this sense all memories are "created" rather than simply "received." No memory or mental image exactly replicates the constellation of nerve impulses associated with the initial sensation. Past experience, encoded in the strength of synaptic connections throughout the activated neural networks, modifies incoming information.

Thoughts and emotions "emerge" from patterns of electrical impulses conducted along the fine processes of nerve cells. Our nerve cells function in much the same manner as do worm nerve cells. But our thoughts differ from worm thoughts because human nerve cells are arranged in more intricate and more adaptable circuits. To understand memory and memory distortion, it is important to understand the anatomy and chemical architecture of neural circuits that are active during the processing of explicit and implicit memories. The time is right. Advances at many levels of analysis have provided new opportunities for relating memory to specific brain functions.

New chemical transmitters have been uncovered, novel mechanisms of transmitter action have been described, and loci within the brain where they act have been identified with unprecedented precision. Plausible models of behavior have emerged from this new chemical architecture. Methods for recording the signals of single neurons or small groups of neurons in unanesthetized, behaving animals have led to important insights regarding the function of nerve cell ensembles that are active during the formation, consolidation, and recall of memories. Large ensembles of neurons can be monitored with imaging techniques based on positron emission or magnetic resonance. These noninvasive techniques have brought the human brain to center stage because they are capable of detecting patterns of neural activity through the intact skull. A remarkable diversity between individuals even when performing simple tasks is one of the most important early findings and one of the most relevant for students of memory distortion.

In the context of memory distortion, it is important to emphasize that the brain's functional architecture is not fixed. The strength of synaptic connections may increase or decrease as a function of past experience. Genes influence behavior, of course, and experience does too. It will be crucial to determine the limits of this remarkable synaptic plasticity. Recent studies have demonstrated a clear relationship between synaptic plasticity and simple forms of learning in invertebrates and vertebrates. These findings have immediate import for more complex phenomena associated with short-term and long-term memory in humans. Can memory distortion, normal and abnormal, be understood at the level of synaptic connections? What mechanisms might account for the recollection of a thought that has not emerged to the level of consciousness for a prolonged period of time?

The human brain need no longer be considered an impenetrable black box. We must crawl into the box and try to understand the brain as it functions in the context of human affairs. This requires that the advances in neuroscience be paralleled by equally creative thinking at the level of psychology and the behavior of societies. The most powerful neurobiological techniques will not be sufficient without clear definitions of important questions to be asked and the levels of understanding that are sought. There is a need for theories that relate neuronal activity to mental life. To understand how memories are formed and stabilized, we must move beyond insights gained about the first stages of sensory input and the final pathways of motor output to consider emotional valence, and the elusive phenomena associated with consciousness. Insights from the psychological level of analysis and from the studies of small groups and whole societies around the globe and through time must be incorporated.

A start must be made. Hence this volume and our choice of contributors, a group of investigators who would not have met one another at a conventional gathering with a more restricted scope. We want to test the premises of the new MBB initiative by exploring the phenomenon of memory distortion at all levels.

We are grateful to our colleagues in MBB for their time and energy and their bold pursuit of important questions. Shawn Bohen is the able administrator who has held the center together and brought us to this important launch. Chrissy Thurmond organized the meeting and kept track of every detail with infectious joy and energy. None of our efforts would have been possible without the generous support of the Dana Foundation and the steadfast commitment of the Foundation's leader, David P. Mahoney.

Gerald D. Fischbach
Joseph T. Coyle

Memory Distortion

Memory Distortion:
History and Current Status

Daniel L. Schacter

Akira Kurosawa's classic film *Rashomon* explores four eyewitness recollections of a violent episode. Even though all four witnesses ostensibly have viewed the same event, each person's recollection of it differs fundamentally from those of the others. All of the recollections are heavily influenced by the specific biases and needs of the individual rememberers, yet each of them expresses complete confidence in the validity of his or her version of what happened. Focusing on any single account of the episode alone, the viewer is easily convinced that a more or less approximate version of the truth is at hand; considering all four together, one is hopelessly confused about what did or did not happen. Indeed, by the film's conclusion, the viewer is left pondering whether and to what extent memories can ever tell us what "actually happened" at a particular time and place in the past.

Kurosawa's film highlights a fundamental observation that is central to this book: the output of human memory often differs—sometimes rather substantially—from the input. Remembering can fail not only because information is forgotten over time, but also because it is changed and distorted. Fortunately, memory operates with a high degree of accuracy across many conditions and circumstances. Indeed, it is possible to create conditions in which people exhibit impressively accurate levels of recollection, recalling hundreds of previously studied words (Mantyla, 1986) or recognizing thousands of previously viewed pictures (Standing, Conezio, and Haber, 1970). The fact that memory is often reliable makes a good deal of sense: just like other biologically based capacities, many features of memory are adaptations that help an organism to survive and prosper in its environment (see Anderson and Schooler, 1991; Rozin, 1976; Sherry and Schacter, 1987). Given the crucial role that memory plays in numerous aspects of everyday life, a memory system that consistently produced seriously distorted outputs would wreak havoc with our very existence. Nevertheless, everyday experience and laboratory research indicate clearly that memory is far from perfect, and that under certain circumstances it can be surprisingly inaccurate.

Memory distortion has long been a fundamental theoretical and empirical problem for cognitive psychologists who are interested in understanding how memories are encoded, stored, and retrieved (e.g., Bartlett, 1932; Neisser, 1967), and for researchers who are interested in such applied problems as the reliability of eyewitness testimony (e.g., Loftus, 1979). Memory distortion has also posed a major challenge for clinical psychologists and psychiatrists who are concerned with reconstructing and understanding the personal histories of their patients (e.g., Freud, 1899; Spence, 1984). These issues and concerns have recently become the focus of intense interest throughout psychology and psychiatry—and in society more generally—as a consequence of discussions and debates concerning the accuracy of recovered or repressed memories of childhood abuse (see Goldstein and Farmer, 1992; Harvey and Herman, 1994; Herman, 1992; Kihlstrom, in press; Lindsay and Read, 1994; Loftus, 1993; Loftus and Ketcham, 1994; Ofshe and Watters, 1994; Pedzek, 1994; Pendergrast, 1995; Read and Lindsay, 1994; Schacter, 1995; Schooler, 1994; Spence, 1994; Terr, 1994; Wright, 1994; Yapko, 1994). During the past several years, there has been an explosion of cases in which adults undergoing psychotherapy claim to have recovered long-repressed memories of sexual abuse at the hands of parents or other family members. Yet the accusations are frequently denied by people who believe that they have been wrongfully accused on the basis of false memories. Although the widespread incidence of child abuse in our society is increasingly recognized (Herman, 1992; Yapko, 1994), it is often difficult to determine whether and in what sense individual memories are true or false. Nevertheless, the extreme emotional stress of both the patients and their families highlights the need to understand more fully the conditions under which accuracy and distortion in memory are most likely to be observed.

Scientific interest in memory distortion is not restricted to cognitive psychologists and clinical psychiatrists. Moving downward from the cognitive/psychological level of analysis to the level of brain cells and systems, neuroscientists have provided relevant observations and ideas about the nature of distorted memory. For example, neuropsychologists have studied patients with certain kinds of brain damage who confabulate about episodes and events that never occurred (e.g., Moscovitch, 1989; Talland, 1965). Moreover, issues concerning memory distortion are related directly to fundamental questions about the biological basis of memory storage: Where and how are memories stored in the brain? How does the neural representation of a memory change over time? And how do hormones and other neuromodulators influence and perhaps alter the storage and retrieval of memories?

Issues and questions concerning memory distortion also arise when we move upward from the cognitive/psychological level of analysis to the level of social or collective memory. During the past decade there has been increasing interest in questions concerning how societies remember—and often misremember—their pasts. A prominent theme in this area of study is that societies often hold beliefs about their pasts that are based on stories and myths that develop and change over time, often bearing little resemblance to the events that initially gave rise to them (e.g., Fentress and Wickham, 1992; Hobsbawm and Ranger, 1983; Kammen, 1991; LeGoff, 1992). Thus, understanding the nature of collective memory is inextricably intertwined with understanding the nature of memory distortion. Yet here, too, issues pertaining to memory distortion are of more than purely academic concern. For example, recent attempts by various fringe groups to deny the occurrence of the Holocaust have alerted scholars and the lay public alike to the extraordinary dangers that are posed by willful distortion of collective memory (see, for example, Lipstadt, 1993; Vidal-Naquet, 1992).

It seems abundantly clear, then, that even though memory distortion traditionally has been viewed as a problem for psychologists, it is relevant to, and can be studied by, a broader range of scientists and scholars. This volume is predicated on the notion that our understanding of memory distortion will be enhanced by—and may even require—investigation and inquiry at several different levels of analysis by scientists and scholars from a variety of disciplines. In the chapters that follow, a distinguished group of psychologists, psychiatrists, neurobiologists, sociologists, and historians address issues and questions concerning the nature of memory distortion at levels of analysis ranging from the most "micro"—the workings of brain cells and synapses—to the most "macro"—the operations of societies and cultures.

The book is divided into five sections, each concerned with a perspective that represents a particular level and type of analysis: cognitive, psychopathological and psychiatric, neuropsychological, neurobiological, and sociocultural. A number of the contributors have worked directly on phenomena of memory distortion, and their work provides examples of, and ideas about, memory distortion in normal adults (Loftus, Feldman, and Dashiell, Chapter 1; McClelland, Chapter 2), children (Ceci, Chapter 3), brain-damaged patients (Moscovitch, Chapter 8), and various psychopathological populations (Krystal, Southwick, and Charney, Chapter 5; Mineka and Nugent, Chapter 6; Spiegel, Chapter 4). The chapters by Assman (Chapter 14), Kammen (Chapter 12), and Schudson (Chapter 13) all consider memory distortion at the level of cultures and societies. The work of other contributors has focused less specifically on memory distortion per se and is concerned with basic memory processes that are central to understanding the mechanisms that underlie distorted memory, such as the architecture of memory systems in the brain (Squire, Chapter 7), hormonal influences on learning and retrieval (McGaugh, Chapter 9), and cellular and synaptic mechanisms of memory (Swain et al., Chapter 10; Abel et al., Chapter 11).

By joining the work of researchers who have focused specifically on memory distortion with those who have been concerned with general issues in the analysis of memory, this volume offers a range of perspectives that place the problem of distortion within a broader context of memory research. Although the focus is on the analysis of distortion, it is important not to lose sight of the fact that memory is often accurate. But when distortion does occur, it can have important theoretical and practical implications. Accordingly, it seems useful to try to understand the nature of memory distortion at the various levels of analysis that are represented in this volume. The major purposes of this introductory chapter are threefold: to provide some historical background concerning approaches that have been taken to the understanding of memory distortion; to identify some of the major themes in the individual chapters that follow; and to highlight issues and problems for future investigation.

Memory Distortion: A Historical Overview

A central premise of this volume is that memory distortion can be usefully approached at different levels of analysis. Historically, however, the bulk of research and theorizing that has specifically addressed memory distortion has focused on the psychological level of analysis, either in laboratory studies of normal individuals or clinical investigations of psychopathology. The history of scientific thinking about memory distortion is therefore to a large extent a history of psychological approaches to the problem. Hence this historical review focuses primarily on psychological perspectives. However, relevant developments at both the neural and the sociocultural levels of analysis will be included in order to delineate some of the background that is relevant to all the perspectives represented in this book.

Late Nineteenth and Early Twentieth Century Perspectives

The latter part of the nineteenth century was an important time for the development of memory research. Although philosophers had offered observations and theories about the nature of memory for centuries, dating back to Aristotle's initial formulation of the laws of association (Sorabji, 1972), there was little or nothing in the way of systematic evidence that could be used as a scientific basis for proposing or rejecting theories concerning the nature of memory. All that changed in 1885, however, when the German psychologist Hermann Ebbinghaus published a now classic treatise in which he described the first application of the experimental method to the analysis of human memory (Ebbinghaus, 1885/1964). Most important with respect to memory distortion, Ebbinghaus introduced a methodological innovation that has proved to be essential to evaluating whether a memory is true or false: he gained control over the input to the memory system. In earlier philosophical and clinical treatises on memory, discussion centered on introspective recollections of past experiences by the writers themselves or by patients whom they observed. The problem with this sort of procedure is that the investigator typically has no reliable way to check the accuracy of a reported recollection. Ebbinghaus solved this problem by creating a set of to-be-remembered materials—his famous nonsense syllables—that he attempted to memorize. When he later tried to relearn these previously studied items, Ebbinghaus could check his remembered output against the actual record of what he initially studied. The importance of exerting experimental control over the input to memory is so widely accepted in most modern research that one easily forgets what a giant step Ebbinghaus took when he invented the procedure. Indeed, it is precisely the absence of control over, or knowledge of, the inputs to memory that has made the current debate over recovered/repressed memories so vexing. When patients claim to remember an episode from their distant past, it is often difficult to obtain unambiguous external corroboration that the alleged event actually occurred.

The first controlled studies that provided evidence of memory distortion were carried out by European investigators who were interested in the reliability and suggestibility of eyewitness testimony, particularly children's testimony. Ceci and Bruck (1993) have reviewed a number of these early studies. The French psychologist Alfred Binet (1900), for instance, exposed children to various objects and then tested their memories in the presence or absence of misleading questions. Binet found that misleading questions produced systematic distortions in children's recollections. In Germany, Stern (1910) described experiments in which the investigator staged an event in front of a group or a class, and later asked them questions about what happened and who did it. Like Binet, Stern reported that misleading questions could induce distorted memories, and he also observed that young children were apt to confuse real and imagined events. Evidence concerning the unreliability of eyewitness memory was summarized in a well-known monograph by the Harvard psychologist Hugo Munsterburg (1908; see also Loftus, 1979).

In addition to these empirical demonstrations of distorted memory, there were a number of relevant theoretical developments in the late nineteenth and early twentieth centuries. In experimental psychology, the predominant account of memory distortion held that stored memories fade, change, and alter spontaneously over time, although it was never specified exactly how such alterations took place (e.g., Kennedy, 1898). An alternative view was advanced in a wide-ranging theory of memory developed by the German biologist Richard Semon (Semon, 1904/1921; 1909/1923). Semon, little known today, invented the term *engram,* which is still sometimes used to refer to the physical change or trace in the brain that represents a memory. He also developed a relatively detailed theory of memory that placed great importance on the nature of, and relation between, encoding processes (what Semon called "engraphy") and retrieval processes (which he called "ecphory"). According to Semon, every act of engraphy (i.e., encoding and storing new information) involves some ecphory of thoughts, images, and memories that are activated by the current situation. Thus, a newly created engram is not a literal replica of reality, but is always an interpretation that includes retrieved information (see Bentley, 1899; Kuhlmann, 1906). If the input to the memory system is not an accurate reflection of reality, then the output will necessarily be distorted. Semon also argued that memory distortion arises because every act of ecphory constitutes an act of engraphy—that is, when we remember a past experience, it is encoded anew into the memory system. However, we may focus on or think about only certain aspects of the retrieved experience, thereby changing its subsequent memory representation. Semon's ideas, though ignored in his time, were prescient in many ways (Schacter, 1982; Schacter, Eich, and Tulving, 1978).

Working in a clinical setting, Sigmund Freud developed a rather different and far more influential approach to memory distortion. Freud's best known ideas about distortion are related to his still controversial notion of repression, which holds that painful memories are defensively excluded from consciousness. Although Freud defined the concept of repression differently at different times (Erdelyi, 1985), he consistently argued that recollection of past experience could be distorted by dynamic and defensive forces. Freud's discussions of the effects of early sexual trauma on adult psychopathology are also related to issues of memory distortion. In his early writings, Freud (1896) argued that repressed memories of sexual abuse and trauma cause persisting pathological symptoms, and contended that the task of psychoanalysis is to allow patients to retrieve lost traumatic memories.

As is now well known, however, Freud soon abandoned this "seduction theory" of early trauma in favor of the view that the "memories" that his patients retrieved were in fact fantasies or confabulations. Some have argued that Freud's turn away from the seduction theory was based on a self-serving need to ensure his own career advancement and involved suppression of relevant data (Masson, 1984). Others, however, have contended that the change of view reflected Freud's growing awareness of the susceptibility of his patients to suggestion, and his growing appreciation of the likelihood of obtaining false recollections with the procedures that he used in his early work (e.g., Erdelyi, 1985; Schimek, 1987). Erdelyi (1985, p. 68), for instance, concluded that Freud's initial formulation of the seduction theory was based on just a handful of cases, and that he changed his position only when confronted with the "implausibility, and in some cases impossibility, of some of these recollected incidents." Whatever the reasons for his change of view, it is clear that many aspects of Freud's later psychoanalytic thought were built on the notion that early memories are highly likely to be distortions that are produced by fantasy-based confabulations. For example, Freud (1910, p. 83) concluded that childhood memories are "only elicited at a later age when childhood is already past; in the process they are altered and falsified, and are put into the service of later trends, so that generally speaking they cannot be distinguished from phantasies." This theme was also evident in Freud's (1899) idea of "screen memories," which holds that recollections of early childhood experiences are often distortions that protect people from a more unpleasant reality hidden behind the superficial "screen" image that is presented to consciousness. As Spence (1984, p. 89) has pointed out, the difficulty with this idea is that "Freud was never able to provide a clear rule that would allow us to separate the 'real' memory— the central, veridical core—from the subsequent distortions." Unlike Ebbinghaus, Freud had no independent means of checking the accuracy of reported recollections, and therefore could never provide an entirely satisfying account of memory distortion.

The French psychiatrist Pierre Janet also made interesting clinical observations concerning memory distortion. Janet (1928) argued that "narrative memories" for everyday experiences are always reconstructed and frequently distorted (see Ross, 1991; van der Kolk and van der Hart, 1991). Like Semon, he contended that new experiences are encoded with respect to, and incorporated into, preexisting knowledge structures; accordingly, individual experiences may be very difficult to retrieve later as separate, distinct entities. Janet contrasted such reconstructive, narrative memories with traumatic memories, which he believed can preserve the exact details of disturbing events over long periods of time (Ellenberger, 1970; Perry and Laurence, 1984; van der Kolk and van der Hart, 1991). The question of whether traumatic experiences are in some way less subject to distortion than nontraumatic ones constitutes a point of great interest to contemporary clinicians and researchers, because it is central to the debates mentioned earlier concerning the accuracy of recovered memories.

Psychiatrists and psychologists also participated in a lively controversy concerning the experience of false recognition that is often referred to as "déjà vu": an intense feeling that we have already experienced an event that is occurring for the first time. Debate focused on whether this memory distortion is normal or pathological, whether it is best described as "false memory," "paramnesia," or "déjà vu," and whether different varieties of the phenomenon could be distinguished (for historical review, see Berrios, 1995).

Clinical observations of memory distortion in brain-damaged patients were also made during the turn-of-the-century period. Korsakoff (1889a,

1889b) described a striking form of amnesia that resulted from alcohol abuse. Known today as Korsakoff's syndrome, the disorder is characterized by a severe impairment of memory for recent and remote events (Butters and Cermak, 1980; Mayes, 1988). Shortly after Korsakoff's initial description of the syndrome, Bonhoeffer (1904) pointed out that such patients often produce extensive and sometimes bizarre confabulations concerning events that never occurred. These memory distortions contrasted sharply with the patients' inability to remember accurately even the simplest episodes from their day-to-day lives. At around the same time, Pick (1903) described the confabulatory phenomenon of reduplicative paramnesia, where patients become convinced that a familiar person or place has been "duplicated." Patients with this disorder, also known as Capgras syndrome, insist that two highly similar people or places exist when in fact there is only one.

1920–1970: Bartlett and Beyond

Although the turn-of-the-century period yielded observations and ideas concerning memory distortion, it did not provide much firm experimental evidence concerning the nature and basis of distortion. During the 1920s and 1930s, such evidence began to appear. A number of experiments were conducted in psychological laboratories that examined the hypothesis that memories change autonomously over time in a manner dictated by Gestalt laws of organization—that is, memories change spontaneously toward becoming "good Gestalts." For example, Wulf (1922) reported that memories of visual forms become more regular and symmetrical with increasing time after initial learning. Some subsequent researchers reported similar observations (e.g., Allport, 1930; Perkins, 1932), and Koffka (1935) cited these autonomous transformation effects as support for his Gestalt theory of memory. Others, however, argued that such effects are largely experimental artifacts (e.g., Gibson, 1929; Zangwill, 1937). Modern researchers have tended to agree with this latter view, and have thus dismissed the Gestalt account of memory distortion (e.g., Baddeley, 1976).

There is little doubt that the single most important development concerning memory distortion during this period was the publication of Sir Frederic Bartlett's (1932) classic monograph, *Remembering*. Bartlett exposed his subjects to an engaging story, an old Indian legend entitled "The War of the Ghosts." After hearing the story, subjects were asked to retell it on several occasions. Bartlett found that people rarely recalled all of the events in the story accurately; they often remembered occurrences that made general sense, or that fit their expectations of what should have happened, even though they were not in fact part of the original story. Bartlett also observed that the recollections of his participants changed—sometimes substantially—across multiple retellings of the story. Curiously, as Roediger,

Wheeler, and Rajaram (1993) point out, Bartlett's original results have not been replicated by others and may have been attributable to the specific test instructions that he gave to his subjects (see Gauld and Stephenson, 1967).

Nevertheless, on the basis of his observations Bartlett concluded that memories are imaginative reconstructions of past events that are heavily influenced by the rememberer's preexisting knowledge structures or *schemas*. The notion of a schema had originally been developed by the British neurologist Henry Head (1926) to refer to an organized mental representation of one's body. Bartlett applied this notion to memory, arguing that schemas influence what is extracted from an experience and determine how it is reconstructed. Bartlett argued further that remembering is a fundamentally social activity that is inevitably distorted by the attitudes and needs of the rememberer (for a precursor of this viewpoint, see Crosland, 1921).

Bartlett's contributions had relatively little impact on memory research in the years following the publication of his book. The experimental study of memory was dominated by stimulus-response–oriented studies of verbal learning, and Bartlett's more naturalistic studies and cognitive theories did not fit well with the reigning behavioristic *Zeitgeist*. However, the theoretical approach to forgetting that prevailed between 1920 and 1970, known as interference theory, did have some interesting things to say about memory distortion. Interference theory held that forgetting is not attributable to passive loss or decay of information over time, but rather to the interfering effects of events that occur after initial learning—the well-known phenomenon of *retroactive interference* (also known as *retroactive inhibition*) that had been discovered early in the twentieth century (Müller and Pilzecker, 1900). Most of the relevant studies were conducted within the relatively narrow context of the "A-B, A-C" paradigm of paired-associate learning, where the same stimulus words are paired with different response words on two different lists; learning the second pairing impairs a person's memory for the first pairing (for a review, see Crowder, 1976). Nevertheless, as Loftus, Feldman, and Dashiell point out in Chapter 1, this research tradition was an important predecessor of modern work on misleading post-event information and memory distortion.

In addition to exploring basic phenomena of interference, research conducted within this tradition yielded other striking demonstrations of memory distortion. For example, Deese (1959) had subjects study a list of words (e.g., bed, pillows, rest, sheets) that are strong associates of a nonstudied critical item (e.g., sleep), and then asked for recall of the list words. He reported that subjects often produced the nonstudied critical items on the recall test—that is, they exhibited false memories for the nonstudied but strongly associated items. Deese thus proposed an associative account of memory distortion as an alternative to the schema theory that had been advocated by Bartlett (1932). Recent work indicates that Deese's procedure is indeed a powerful method for inducing subjectively compelling false recollections (Read, 1993; Roediger and McDermott, 1995). Underwood (1965) reported a similar phenomenon in the domain of recognition memory. After studying a list of familiar words, subjects who were given a yes/no recognition test frequently responded with false alarms to nonstudied words that were associatively related to words that had been presented on the original list. Underwood argued that these false recognitions arise from "implicit associative responses" that occur during initial study of the list items.

The publication of Neisser's (1967) important monograph on cognitive psychology rekindled interest in Bartlett's ideas about schemas and reconstructive memory. According to Neisser, remembering the past is not a simple matter of reawakening a dormant engram or memory trace; past events are constructed by using preexisting knowledge and schemas to piece together whatever fragmentary remains of the initial episode are available in memory. Neisser, using an analogy initially developed by Hebb (1949) to characterize perception, likened the rememberer to a paleontologist who attempts to reconstruct a dinosaur from fragmentary fossil remains: "out of a few stored bone chips, we remember a dinosaur" (1967, p. 285). In this view, all memories are constructions because they include general knowledge that was not part of a specific event, but is necessary to reconstruct it. The fundamentally constructive nature of memory in turn makes it susceptible to various kinds of distortions and inaccuracies. Not surprisingly, Neisser embraced Bartlett's observations and ideas about the nature of memory.

These developments in experimental/cognitive psychology were paralleled by a number of noteworthy ideas and findings in other fields. With the death of Freud in 1939, psychiatry and psychoanalysis entered the post-Freudian era. Perhaps the most significant post-Freudian hypotheses regarding memory distortion were put forward by the psychoanalyst Ernst Kris. Kris's central idea was his notion of the "personal myth": a highly accessible but fundamentally distorted narrative of self or life story (Kris, 1956). As Ross (1991) points out, Kris's personal myth is conceptually similar to Freud's screen memory, except that it applies to a person's entire autobiography rather than merely a single event. Thus, Kris stated that even the most confident and detailed telling of a person's life story may be fundamentally distorted because "the firm outline and richness in detail are meant to cover significant omissions and distortions" (cited in Ross, 1991, p. 85). Kris traced the roots of the personal myth to early childhood, where fantasy and reality are difficult to separate and become inextricably merged in memory. Kris believed that apparent childhood memories of single events are in all likelihood composites of repeated events. These ideas led him to conclude that therapeutic reconstructions of the past are "regularly concerned with some thought processes and feelings that did not necessarily 'exist' at the time the 'event' took place" (Ross, 1991, p. 86). There is a clear resemblance between Kris's ideas and the cognitive perspectives of Bartlett and Neisser.

In the neurological and neuropsychological literatures, scattered clinical observations of confabulation in Korsakoff patients continued to appear, together with a variety of new theoretical accounts of the phenomenon (e.g., Talland, 1961, 1965; Williams and Rupp, 1938; Wyke and Warrington, 1960). For instance, Talland (1961) distinguished between two major forms of memory distortion in Korsakoff amnesics: *confabulation,* where patients misremember the time and other contextual aspects of actual events; and *fabrication,* where patients concoct improbable and bizarre scenarios that could not have in fact occurred. (Although the use of the term *confabulation* in the memory literature has traditionally been restricted to clinical populations with neurological or psychiatric histories, it has recently come to be used much more widely to describe memory distortions in normal children and adults; see Ceci, Chapter 3; Goldstein and Farmer, 1992; Roediger, Wheeler, and Rajaram, 1993; Yapko, 1994. Despite this broader application, I will use the term *confabulation* only in reference to the distorted narrative productions of neurological or psychiatric patients, and will use the term *false memories* when discussing normal populations; see Kopelman, 1987.) In addition, Whitty and Lewin (1957) reported that patients who had undergone surgical removal of the anterior cingulate for relief of intractable obsessional neurosis exhibited spontaneous confabulations even though they did not exhibit amnesia, thereby suggesting that the presence of severe memory disorder is not a necessary condition for the occurrence of confabulation. Other non-Korsakoff amnesic patients were described, such as the famous case of H. M. (Scoville and Milner, 1957), who displayed a profound loss of memory for recent events after bilateral resection of the medial temporal lobes. H. M. did not exhibit extensive confabulation, which indicates that severe memory disorder is also not a sufficient condition for confabulation (see Johnson, 1991; McGlynn and Schacter, 1989; Moscovitch, Chapter 8). These kinds of observations suggest that confabulation is based on brain structures that are different from the structures that are damaged in cases of severe amnesia.

Issues concerning the brain and memory distortion were also raised by the studies of Wilder Penfield and his associates. They reported that electrical stimulation of specific areas in the temporal lobes of surgical patients often elicits the retrieval of vivid, detailed recollections of specific episodes, including apparently long-forgotten experiences from the patient's past (e.g., Penfield, 1958; Penfield and Perot, 1963). On the basis of these observations, Penfield suggested that the temporal lobes retain highly detailed memories of virtually all experiences, which can be brought to consciousness with appropriate stimulation. However, Penfield's hypothesis is problematic because vivid recollective experiences were elicited only rarely by electrical stimulation, and there is little reason to believe that patients' subjective experiences were accurate memories of particular events; rather, it seems more likely that they were generic descriptions of past experience or outright false memories (see Loftus and Loftus, 1980; Squire, 1987).

Penfield's data led him to believe that memories are stored in highly localized areas of the temporal lobes. By contrast, Karl Lashley (1950) came to a quite different conclusion based on the results of brain lesion experiments that failed to reveal a specific site of memory storage. Lashley argued that memories are distributed throughout the brain, rather than being retained in a single place. However, Lashley's extreme anti-localizationist views were problematic for a variety of reasons (see, e.g., Kandel, Schwartz, and Jessell, 1991, pp. 11–12), and modern views of distributed memory storage differ markedly from Lashley's in many ways. In particular, they rely heavily on the idea that specific cortical areas participate in the storage of particular kinds of information (for a historical discussion see Polster, Nadel, and Schacter, 1991; Squire, 1987). This general idea—that different aspects of memories are stored in distinct brain regions, with distributed representation within each region—is essential to understanding various aspects of memory distortion (McClelland, Chapter 2; Squire, Chapter 7).

One further development from this time period deserves mention. In 1925, the French sociologist Maurice Halbwachs published a book entitled *The Social Framework of Memory (Les Cadres Sociaux de la Mémoire)*. In this book and a subsequent posthumous volume entitled *The Collective Memory* (1950/1980), Halbwachs provided an extensive analysis of how social groups remember and perpetuate their collective pasts, with a strong emphasis on the distortions that are an inevitable part of collective memory (for discussion, see Ross, 1991). In addition, Halbwachs believed that social groups exert a profound influence on the content of individual memories, and help to create various illusions, condensations, and distortions. Although Halbwachs's views are extreme in a number of respects—he believed that all memories are in some sense collective rather than individual—his ideas are important because they represent a first attempt to systematically discuss sociocultural factors as a source of memory distortion. Indeed, Halbwachs's ideas were cited by Bartlett (1932, pp. 294–296) in his classic monograph.

The 1970s: The Rise of Constructivism

Stimulated in part by Neisser's (1967) constructive account of memory and the ensuing rediscovery of Bartlett's work, cognitive psychologists during the 1970s exhibited increased interest in memory reconstruction and distortion. A number of compelling experimental demonstrations of distorted memory were reported, usually involving paradigms that elicited false recognition of novel materials. For instance, in a study by Sulin and Dooling (1974), subjects read brief passages about a wild and unruly girl; some were told that the passage was about Helen Keller, and others were told that the passage concerned Carol Harris. After a week's delay, the former group of subjects were much more likely than the latter to claim that they had read the sentence "She was deaf, dumb, and blind," even though the sentence had not been presented in the initial passage. Other compelling demonstrations of false recognition that involved constructive processes such as abstraction and integration were also reported (e.g., Bransford and Franks, 1971; Bransford, Barclay, and Franks, 1972; Brewer, 1977; Johnson, Bransford, and Solomon, 1973; Posner and Keele, 1968; Snyder and Uranowitz, 1978; for a review, see Alba and Hasher, 1983). Developmental researchers who adapted some of the paradigms used in these studies reported evidence of false recognition in children (e.g., Johnson and Scholnick, 1979; Liben and Posansky, 1977; Paris and Carter, 1973; for related developmental memory distortions, see Furth, Ross, and Youniss, 1974; Liben, 1974).

At around the same time, Loftus and her colleagues published a series of pioneering studies that demonstrated both that leading questions can systematically alter memory reports (e.g., Loftus and Palmer, 1974), and that post-event misinformation can alter memory for an original event (e.g., Loftus, Miller, and Burns, 1978). These experiments served to heighten interest in issues concerning the suggestibility of eyewitness testimony, and led to a great deal of subsequent research indicating that the memory of eyewitnesses can be distorted by numerous sources of influence (e.g., Loftus, Feldman, and Dashiell, Chapter 1; Wells and Loftus, 1984).

Although the major developments concerning memory distortion during the 1970s emerged from cognitive psychology, contributions from other fields are worth noting. In psychoanalysis, Fine, Joseph, and Waldhorn (1971) published a monograph describing the deliberations and ideas of the Kris Study Group, a collection of psychoanalysts who were interested in the nature of reconstruction, the relation between memories and fantasies, the basis and functions of screen memories, and other aspects of memory distortion that had been central to Kris's thought (Ross, 1991). This monograph touches on many issues that are quite relevant to contemporary debates concerning false memories and traumatic experience. In neuropsychology, new evidence pointed toward a link between frontal lobe dysfunction and confabulation (Alexander, Stuss, and Benson, 1979; Stuss, Alexander, Lieberman, and Levine, 1978), and the theoretical implications of confabulation for theories of memory began to be appreciated (Luria, 1976; Mercer, Wapner, Gardner, and Benson, 1977).

The 1980s and 1990s: New Knowledge, New Controversy

The past fifteen years have been an extraordinarily fruitful period for memory research, with some of the most exciting developments occurring at the interfaces between neuroscience, neuropsychology, and cognitive psychology (see Gazzaniga, 1995; Kosslyn and Koenig, 1992; LeDoux and Hirst, 1986; Schacter, 1992; Schacter and Tulving, 1994; Squire, 1987, 1992). Many of these developments have direct or indirect implications for understanding memory distortion.

One recent research development with important implications for distortion involves the analysis of *source memory*. Source memory, also known as source monitoring (Johnson, Hastroudi, and Lindsay, 1993), refers to the processes that allow people to remember when, where, and how a memory was acquired. Interest in this issue was sparked by several developments. Johnson and colleagues (e.g., Johnson and Raye, 1981; Johnson, Foley, Suengas, and Raye, 1988) reported an important series of experiments and ideas concerning the processes involved in distinguishing between memories of actual events and memories of prior imaginings and fantasies ("reality monitoring"). Subsequent studies delineated conditions under which recollections of external events and internal imaginings can be confused, thereby producing distorted memories (e.g., Johnson and Suengas, 1989). This line of research also began to yield evidence that young children have difficulties distinguishing between memories of real and imagined events (e.g., Foley and Johnson, 1985; Johnson and Foley, 1984), a finding that has been confirmed and extended in various studies that are summarized by Ceci (Chapter 3).

At around the same time, neuropsychological research revealed that brain-damaged patients sometimes exhibit a dramatic phenomenon known as *source amnesia*, which had been initially observed in studies of hypnosis (Evans and Thorn, 1966). Schacter, Harbluk, and McLachlan (1984) reported that amnesic patients could occasionally learn new fictitious facts, such as "Bob Hope's father was a fireman." However, even when they could recall a fact, the patients were often unable to remember that the experimenter had just told it to them minutes earlier. Instead, they frequently invented a plausible source, claiming that they had read the fact in a newspaper or heard about it on the radio. Significantly, amnesics who showed signs of frontal lobe damage were more vulnerable to source amnesia than amnesics who did not exhibit frontal signs (Schacter et al., 1984; Shimamura and Squire, 1987); indeed, subsequent research indicated that source amnesia could be observed in patients with restricted frontal lobe lesions (Janowsky, Shimamura, and Squire, 1989; see Squire, Chapter 7). Source memory deficits have also been documented in elderly adults, particularly those with neuropsychological signs of frontal impairment (Craik, Morris, Morris, and

Loewen, 1990; McIntyre and Craik, 1987; Schacter, Kaszniak, Kihlstrom, and Valdiserri, 1991; Schacter, Osowiecki, Kaszniak, Kihlstrom, and Valdiserri, 1994), and in young children (Ceci, Chapter 3; Ceci, Crotteau Huffman, Smith, and Loftus, 1994; Gopnick and Graf, 1988; Lindsay, Johnson, and Kwon, 1991; Schacter, Kagan, and Leichtman, 1995).

Source amnesia became more directly linked to memory distortion in several different ways. Neuropsychological studies suggested that failures of source memory and reality monitoring are implicated in the confabulations of brain-damaged patients, and also provided increasing evidence that frontal lobe pathology is often associated with confabulation (DeLuca and Cicerone, 1991; Kapur and Coughlan, 1980; Johnson, 1991; Moscovitch, 1989, Chapter 8). Cognitive research revealed that failures of source memory play a key role in the kind of post-event misinformation effects that were initially studied by Loftus and colleagues (e.g., Belli, Lindsay, Gales, and McCarthy, 1994; Cohen and Faulkner, 1989; Lindsay, 1990; Lindsay and Johnson, 1989; Zaragoza and Koshmider, 1989; Zaragoza and Lane, 1994). These experiments indicated that when people witness a particular event (e.g., a car stopped at a stop sign) and are later given misleading information about it (e.g., the car stopped at a yield sign), they often fail to remember whether the critical information was part of the original event or was only suggested to them later. In light of other experiments showing that post-event information does not necessarily eliminate the original memory (McCloskey and Zaragoza, 1985), it is now clear that failures of source memory are a major contributor to memory distortions that are produced by post-event misinformation. Ceci (Chapter 3) describes recent developmental evidence indicating that distorting influences of post-event suggestion in young children are closely linked with deficient source memory (see also Bruck and Ceci, 1995).

Another important line of research has revealed that when people forget the source of their knowledge, they become susceptible to various other kinds of memory distortions and illusions. For instance, Jacoby, Kelley, Brown, and Jasechko (1989) found that people who had been exposed to a nonfamous name (e.g., Sebastian Weisdorf) would later call that name "famous" if they were tested after a long delay and no longer recollected that they had seen the name in a previous experimental session. The name may have seemed like a familiar one when it was exposed a second time, but because people failed to recollect the source of their knowledge they mistakenly attributed the name's familiarity to the "fame" of the nonfamous person. This result, along with other similar memory biases and illusions (e.g., Jacoby and Whitehouse, 1989; Whittlesea, 1994), highlights the fact that people often make inferences and attributions concerning the source of retrieved knowledge, and that these source attributions are quite prone to error (e.g., Kelley and Jacoby, 1990; Kelley and Lindsay, 1993).

During the 1980s, cognitive psychologists exhibited increasing interest in everyday manifestations of memory for real-life experiences outside the confines of the laboratory (e.g., Rubin, 1986). One relevant example is provided by Neisser's (1982) analysis of John Dean's recollections of conversations related to the Watergate cover-up. Comparing Dean's courtroom testimony with Nixon's tapes of the actual conversations, Neisser concluded that Dean did not possess the photographic memory that some ascribed to him; his recollections of specific incidents and episodes were riddled with errors and distortions, often of a self-serving variety. Yet Neisser also observed that Dean's retention of the general character and gist of events was quite accurate. Neisser argued more generally that memories for details of individual episodes are typically not retained fully or accurately; rather, people tend to remember the recurring themes and summary features of repeated episodes—what Neisser termed "repisodic" memories. Barclay (1986) came to a similar conclusion on the basis of naturalistic experiments that examined memories for salient real-life events (Barclay and Wellman, 1986). With the passage of time, individual episodes tended to merge together; consequently, people became more likely to make false alarms when asked about made-up events that could have occurred and were similar to events that had occurred. Barclay referred to this process as the "schematization" of autobiographical memory (see also Linton, 1986).

A related set of recent ideas and findings concerns the contribution of retrieval processes to memory distortion. Following Bartlett (1932) and Neisser (1967), a number of theorists in both cognitive psychology (e.g., Tulving, 1983) and psychoanalysis (e.g., Spence, 1984) have contended that memories are not simply "awakened" from storage by a retrieval cue; rather, information in the retrieval environment contributes to, and is often part of, the subjective experience of remembering. Therefore, the retrieval environment probably plays a role in distorted remembering. Tulving (1983), for example, argued that "recollective experience and measured aspects of recollective experience do not provide evidence about the properties of information stored about the event, but rather about the joint (synergistic) effects of both the stored information and the retrieval information" (p. 180). Tulving went on to hypothesize that "memory distortions, rememberers 'remembering' things that did not occur, could be attributed to the constructive role of retrieval information" (p. 181). Spence (1984), reflecting an acute awareness regarding the influence of the retrieval environment in psychoanalytic therapy, pointed out that the exact wording of a question by the analyst may have a powerful influence on the recollective experience of the patient. Spence reflected that "we have come a long way from the naive illusion that recalling the past is a simple act of going back to an earlier time and place and reading off the content of the scene that emerges" (p. 93).

Rather, Spence conceded, "More than we realized, the past is continuously being reconstructed in the analytic process" (p. 93).

Loftus's experiments on the distorting effects of leading questions (Loftus and Palmer, 1974) support these suggestions. Other evidence that is broadly consistent with these ideas is provided by what Dawes (1988, 1991) has called "biases of retrospection." For example, in a study by Marcus (1986), people were asked in 1973 to rate their attitudes toward several salient social issues. In 1982, they were asked to make the same ratings, and were also asked to indicate what their attitudes had been in 1973. The key finding was that memory for the 1973 attitudes was much more closely related to the subjects' present (i.e., 1982) views than to their past (i.e., 1973) views. In this and other similar studies (e.g., Collins, Graham, Hansen, and Johnson, 1985; Nisbett and L. Ross, 1980; M. Ross, 1989), salient information in the present retrieval environment (subjects' current attitudes) helps to distort their recollections of what they once believed. A similar sort of retrospective bias has been reported in studies of chronic pain patients: recollection of past pain experiences is heavily biased by current pain levels (Eich, Reeves, Jaeger, and Graff-Radford, 1985). Research on depressed patients has also yielded evidence for retrospective bias (e.g., Lewinsohn and Rosenbaum, 1987). Retrospective bias appears to be most pronounced when people attempt to remember specific episodes and least pronounced when they reflect on the general features of their autobiography (Brewin, Andrews, and Gotlib, 1993).

Additional recent evidence for the contribution of retrieval processes to memory distortion comes from experiments that indicate that the act of retrieval itself can create false memories. For example, Roediger, Wheeler, and Rajaram (1993) found that when people were forced to make guesses about what items had appeared in a study list, they later came to believe that many of their incorrect guesses were actual memories of objects they had seen previously (see Hastie, Landsman, and Loftus, 1978; Schooler, Foster, and Loftus, 1988).

The foregoing considerations apply to another important area of recent research: hypnosis and memory distortion. Although there is a fairly widespread belief among clinicians and law enforcement agents that hypnosis can increase the accuracy of memory (e.g., Kroger and Douce, 1979; Yapko, 1994), controlled studies indicate otherwise (Lynn and Nash, 1994; Smith, 1983; Spiegel, Chapter 4). The evidence suggests that hypnosis creates a retrieval environment in which people are more willing than usual to call a mental experience a "memory," and in which they express a great deal of confidence in both their true and false memories (e.g., Barnier and McConkey, 1992; Dywan and Bowers, 1983; Klatzky and Erdelyi, 1985; Laurence and Perry, 1983; Lynn, Milano, and Weekes, 1991; Orne, Soskis, Dinges, and Orne, 1984; Sheehan, 1988; Sheehan, Green, and Truesdale, 1992). Because hypnotized subjects appear to be quite susceptible to source amnesia (Evans and Thorn, 1966; Evans, 1979), it is especially difficult for them to distinguish between memories of real events and imaginary events that were suggested during hypnosis (Whitehouse, Orne, Orne, and Dinges, 1991). Thus, hypnosis appears to be a potent technique for inducing false memories.

The 1980s and 1990s also produced a good deal of research concerning the relation between emotion and memory distortion. One line of investigation has focused on *flashbulb memories*—vivid recollections of the circumstances surrounding a highly arousing or emotional event, such as remembering how you heard about the assassination of John F. Kennedy. In their seminal paper that introduced the flashbulb concept, Brown and Kulick (1977) argued that flashbulb memories are mediated by a special mechanism that "freezes" the exact details of a scene in memory. Subsequently, a number of studies investigated the accuracy of flashbulb memories by probing people's recollections of salient public events (e.g., the Challenger explosion) soon after they occurred, and again after a long delay. Some evidence indicates that flashbulb events can be remembered quite accurately (Conway et al., 1994), or at least more accurately than more mundane events (Christianson, 1989), but it is also clear that they are subject to decay and distortion (Christianson, 1989; McCloskey, Wible, and Cohen, 1988; Neisser and Harsch 1992; Weaver, 1993). Perhaps the most salient feature of flashbulb memories is that people express a great deal of confidence in them even when they are inaccurate (Neisser and Harsch, 1992; Weaver, 1993). Neisser and Harsch (1992) also reported evidence suggesting that failures of source memory played a role in many of the distortions that occurred in college students' recollections of the Challenger disaster (for extensive discussion of Challenger flashbulb memories, see the chapters in Winograd and Neisser, 1992). More recently, developmental studies have begun to examine the accuracy of children's memories for traumatic experiences in everyday life (Goodman, Quas, Batterman-Faunce, Riddlesberger, and Kuhn, 1994; Howe, Courage, and Peterson, 1994).

There has also been a growing body of laboratory research on memory for emotionally arousing events, which indicates that emotional arousal typically enhances the accuracy of memory for the central aspects of an event and impairs memory for more peripheral details (e.g., Christianson and Loftus, 1991; Heuer and Risberg, 1992). In addition, research on mood and memory during the 1980s began to reveal that a person's mood can exert biasing effects on memory, in such a way that information that is congruent with a current mood tends to be well remembered, and information that is incongruent with a current mood tends to be more poorly remembered (Bower, 1981, 1992). These effects have been observed in college students, and also in patients suffering from depression and other affective disorders (see Mineka and Nugent, Chapter 6).

Several other general developments in memory research during recent years are also pertinent to specific aspects of distortion. First, theoretical models of memory have been increasingly based on the principles of connectionism and parallel distributed processing (PDP; see McClelland and Rumelhart, 1986). In PDP models, memories are not stored as discrete traces but rather are superimposed on preexisting memories in a composite representation. This kind of model is consistent with, and predicts the occurrence of, various kinds of memory distortions (McClelland, Chapter 2; Metcalfe, 1990). Second, there has been growing awareness that memory is not a unitary or monolithic entity, but is composed of separate yet interacting systems and subsystems (for a recent review, see Schacter and Tulving, 1994). A good deal of this research has centered on the distinction between explicit and implicit memory (Schacter, 1987), also sometimes referred to as declarative and nondeclarative memory (Squire, 1992, Chapter 7). Explicit memory involves conscious recollection of past experiences, whereas implicit memory involves nonconscious effects of past experiences on subsequent behavior and performance, such as skill learning and priming effects that are preserved in amnesic patients who lack explicit memory. Explicit memory appears to depend heavily on memory systems involving the medial temporal lobes, diencephalic structures, and frontal lobes, which function to bind together representations at various cortical sites into a coherent memory. By contrast, various kinds of implicit memory reflect changes in different brain regions—priming, for instance, appears to depend on changes in individual cortical systems, whereas skill learning relies heavily on subcortical structures such as the basal ganglia (e.g., Schacter, 1994; Squire, 1992, Chapter 7).

The implications of research on multiple forms of memory for distortion-related issues are severalfold. First, the availability of implicit memory tests provides new ways to assess memory distortion (Loftus, Feldman, and Dashiell, Chapter 1). Second, because implicit memories do not involve recollection of source information, they may give rise to vague sensations or feelings for which people attempt to generate a plausible—but possibly inaccurate—source or cause. Third, the idea that storage and retrieval of explicit memories involves binding together different kinds of information from diverse cortical sites provides a biological basis for the notion that retrieval of a memory is a complex construction involving many different sources of information—not a simple playback of a stored image (see Squire, Chapter 7). Fourth, the existence of multiple forms of memory reminds us that memory is not a unitary entity and that it is necessary to qualify general statements about "memory distortion" with respect to particular kinds of memory. Most cognitive, neuropsychological, and psychiatric research on memory distortion focuses on the episodic memory system that is most central to explicit recollection of past experiences. However, questions about distortion could also be raised about other memory systems, including working memory, which is involved in short-term retention of various kinds of information; semantic memory, which handles conceptual and factual knowledge; procedural memory, which underlies the acquisition of skills and habits; and perceptual representation systems, which represent information about the form and structure of words and objects (see Schacter and Tulving, 1994).

The developments of the 1980s and 1990s discussed thus far are the products of laboratory research, but memory distortion has also become a topic of sociocultural relevance during recent years. The study of social and collective memory, with its emphasis on cultural processes of myth and distortion, has grown explosively during the past decade (e.g., Kammen, 1991; Maier, 1988; Schudson, 1992). And, as noted earlier in the chapter, the accuracy of recovered memories of sexual abuse has emerged during the past few years as an issue with major social implications, accompanied by heated discussion and debate. Widespread public awareness of repressed and recovered memories developed in 1990 when a jury convicted George Franklin of the 1969 murder of a nine-year-old girl, based largely on the recovered memories of Franklin's daughter Eileen (Loftus and Ketcham, 1994; MacLean, 1993; Terr, 1994). There soon followed a spate of lawsuits, often pitting the recovered abuse memories of accusing children against the denials of their parents. In 1992, a group of such parents helped to form the False Memory Syndrome Foundation, which grew to more than 13,000 members within two years (Pendergrast, 1995). In 1994, a jury awarded $500,000 in damages to Gary Ramona, who had sued his daughter's therapist for implanting false memories of sexual abuse (see Pope and Hudson, 1994b). At the same time, concerned clinicians pointed toward the widespread incidence of child abuse and warned of an undesirable backlash against genuine victims of abuse (e.g., Herman and Harvey, 1993). Although the debate concerning recovered memories remains unresolved, these developments remind us that achieving a better scientific understanding of memory distortion is not merely a matter of theoretical concern, but has significant implications for the day-to-day lives of many members of our society.

Looking to the Future: Understanding Memory's Fragile Power

At the conference on which this volume is based, various works of art were displayed that depict, explore, or comment on particular aspects of memory. A major theme in many of the works is that memory is simultaneously *fragile* and *powerful*: memories are often ephemeral and distorted, on the one hand,

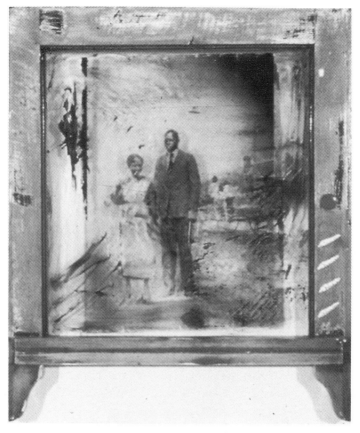

Figure I.1 Cedar Lane, by Mildred Howard. Mixed media on window frame, 21 × 17¾ × 1½″, 1992. Collection of Daniel L. Schacter and Susan McGlynn. Reproduced courtesy of Nielsen Gallery.

yet subjectively compelling and influential, on the other (Schacter, in press). This theme is evident in Mildred Howard's *Cedar Lane* (Figure I.1), where the artist reprints an old family photograph on an antique window frame that is decorated with family memorabilia. The image—like a memory—is evanescent and incomplete, but at the same time exudes a strong emotional resonance.

The coexistence of fragility and power in memory is also starkly evident in some of the testimonies of Holocaust survivors that are eloquently described and discussed by Langer (1991). On the one hand, some survivors report that their memories of the Holocaust seem distant and removed from their present selves. One survivor of Auschwitz, for instance, commented that "I have the feeling that the 'self' who was in camp isn't me . . . No, it's too unbelievable. And everything that happened to this other 'self,' the one from Auschwitz, doesn't touch me now" (Langer, 1991, p. 5). Yet at another level, these distant recollections have a profound and persisting influence on the life of the survivor. As one of them put it, "I can't take full satisfaction in the achievements of my children today because part of my present life is my remembrance, my memory of what happened then, and it casts a shadow over my life today" (p. 34).

The "fragile power" theme also captures an important feature of memory distortion, one that is well illustrated by various chapters in this volume: even when memories are vivid and subjectively compelling, there is still no guarantee that they are accurate. Even though vivid memories are often veridical (e.g., Conway et al., 1994), it is striking that a variety of conditions exist in which subjectively compelling memories are grossly inaccurate. Moscovitch's discussion of confabulation (Chapter 8) highlights the fact that patients believe that their fabricated memories are real even in the face of contrary evidence, and even when they acknowledge intellectually that the memories are indeed rather peculiar (see also Dalla Barba, 1993a). The developmental experiments of Ceci and collaborators (Chapter 3) indicate quite clearly that some young children can be influenced by misleading suggestions and stereotypes to remember events that never happened, and that a significant minority of them find their false memories so subjectively compelling that they are not convinced by debriefing that the memories are incorrect (see Pezdek and Roe, 1994; Saywitz and Moan-Hardie, 1994). Indeed, Ceci reports that these false recollections are so detailed and convincing that skilled professionals are unable to distinguish them from veridical recollections. Loftus, Feldman, and Dashiell (Chapter 1) review their recent work indicating that even some normal adults can be induced to produce detailed, subjectively compelling false memories when asked about childhood events that never occurred, such as becoming lost in a shopping mall. Hyman, Husband, and Billings (in press) have reported similar results in a study in which college students were asked about various childhood events that never happened, including an overnight hospitalization for an ear infection, and releasing the parking brake on a car after having been left alone in it.

What accounts for the strong subjective convictions that can accompany these and other false memories? A variety of factors are no doubt involved, but source amnesia is likely a major contributor. Moscovitch argued that the confabulations exhibited by his patient and by others exemplify source amnesia extended across an entire lifetime, in the sense that the confabulations are often based on memories of actual happenings from a patient's life that were mistakenly placed in the wrong context. Ceci and colleagues have provided direct evidence that the inaccurate memories produced by suggestion in young children often involve deficient source memory. Loftus and her colleagues suggest that the false memories exhibited by adults in their studies often include bits and pieces of real memories that are melded together into a false one. In these and other situations reviewed earlier, the content of a past event or imagining becomes "unglued" from its original source and mistakenly connected to another one. Thus, there is both source amnesia and source confusion. When a false memory contains remnants of actual past experiences—contents and sources of past experiences mistakenly put together—it is easy to see how it could give rise to a strong subjective conviction that the memory is real (see Moscovitch, Chapter 8; Squire, Chapter 7).

In view of the evidence noted previously that links source amnesia with frontal lobe dysfunction, an important area for future investigation would be to examine the relations among source amnesia, memory distortion, and frontal function. It is worth pointing out in this regard that Moscovitch's confabulating patient has frontal lobe damage, as do many other (but not all) confabulating patients (see DeLuca and Cicerone, 1991; Kapur and Coughlan, 1980; Moscovitch, 1989, Chapter 8; Stuss et al., 1978). Reduplicative paramnesia (duplication of familiar people and places) also appears to be linked with frontal lobe damage (Alexander et al., 1979; Stuss, 1991). Moreover, recent observations indicate that in standard laboratory memory tests of recognition memory, patients with frontal damage make abnormally large numbers of false alarms to novel items, and express undue confidence in these false memories (Delbecq-Derouesne, Beauvois, and Shallice, 1990; Parkin, Bindschaedler, Harsent, and Metzler, 1994; Schacter and Curran, in press). Frontal regions may also be implicated in the source amnesia and memory distortion exhibited by young children in the studies of Ceci and colleagues, because frontal functions mature relatively late in development (e.g., Schacter et al., 1995; Smith, Kates, and Vriezen, 1992).

In light of these linkages, the next step is to explore in more detail what aspects of the frontal region and other brain structures are implicated in the production of false memories. Recent neuroimaging evidence from experiments using positron emission tomography (PET) suggests that regions of the right prefrontal cortex may be especially involved in explicit retrieval of episodic memories (Shallice, Fletcher, Frith, Grasby, Frackowiak, and Dolan, 1994; Squire, Ojemann, Miezin, Petersen, Videen, and Raichle, 1992; Tulving, Kapur, Craik, Moscovitch, and Houle, 1994). Indeed, it has been suggested that the right prefrontal region is specifically involved in monitoring and verification of memories (Shallice et al., 1994). Consistent with this idea, damage to right frontal regions has been observed in some neuropsychological cases of confabulation and false recognition (e.g., Delbecq-Derouesne et al., 1990; DeLuca and Cicerone, 1991; Schacter and Curran, in press). It is thus conceivable that right prefrontal regions are implicated in some instances of false memory in normal, non-brain-damaged people. The availability of modern brain imaging techniques, such as positron emission tomography and functional magnetic resonance imaging, provides a potentially powerful tool for evaluating this hypothesis and exploring the neuroanatomical basis of false memories in normal populations. To accomplish this objective, it will be necessary to develop and refine experimental paradigms that can reliably induce false memories in the laboratory setting.

The foregoing observations also point to the need to appreciate more fully, and explore more systematically, an important insight noted earlier: that the subjective experience of remembering does not correspond in any simple way to the reawakening or reactivation of a dormant picture in the mind. Rather, information available in the present retrieval environment combines with stored information to yield an emergent pattern of activity that we experience as a "memory." Although evidence reviewed earlier provides some information concerning the contribution of the retrieval environment to the experience of remembering, the issue is sorely in need of systematic research (for a recent example, see Ochsner, Schacter, and Edwards, 1995). This point is particularly relevant to the current debate on recovered memories of childhood abuse, where it has been argued that therapists who are too eager to infer a history of abuse on the basis of ambiguous symptoms may engage in suggestive questioning that creates a false memory of abuse, rather than eliciting a true memory of an actual traumatic event (see Ceci and Loftus, 1994; Kihlstrom, in press; Lindsay and Read, 1994; Loftus and Ketcham, 1994; Ofshe and Watters, 1994; Pendergrast, 1995; Yapko, 1994; Wright, 1994).

The general idea that memories are always complex constructions fits well with recent ideas about how the brain encodes, stores, and retrieves memories. McClelland (Chapter 2) points out that in connectionist models, which attempt to capture important features of brain-style computation, the very nature of distributed representations precludes any simple notion of a stored snapshot of an event: memories are stored as patterns of activation across numerous units and connections that are involved with the storage of many different memories. Because memories are necessarily superimposed on one another, the output that a connectionist model produces as a "memory" of a particular event always contains some influence from other memories; that is, to a greater or lesser degree, the output of a connectionist model reflects a composite construction of individual underlying representations. McClelland describes a computational model in which the hippocampus and related structures in the medial temporal lobe perform the crucial function of separating individual memories from one another, thereby allowing accurate recall of individual episodes. Squire (Chapter 7) summarizes evidence supporting a similar idea that medial temporal lobe structures bind together various elements or components of a memory. The medial temporal system stays involved in binding a memory for a limited time period, and then it is no longer needed to maintain the memory. This changing role of the medial temporal region over time is thought to reflect a consolidation process that continues for long periods of time after the initial encoding of a memory (see also McGaugh, Chapter 9).

These ideas about the constructive nature of memories are compatible with, and suggest a basis for, the occurrence of distortion. To progress further, more specific links between hypothesized brain mechanisms of memory and particular phenomena of memory distortion are needed. The same can be said of the research concerning neural plasticity and cellular mechanisms of memory that is presented by Swain and colleagues (Chapter 10). They describe evidence for ongoing change, reorganization, and plasticity in the brain at the level of cells and synapses. Such evidence suggests that basic properties of cellular and synaptic mechanisms could provide a fertile substrate for distortion to occur, while at the same time providing the substrate that ensures a reasonable degree of accuracy. Indeed, Abel and his colleagues (Chapter 11) delineate some of the key properties of basic cellular mechanisms that provide a foundation for veridical memory and that may also underlie distortion. But exactly how such processes are related to cognitive and behavioral evidence of distortion and accuracy in human memory remains to be determined.

These issues lead naturally to another critical question that is raised in a number of the chapters: Under what conditions is memory largely accurate, and under what conditions is distortion most likely to occur? Although this volume is concerned primarily with understanding distortion, it must be emphasized again that memory is quite accurate in many situations. It is unlikely that a memory system that consistently produced seriously distorted outputs would possess the adaptive characteristics necessary to be preserved by natural selection. Therefore, the key issue is not whether memory is "mostly accurate" or "mostly distorted"; rather, the challenge is to specify the conditions under which accuracy and distortion are most likely to be observed.

One idea suggested in a number of chapters (see Ceci, Chapter 3; McClelland, Chapter 2; McGaugh, Chapter 9; Squire, Chapter 7) is that "strong" memories—well encoded or frequently rehearsed information, for example—are less likely to exhibit distortion than are "weak" memories. Stated in slightly different terms, when a stored representation or engram is held together by strong connections among its constituent features, it may be less susceptible to distorting influences than when the connections are weak. Thus, distortion might be particularly pronounced when recall is attempted long after a single experience that has not been retrieved or thought about in the interim, or when an experience was not particularly well encoded at the outset (for a related idea, see Brainerd, Reyna, and Kneer, in press; Reyna and Kiernan, 1994). Some evidence along these lines exists. As noted earlier, in a study of memory for real-life experiences, Barclay and Wellman (1986) found that the incidence of false recollections increased systematically with the passage of time. Brainerd and colleagues (in press) and Reyna and Kiernan (1994) have recently provided similar evidence in a developmental study of false recognition (see also Pezdek and Roe, 1994). In addition, source amnesia is observed more frequently after long delays than after short delays (Schacter et al., 1984, 1991; Shimamura and Squire, 1991), and memory distortions that are attributable to source amnesia are observed most readily at long delays (e.g., Ceci, Chapter 3; Lindsay, 1990). Distortions that reflect the undue influence of preexisting semantic knowledge are also most apparent after long retention intervals (e.g., Sulin and Dooling, 1974). Moreover, in a connectionist simulation described by McClelland (Chapter 2), distortion was heightened as a result of weak encoding of inputs that made newly formed memories particularly susceptible to "leakage" from preexisting knowledge. It is interesting to note in this regard that the memory biases of depressed patients described by Mineka and Nugent (Chapter 6) appear to reflect the excessive influence of preexisting knowledge. Activation of preexisting knowledge at the time of encoding is also implicated in various other memory illusions and biases (e.g., Alba and Hasher, 1983; Bransford and Franks, 1971; Roediger and McDermott, 1995). Further research is now needed that explores the neural underpinnings of the relations among encoding processes, activation of preexisting knowledge, and memory distortion.

These considerations also apply to the question of whether emotionally arousing, traumatic memories are less susceptible to distortion than are "ordinary" memories. There is abundant evidence indicating that emotionally arousing and traumatic experiences can be extremely well retained (e.g., Christianson and Loftus, 1991; McGaugh, Chapter 9; Spiegel, Chapter 4). Indeed, in cases of post-traumatic stress disorder, intrusive recollections of traumatic experiences are experienced by most patients (Krystal et al., Chapter 5). McGaugh (Chapter 9) argues that the memory-enhancing effects of emotion may be modulated by the endogenous release of stress-related and other hormones that operate through the amygdala. By this view, the amygdala may modulate the formation of new memories and supply some of the hormonal "glue" that helps to bind them.

Although it seems clear that emotional memories are often well retained, there is relatively little direct evidence concerning whether they are less susceptible to distortion than are nonemotional memories. For example, the claim has been made that traumatic memories are retained in pristine, unchanged form over long periods of time, and therefore differ fundamentally from nontraumatic, narrative memories that are susceptible to decay and distortion (e.g., van der Kolk, 1994). Such a claim may turn out to have some merit, but the main evidence for it is the vivid and detailed nature of flashbacks and other traumatic memories reported by trauma survivors, which seem to preserve the exact details of the original scene even years or decades after the event occurred. However, it is rarely possible to check these vivid recollections against an independent record of what actually happened, and there are good reasons to believe that flashbacks are not necessarily veridical (Frankel, 1994). The fact that a memory is vivid and detailed need not mean that it is entirely accurate, and there is evidence that the same is true of at least some emotionally traumatic memories (Ceci, Chapter 3; Ceci and Loftus, 1993; Frankel, 1994; Good, 1994; Lipinski and Pope, 1994; Loftus, Feldman, and Dashiell, Chapter 1; Neisser and Harsch, 1992; Ofshe and Watters, 1994; Spiegel, Chapter 4). What is abundantly clear, however, is that we lack a firm base of scientific knowledge that allows systematic evaluation of the hypothesis that emotionally traumatic memories are relatively immune to decay and distortion, even at long delays after the original experience. Evidence from the study of nonhuman animals points toward a long-lasting and perhaps indelible persistence of emotional memories, as exemplified by long-term retention of fear-conditioned responses (e.g., LeDoux, 1992; see Krystal, Southwick, and Charney, Chapter 5). But even in studies of laboratory rats, some data suggest that fearful memories are malleable and subject to reconstruction (Henderson, 1985).

The state of the evidence becomes even murkier when we consider the potential accuracy of memories that have allegedly been subject to repression and then recovered years later—the phenomenon that is at the center of the recovered memories controversy. It is important to keep in mind when discussing this controversy that several different issues need to be distinguished and considered (Schacter, 1995). First is the factual question of whether repeated traumatic experiences can be effectively excluded from conscious awareness for years and then recovered. There is a large clinical literature on functional amnesias, in which emotionally traumatic events can produce extensive amnesia for much or all of a patient's personal past (Schacter and Kihlstrom, 1989; Spiegel, Chapter 4). However, these cases involve situations in which a single traumatic event produces retrograde amnesia for both traumatic and nontraumatic events, and do not speak directly to the issue of whether people can block out ongoing, repeated traumatic experiences. Several studies have provided evidence on this point, and they all suggest that some adult women can exhibit varying degrees of forgetting of childhood abuse episodes (Briere and Conte, 1993; Herman and Schatzow, 1987; Loftus, Polonsky, and Fullilove, 1993; Williams, 1994). But the methodological limitations of these studies do not allow them to distinguish between (1) "ordinary" forgetting of single episodes from childhood that would be expected to occur for both traumatic and nontraumatic events—forgetting that is attributable to normal processes such as decay, interference, inhibition, and intentional or unintentional failure to rehearse an event; and (2) massive repression of repeated traumatic experiences that is based on a special defensive mechanism that produces profound amnesia (for discussion, see Berliner and Williams, 1994; Freyd, in press; Kihlstrom, in press; Lindsay and Read, 1994; Loftus, 1993; Loftus, Feldman, and Dashiell, Chapter 1; Ofshe and Watters, 1994; Pendergrast, 1995; Pope and Hudson, 1994b; Schacter, 1995; Spiegel, Chapter 4). It seems clear that more detailed and systematic investigations that examine the nature of forgetting of abusive episodes are required to distinguish between these possibilities. Existing research on functional retrograde amnesia (Schacter and Kihlstrom, 1989) and organic retrograde amnesia (Squire, Chapter 7) could provide useful methods and concepts for such investigations.

Whatever the cause of memory loss—ordinary forgetting or defensive repression—another issue concerns whether people can recover accurate memories of traumatic episodes that have been inaccessible for long periods of time. There is as yet little scientifically compelling evidence that bears on this question. There are several credible reports of individuals who have forgotten and later recovered specific incidents of sexual trauma, including Brown University ethics professor Ross Cheit (Horn, 1993) and a patient described by Nash (1994). In addition, a study of people who reported abuse by Father James Porter, a priest from Massachusetts, indicates that approximately 15 percent of them had never thought about their abuse until the case became publicized in the media, when they remembered it (Stuart Grassian, personal communication, December 2, 1994). However, there is as yet no evidence beyond informal anecdotes (e.g., Terr, 1994) that people can forget and then recover years of repeated, horrific abuse of the kind that is frequently described in recovered memory cases (e.g., Loftus and Ketcham, 1994; Ofshe and Watters, 1994).

A further question concerns whether people can falsely create an entire history of traumatic sexual abuse when none occurred. There is no hard scientific evidence that shows such a phenomenon unequivocally. Moreover, a direct experimental demonstration along these lines is precluded because of ethical considerations. Nevertheless, it has been shown that when hypnotized subjects who are regressed to a "past life" are given suggestions that they were abused in their past life, many subsequently "remember" the abuse (Spanos, Menary, Gabora, DuBreuil, and Dewhirst, 1991). Other observations also indicate that it is quite likely that therapeutic implantation of false memories has occurred, including the use of suggestive techniques by therapists (Lindsay and Read, 1994; Loftus and Ketcham, 1994; Ofshe and Watters, 1994; Yapko, 1994), personal testimonies from former therapy patients who have retracted their claims of abuse (Goldstein and Farmer, 1993; Pendergrast, 1995), and frequent reports of therapeutically-induced recovered memories of satanic ritual abuse despite repeated failures by law enforcement officials to find any evidence for the occurrence of such abuse (Lanning, 1989; Ofshe and Watters, 1994). In view of the scientific importance of questions concerning the accuracy of recovered memories, and the associated emotional stakes for patients, therapists, and families, it seems prudent to call for systematic studies to explore these issues with the best methods available.

The recovered memories controversy also highlights the existence of other fundamental gaps in our scientific knowledge concerning memory distortion. Regardless of whether true traumatic memories are especially accurate, questions remain concerning the conditions under which false memories can be suggested and implanted. Several chapters in this volume highlight the fact that under the conditions that prevail in controlled research studies, only a minority of healthy children and adults are prone to producing extensive false memories (Ceci, Chapter 3; Loftus, Feldman, and Dashiell, Chapter 1; Spiegel, Chapter 4). What differentiates those people who are susceptible to such suggestion-induced false memories and those who are not? As Spiegel points out, hypnotic suggestibility is a highly reliable individual characteristic, and it could well be related to a person's degree of proneness to memory distortion, with more suggestible individuals being more likely than non-suggestible ones to produce false memories in response to suggestive or leading questions. Indeed, several studies have provided evidence that medium- and high-hypnotizable subjects are especially prone to produce false memories in response to suggestion (see Lynn and Nash, 1994). It is also noteworthy that an individual's degree of suggestibility in response to leading questions outside the context of hypnosis, referred to as interrogative suggestibility (Gudjonsson, 1991), appears to be unrelated to hypnotizability (Register and Kihlstrom, 1988) and may be an important characteristic of individuals who are prone to distorted recollections. Other possibilities also need to be considered. It is conceivable, for instance, that studies using functional neuroimaging techniques might provide insights into patterns of brain activation that distinguish between those who are more and less susceptible to producing detailed false memories.

A related and poorly understood issue concerns the potential sources of suggestive influence that lead to the production of false memories. In the recovered memories controversy, attention has focused on therapists who are convinced that a client has been abused even when he or she has no recollection of it, and therefore engage in suggestive probing and questioning that eventually leads to the production of a false memory. Consider, however, Halbwachs's (1950/1980) idea that social and cultural factors can influence and perhaps distort the content of an individual's recollection. Could a widespread cultural belief in the recoverability of repressed memories create an atmosphere that is conducive to the creation of false memories in highly suggestible individuals? There is no scientific evidence that bears directly on this question. Nevertheless, it has been argued that one reason for the recent explosion of recovered memories of sexual abuse involves a widespread "culture of victimization" that influences people to see themselves as victims, and media depictions that encourage the belief that repression and recovery of traumatic memories is a common occurrence and established fact (Pendergrast, 1995; Yapko, 1994). It is at least conceivable that such sociocultural influences could facilitate the production of false memories by suggestible individuals.

Systematic study of the "top-down" influences of culture on the individual brain/mind faces significant methodological obstacles. However, consideration of the matter brings into sharp focus the important question of how individual memories are shaped and perhaps distorted by social and cultural influences. This question lies at the heart of the chapters in Part V of this book, by Assmann, Kammen, and Schudson. All three chapters provide compelling examples of how psychological, social, and political forces can conspire to create distorted collective memories of significant events in a society's past; indeed, these authors suggest that at the collective level, memory distortion is pervasive and perhaps inevitable. Yet these collective myths have powerful effects on how a society views its past, present, and future—precisely because they influence what is acquired and retained by the individual rememberers in the society. Kammen's discussion of attempts to induce "cultural amnesia" in newly-arriving American immigrants (Chapter 12), Schudson's analysis of depictions of Watergate and other public events by the media and by politicians (Chapter 13), and Assmann's consideration of the roots of anti-Semitism (Chapter 14) all illustrate how cultural myths can exert a profound influence on the minds and behaviors of the individuals in a society. And just as source amnesia operates at the individual level, it is also evident at the collective level: cultural myths typically become so embedded in the cognitive fabric of a society that it becomes virtually impossible to discern their origin. Can these cultural distortions ultimately be understood in terms of the properties of the individual brains that are influenced by and give rise to them? Only time will tell, but it seems clear that interdisciplinary approaches will be required to achieve such an understanding.

At the sociocultural level, then, we see ample evidence for both the fragility and the power of memory. As Schudson emphasizes, however, observations of distortion in collective memory need not and must not lead to an extreme form of historical relativism that asserts that all versions of the past have some validity. Attempts to deny the occurrence of the Holocaust, for instance, highlight the necessity of acknowledging that an objectively knowable past exists, and that memory is not infinitely malleable. Understanding distortion in collective memory thus becomes an essential task in order to preserve and defend those accounts of the past that are grounded in objective reality. Analogously, it is crucial to understand the nature of memory distortion at the individual level in order to preserve the integrity and believability of memories that are based on real events that actually occurred. One potentially tragic consequence of the recovered memories controversy, for example, is that the existence of false memories in some cases could cast doubt on the validity of true recollections in others (Loftus, 1993). Given the widely acknowledged enormity of the child abuse problem in our society (e.g., Herman, 1992; Herman and Harvey, 1993; Yapko, 1994), this kind of doubt represents an unacceptable outcome that highlights the need for greater understanding of the similarities and differences between true and false memories. These are some of the reasons why the study of memory distortion is both an intriguing scientific enterprise and a pressing social concern. It is our hope that the chapters in this volume can help to provide a foundation for understanding memory distortion that will serve the purposes of both science and society.

References

Alba, J. W. and L. Hasher. 1983. "Is memory schematic?" *Psychological Bulletin*, 93: 203–231.

Alexander, M. P., D. T. Stuss, and D. F. Benson. 1979. "Capgras syndrome: A reduplicative phenomenon." *Neurology*, 29: 334–339.

Allport, G. 1930. "Change and delay in the visual memory image." *British Journal of Psychology*, 21: 138–148.

Anderson, J. R. and L. J. Schooler. 1991. "Reflections of the environment in memory." *Psychological Science*, 2: 396–408.

Baddeley, A. D. 1976. *The psychology of memory*. New York: Basic Books.

Barclay, C. R. 1986. "Schematization of autobiographical memory." In D. C. Rubin (Ed.), *Autobiographical memory* (pp. 82–99). Cambridge: Cambridge University Press.

Barclay, C. R. and H. M. Wellman. 1986. "Accuracies and inaccuracies in autobiographical memories." *Journal of Memory and Language*, 25: 93–103.

Barnier, A. J. and K. M. McConkey. 1992. "Reports of real and false memories: The relevance of hypnosis, hypnotizability, and the context of memory test." *Journal of Abnormal Psychology*, 101: 521–527.

Bartlett, F. C. 1932. *Remembering*. Cambridge: Cambridge University Press.

Belli, R. F., D. S. Lindsay, M. S. Gales, and T. T. McCarthy. 1994. "Memory impairment and source misattribution in postevent misinformation experiments with short retention intervals." *Memory and Cognition*, 22: 40–54.

Bentley, I. M. 1899. "The memory image and its qualitative fidelity." *American Journal of Psychology*, 11: 1–48.

Berliner, L. and L. M. Williams. 1994. "Memory of child sexual abuse: A response to Lindsay and Read." *Applied Cognitive Psychology*, 8: 379–387.

Berrios, G. 1995. "Déjà vu in France during the 19th century: A conceptual history." *Comprehensive Psychiatry*, 36: 123–129.

Binet, A. 1900. *La suggestibilité*. Paris: Schleicher Freres.

Bonhoeffer, K. 1904. "Die Korsakowsche Symptomenkomplex in seinen Beziehungen zu den verschiedenen Krankheitsformen." *Allg. Z. Psychiat.*, 61: 744.

Bower, G. H. 1981. "Mood and Memory." *American Psychologist*, 36: 129–148.

Bower, G. H. 1992. "How might emotions affect learning?" In S.-Å. Christianson (Ed.). *The handbook of emotion and memory: Research and theory* (pp. 3–31). Hillsdale, N.J.: Lawrence Erlbaum Associates.

Brainerd, C. J., V. F. Reyna, and R. Kneer. In press. "False-recognition reversal: When similarity is distinctive." *Journal of Memory and Language*.

Bransford, J. D., J. R. Barclay, and J. J. Franks. 1972. "Sentence memory: A constructive versus interpretative approach." *Cognitive Psychology*, 3: 193–209.

Bransford, J. D. and J. J. Franks. 1971. "The abstraction of linguistic ideas." *Cognitive Psychology*, 2: 331–350.

Brewer, W. F. 1977. "Memory for the pragmatic implications of sentences." *Memory and Cognition*, 5: 673–678.

Brewin, C. R., B. Andrews, and I. H. Gotlib. 1993. "Psychopathology and early experience: A reappraisal of retrospective reports." *Psychological Bulletin*, 113: 82–98.

Briere, J. and J. Conte. 1993. "Self-reported amnesia for abuse in adults molested as children." *Journal of Traumatic Stress*, 6: 21–31.

Brown, R. and J. Kulik. 1977. "Flashbulb memories." *Cognition*, 5: 73–99.

Bruck, M. L. and S. Ceci. 1995. "Brief on behalf of Amicus developmental, social, and psychological researchers, and scholars in *State v. Michaels* and commentaries." *Psychology, Public Policy and Law*, 1: 272–322.

Butters, N. and L. S. Cermak. 1980. *Alcoholic Korsakoff's syndrome: An information processing approach*. New York: Academic Press.

Ceci, S. J. and M. Bruck. 1993. "Suggestibility of the child witness: A historical review and synthesis." *Psychological Bulletin*, 113: 403–439.

Ceci, S. J., M. L. Crouteau Huffman, E. Smith, and E. F. Loftus. 1994. "Repeatedly thinking about non-events: Source misattributions among preschoolers." *Consciousness and Cognition*, 3: 388–407.

Ceci, S. J. and E. F. Loftus. 1994. " 'Memory work': A royal road to false memories?" *Applied Cognitive Psychology*, 8: 351–364.

Christianson, S.-Å. 1989. "Flashbulb memories: Special, but not so special." *Memory and Cognition*, 17: 435–443.

Christianson, S.-Å. and E. Loftus. 1991. "Remembering emotional events: The fate of detailed information." *Cognition and Emotion*, 5: 81–108.

Cohen, G. and D. Faulkner. 1989. "Age differences in source forgetting: Effects on reality monitoring and eyewitness testimony." *Psychology and Aging*, 4: 10–17.

Collins, L. N., J. W. Graham, W. B. Hansen, and C. A. Johnson. 1985. "Agreement between retrospective accounts of substance use and earlier reported substance use." *Applied Psychological Measurement*, 9: 301–309.

Conway, M. A., S. J. Anderson, S. F. Larsen, C. M. Donnelly, M. A. McDaniel, A. G. R. McClelland, R. E. Rawles, and R. H. Logie. 1994. "The formation of flashbulb memories." *Memory and Cognition*, 22: 326–343.

Craik, F. I. M., L. W. Morris, R. G. Morris, and E. R. Loewen. 1990. "Relations between source amnesia and frontal lobe functioning in older adults." *Psychology and Aging,* 5: 148–151.

Crosland, H. A. 1921. "A qualitative analysis of forgetting." *Psychological Monographs,* 29: Whole No. 130.

Crowder, R. 1976. *Principles of learning and memory.* Hillsdale, N.J.: Lawrence Erlbaum Associates.

Dalla Barba, G. 1993. "Confabulation: Knowledge and recollective experience." *Cognitive Neuropsychology,* 10: 1–20.

Dawes, R. 1988. *Rational choice in an uncertain world.* San Diego: Harcourt, Brace and Jovanovich.

Dawes, R. M. 1991. "Biases of retrospection." *Issues in Child Abuse Accusations,* 1: 25–28.

Deese, J. 1959. "On the prediction of occurrence of particular verbal intrusions in immediate recall." *Journal of Experimental Psychology,* 58: 17–22.

Delbecq-Derouesné, J., M. F. Beauvois, and T. Shallice. 1990. "Preserved recall versus impaired recognition." *Brain,* 113: 1045–1074.

DeLuca, J. and K. D. Cicerone. 1991. "Confabulation following aneurysm of the anterior communicating artery." *Cortex,* 27: 417–423.

Dywan, J. and K. S. Bowers. 1983. "The use of hypnosis to enhance recall." *Science,* 222: 1184–1185.

Ebbinghaus, H. 1885/1964. *Memory: A contribution to experimental psychology.* New York: Dover.

Eich, E., J. L. Reeves, B. Jaeger, and S. B. Graff-Radford. 1985. "Memory for pain: Relation between past and present pain intensity." *Pain,* 23: 375–379.

Ellenberger, H. F. 1970. *The discovery of the unconscious.* New York: Basic Books.

Erdelyi, M. H. 1985. *Psychoanalysis: Freud's cognitive psychology.* New York: W. H. Freeman and Company.

Evans, F. J. 1979. "Posthypnotic source amnesia." *Journal of Abnormal Psychology,* 88: 556–563.

Evans, R. and W. A. F. Thorn. 1966. "Two types of posthypnotic amnesia: Recall amnesia and source amnesia." *International Journal of Clinical and Experimental Hypnosis,* 14: 162–179.

Fentress, J. and C. Wickham. 1992. *Social memory.* Oxford: Blackwell.

Fine, B. D., E. D. Joseph, and H. F. Waldhorn. 1971. *Recollection and reconstruction in psychoanalysis.* New York: International Universities Press.

Foley, M. A. and M. K. Johnson. 1985. "Confusions between memories for performed and imagined actions." *Child Development,* 56: 1145–1155.

Frankel, F. H. 1994. "The concepts of flashbacks in historical perspective." *International Journal of Clinical and Experimental Hypnosis,* 42: 321–336.

Freud, S. 1896. "The aetiology of hysteria." In J. Strachey (Ed.), *The standard edition of the complete psychological works of Sigmund Freud.* London: Hogarth Press.

Freud, S. 1899. "Screen Memories." In J. Strachey (Ed.), *The standard edition of the complete psychological works of Sigmund Freud* (p. 301). London: Hogarth Press.

Freud, S. 1910. "Leonardo da Vinci and a memory of his childhood." In J. Strachey (Ed.), *The standard edition of the complete psychological works of Sigmund Freud* (11: 59). London: Hogarth Press.

Freyd, J. J. In press. "Betrayal-trauma: Traumatic amnesia as an adaptive response to childhood abuse." *Ethics and Behavior.*

Furth, H., B. Ross, and J. Youniss. 1974. "Operative understanding in children's immediate and long-term reproductions of drawings." *Child Development,* 45: 63–70.

Gauld, A. and G. M. Stephenson. 1967. "Some experiments related to Bartlett's theory of remembering." *British Journal of Psychology,* 58: 39–49.

Gazzaniga, M. 1995. *The cognitive neurosciences.* Cambridge, Mass.: MIT Press.

Gibson, J. J. 1929. "The reproduction of visually perceived forms." *Journal of Experimental Psychology: Human Learning and Memory,* 12: 1–39.

Goldstein, E. and K. Farmer. 1992. *Confabulations: Creating false memories, destroying families.* Boca Raton, Fla: SIRS Books.

Goldstein, E. and K. Farmer. 1993. *True stories of false memories.* Boca Raton, Fla: SIRS Books.

Good, M. I. 1994. "The reconstruction of early childhood trauma: Fantasy, reality, and verification." *Journal of the American Psychoanalytic Association,* 42: 79–101.

Goodman, G. S., J. A. Quas, J. M. Batterman-Faunce, M. M. Riddlesberger, and J. Kuhn. 1994. "Predictors of accurate and inaccurate memories of traumatic events experienced in childhood." *Consciousness and Cognition,* 3: 269–294.

Gopnick, A. and P. Graf. 1988. "Knowing how you know: Young children's ability to identify and remember the sources of their beliefs." *Child Development,* 59: 1366–1371.

Gudjonsson, G. H. 1991. "The application of interrogative suggestibility to police interviewing." In J. F. Schumaker (Ed.), *Human suggestibility: Advances in theory, research, and application* (pp. 279–288). New York: Routledge.

Halbwachs, M. 1950/1980. *The collective memory.* New York: Harper and Row.

Harvey, M. R. and J. L. Herman, 1994. "Amnesia, partial amnesia, and delayed recall among adult survivors of childhood trauma." *Consciousness and Cognition,* 3: 295–306.

Hastie, R., R. Landsman and E. F. Loftus. 1978. "Eyewitness testimony: The dangers of guessing." *Jurimetrics Journal,* 19: 1–8.

Head, H. 1926. *Aphasia and kindred disorders of speech.* Cambridge: Cambridge University Press.

Hebb, D. O. 1949. *The organization of behavior.* New York: Wiley.

Hendersen, R. W. 1985. "Fearful memories: The motivational significance of forgetting." In F. R. Brush and J. B. Overmier (Eds.), *Affect, conditioning, and cognition: Essays on the determinants of behavior* (pp. 42–53). Hillsdale, N.J.: Lawrence Erlbaum Associates.

Herman, J. L. 1992. *Trauma and recovery.* New York: Basic Books.

Herman, J. L. and M. R. Harvey. 1993. "The false memory debate: Social science or social backlash?" *Harvard Medical School Mental Health Letter,* 9: 4–6.

Herman, J. L. and E. Schatzow. 1987. "Recovery and verification of memories of childhood sexual trauma." *Psychoanalytic Psychology,* 4: 1–14.

Heuer, F. and D. Reisberg. 1992. "Emotion, arousal, and memory for detail." In S.-Ä. Christianson (Ed.), *The handbook of emotion and memory: Research and theory* (pp. 151–180). Hillsdale, N.J.: Lawrence Erlbaum Associates.

Hobsbawm, E. and T. Ranger. 1983. *The invention of tradition*. New York: Cambridge University Press.

Horn, M. Nov. 29, 1993. "Memories, lost and found." *U.S. News and World Report*, pp. 52–63.

Howe, M. L., M. L. Courage, and C. Peterson. 1994. "How can I remember when 'I' wasn't there: Long-term retention of traumatic experiences and emergence of the cognitive self." *Consciousness and Cognition*, 3: 327–355.

Hyman, I. E., T. H. Husband, and F. J. Billings. In press. "False memories of childhood experiences." *Applied Cognitive Psychology*.

Jacoby, L. L., C. M. Kelley, J. Brown, and J. Jasechko. 1989. "Becoming famous overnight: Limits on the ability to avoid unconscious influences of the past." *Journal of Personality and Social Psychology*, 56: 326–338.

Jacoby, L. L. and K. Whitehouse. 1989. "An illusion of memory: False recognition influenced by unconscious perception." *Journal of Experimental Psychology: General*, 118: 126–135.

Janet, P. 1928. *L'évolution de la mémoire et de le notion du temps*. Paris: Chahine.

Janowsky, J. S., A. P. Shimamura, and L. R. Squire. 1989. "Source memory impairment in patients with frontal lobe lesions." *Neuropsychologia*, 27: 1043–1056.

Johnson, J. W. and E. K. Scholnick. 1979. "Does cognitive development predict semantic integration?" *Child Development*, 50: 73–78.

Johnson, M. K. 1991. "Reality monitoring: Evidence from confabulation in organic brain disease patients." In G. P. Prigatano and D. L. Schacter (Eds.), *Awareness of deficit after brain injury: Clinical and theoretical issues* (pp. 176–197). New York: Oxford University Press.

Johnson, M. K., J. D. Bransford, and S. K. Solomon. 1973. "Memory for tactic implications of sentences." *Journal of Experimental Psychology*, 98: 203–205.

Johnson, M. K. and M. A. Foley. 1984. "Differentiating fact from fantasy: The reliability of children's memory." *Journal of Social Issues*, 40: 33–50.

Johnson, M. K., M. A. Foley, A. G. Suengas, and C. L. Raye. 1988. "Phenomenal characteristics of memories for perceived and imagined autobiographical events." *Journal of Experimental Psychology: General*, 117: 371–376.

Johnson, M. K., S. Hastroudi, and D. S. Lindsay. 1993. "Source monitoring." *Psychological Bulletin*, 114: 3–28.

Johnson, M. K. and C. L. Raye. 1981. "Reality monitoring." *Psychological Review*, 88: 67–85.

Johnson, M. K. and A. G. Suengas. 1989. "Reality monitoring judgments of other people's memories." *Bulletin of the Psychonomic Society*, 27: 107–110.

Kammen, M. 1991. *Mystic chords of memory: The transformation of tradition in American culture*. New York: Alfred A. Knopf.

Kandel, E. R., J. H. Schwartz, and T. M. Jessell. 1991. *Principles of neural science*. New York: Elsevier.

Kapur, N. and A. K. Coughlan. 1980. "Confabulation and frontal lobe dysfunction." *Journal of Neurology, Neurosurgery and Psychiatry*, 43: 461–463.

Kelley, C. M. and L. L. Jacoby. 1990. "The construction of subjective experience: Memory attributions." *Mind and Language*, 5: 49–68.

Kelley, C. M. and D. S. Lindsay. 1993. "Remembering mistaken for knowing: Ease of retrieval as a basis for confidence in answers to general knowledge questions." *Journal of Memory and Language, 32*: 1–24.

Kennedy, F. 1898. "On the experimental investigation of memory." *Psychological Review, 5*: 477–499.

Kihlstrom, J. F. In press. "Exhumed memory." In S. J. Lynn and N. P. Spanos (Eds.), *Truth in memory.* New York: Guilford Press.

Klatzky, R. L. and M. H. Erdelyi. 1985. "The response criterion problem in tests of hypnosis and memory." *The International Journal of Clinical and Experimental Hypnosis, 33*: 246–257.

Koffka, K. 1935. *Principles of Gestalt psychology.* New York: Harcourt, Brace and World.

Kopelman, M. D. 1987. "Two types of confabulation." *Journal of Neurology, Neurosurgery, and Psychiatry, 50*: 1482–1487.

Korsakoff, S. S. 1889a. "Etude medico-psychologique sur une forme des maladies de la memoire [Medical-psychological study of a form of diseases of memory]." *Revue Philosophique, 28*: 501–530.

Korsakoff, S. S. 1889b. "Über eine besondere Form psychischer Storung, Kombiniert mit multiplen Neuritis." *Archiv für Psychiatrie und Nervenkrankheiten, 21*: 669–704. Trans. M. Victor and P. I. Yakolev. 1955. *Neurology, 5*: 384–406.

Kosslyn, S. M. and O. Koenig. 1992. *Wet mind: The new cognitive neuroscience.* New York: Free Press.

Kris, E. 1956. "The personal myth: A problem in psychoanalytic technique." In *The selected papers of Ernst Kris.* New Haven: Yale University Press.

Kroger, W. S. and R. G. Douce. 1979. "Hypnosis in criminal investigation." *International Journal of Clinical and Experimental Hypnosis, 27*: 358–374.

Kuhlmann, F. 1906. "On the analysis of the memory consciousness: A study in the mental imagery and memory of meaningless visual forms." *Psychological Review, 5*: 316–348.

Langer, L. L. 1991. *Holocaust testimonies: The ruins of memory.* New Haven: Yale University Press.

Lanning, K. V. October, 1989. "Satanic, occult, ritualistic crime: A law enforcement perspective." *The Police Chief,* pp. 62–83.

Lashley, K. 1950. "In search of the engram." Symposium Society of Experimental Psychology (no. 4), Cambridge.

Laurence, J. R. and C. Perry. 1983. "Hypnotically created memory among highly hypnotizable subjects." *Science, 222*: 523–524.

LeDoux, J. and P. Hirst. 1986. *Mind and Brain: Dialogues in Cognitive Neuroscience.* New York: Cambridge University Press.

LeDoux, J. E. 1992. "Emotion as memory: Anatomical systems underlying indelible neural traces." In S.-Ä. Christianson (Ed.), *The handbook of emotion and memory: Research and theory* (pp. 269–288). Hillsdale, N.J.: Lawrence Erlbaum Associates.

LeGoff, J. 1992. *History and memory.* Trans. S. Rendall and E. Claman. New York: Columbia University Press.

Lewinsohn, P. M. and M. Rosenbaum. 1987. "Recall of parental behavior by acute depressives, remitted depressives and nondepressives." *Journal of Personality and Social Psychology, 52*: 611–619.

Liben, L. S. 1974. "Operative understanding of horizontality and its relation to long-term memory." *Child Development*, 45: 416–424.

Liben, L. S. and C. J. Posnansky. 1977. "Inferences on inference: The effects of age, transitive ability, memory load, and lexical factors." *Child Development*, 48: 1490–1497.

Lindsay, D. S. 1990. "Misleading suggestions can impair eyewitnesses' ability to remember event details." *Journal of Experimental Psychology: Learning, Memory, and Cognition*, 16: 1077–1083.

Lindsay, D. S. and M. K. Johnson. 1989. "The eyewitness suggestibility effect and memory for source." *Memory and Cognition*, 17: 349–358.

Lindsay, D. S., M. K. Johnson, and P. Kwon. 1991. "Developmental changes in memory source monitoring." *Journal of Experimental Child Psychology*, 52: 297–318.

Lindsay, D. S. and J. D. Read. 1994. "Psychotherapy and memories of childhood sexual abuse: A cognitive perspective." *Applied Cognitive Psychology*, 8: 281–338.

Linton, M. 1986. "Ways of searching and the contents of memory." In D. C. Rubin (Ed.), *Autobiographical memory* (pp. 50–67). Cambridge: Cambridge University Press.

Lipinski, J. F. and H. G. J. Pope. 1994. "Do 'flashbacks' represent obsessional imagery?" *Comprehensive Psychiatry*, 35: 245–247.

Lipstadt, D. 1993. *Denying the Holocaust: The growing assault on truth and memory*. New York: Free Press.

Loftus, E. F. 1979. *Eyewitness testimony*. Cambridge, Mass.: Harvard University Press.

Loftus, E. F. 1993. "The reality of repressed memories." *American Psychologist*, 48: 518–537.

Loftus, E. and K. Ketcham. 1994. *The myth of repressed memory: False memories and allegations of sexual abuse*. New York: St. Martin's Press.

Loftus, E. F. and G. R. Loftus. 1980. "On the permanence of stored information in the human brain." *American Psychologist*, 35: 409–420.

Loftus, E. F., D. G. Miller, and H. J. Burns. 1978. "Semantic integration of verbal information into a visual memory." *Journal of Experimental Psychology: Human Learning and Memory*, 4: 19–31.

Loftus, E. F. and J. C. Palmer. 1974. "Reconstruction of automobile destruction: An example of the interaction between language and memory." *Journal of Verbal Learning and Verbal Behavior*, 13: 585–589.

Loftus, E. F., S. Polonsky, and M. T. Fullilove. 1994. "Memories of childhood sexual abuse: Remembering and repressing." *Psychology of Women*, 18: 67–84.

Luria, A. 1976. *The neuropsychology of memory*. New York: Wiley.

Lynn, S. J., M. Milano, and J. R. Weekes. 1991. "Hypnosis and pseudomemories: The effects of prehypnotic expectancies." *Journal of Abnormal Psychology*, 60: 318–326.

Lynn, S. J. and M. R. Nash. 1994. "Truth in memory: Ramifications for psychotherapy and hypnotherapy." *American Journal of Hypnosis*, 36: 194–208.

MacLean, H. N. 1993. *Once upon a time: A true story of memory, murder, and the law*. New York: Harper Collins.

Maier, C. S. 1988. *The unmasterable past: History, Holocaust, and German national identity.* Cambridge, Mass.: Harvard University Press.

Mantyla, T. 1986. "Optimizing cue effectiveness: Recall of 500 and 600 incidentally learned words." *Journal of Experimental Psychology: Learning, Memory, and Cognition,* 12: 66–71.

Marcus, G. B. 1986. "Stability and change in political attitudes: Observe, recall, and 'explain.'" *Political Behavior,* 8: 21–44.

Masson, J. M. 1984. *The assault on truth: Freud's suppression of the seduction theory.* New York: Farrar, Straus and Giroux.

Mayes, A. R. 1988. *Human organic memory disorders.* New York: Cambridge University Press.

McClelland, J. L. and D. E. Rumelhart. 1986. *Parallel distributed processing: Explorations in the microstructure of cognition.* Cambridge, Mass.: MIT Press.

McCloskey, M., C. G. Wible, and N. J. Cohen. 1988. "Is there a special flashbulb-memory mechanism?" *Journal of Experimental Psychology: General,* 117: 171–181.

McCloskey, M. and M. Zaragoza. 1985. "Misleading postevent information and memory for events: Arguments and evidence against memory impairment hypotheses." *Journal of Experimental Psychology: General,* 114: 1–16.

McGlynn, S. M. and D. L. Schacter. 1989. "Unawareness of deficits in neuropsychological syndromes." *Journal of Clinical and Experimental Neuropsychology,* 11: 143–205.

McIntyre, J. S. and F. I. M. Craik. 1987. "Age differences in memory for item and source information." *Canadian Journal of Psychology,* 41: 175–192.

Mercer, B., W. Wapner, H. Gardner, and D. F. Benson. 1977. "A study of confabulation." *Archives of Neurology,* 34: 429–433.

Metcalf, J. 1990. "Composite holographic associative recall model (CHARM) and blended memories in eyewitness testimony." *Journal of Experimental Psychology: General,* 119: 145–160.

Moscovitch, M. 1989. "Confabulation and the frontal systems: Strategic versus associative retrieval in neuropsychological theories of memory." In H. L. Roediger III and F. I. M. Craik (Eds.). *Varieties of Memory and Consciousness* (pp. 133–160). Hillsdale, N.J.: Lawrence Erlbaum Associates.

Müller, G. E. and Pilzecker, A. 1900. "Experimentelle beitrage zur lehre vom Gedachtniss [Experimental contributions to the theory of memory]." *Zeitschrift fur Psychologie,* 1: 1–288.

Munsterberg, H. 1908. *On the witness stand: Essays on psychology and crime.* New York: Clark, Boardman, Doubleday.

Nash, M. R. 1994. "Memory distortion and sexual trauma: The problem of false negatives and false positives." *The International Journal of Clinical and Experimental Hypnosis,* 42: 346–362.

Neisser, U. 1967. *Cognitive psychology.* New York: Appleton-Century-Crofts.

Neisser, U. 1982. "John Dean's memory: A case study." In U. Neisser (Ed.). *Memory observed: Remembering in natural contexts* (pp. 139–159). San Francisco: Freeman and Co.

Neisser, U. and N. Harsch. 1992. "Phantom flashbulbs: False recollections of hearing the news about Challenger." In E. Winograd and U. Neisser (Eds.). *Affect and accuracy in recall: Studies of "flashbulb memories"* (pp. 9–31). Cambridge: Cambridge University Press.

Nisbett, R. and L. Ross. 1980. *Human inference: Strategies and shortcomings of social judgement.* Englewood Cliffs, N.J.: Prentice-Hall.

Ochsner, K., D. L. Schacter, and K. Edwards. 1995. "Illusory recall of vocal affect." Submitted for publication.

Ofshe, R. and E. Watters. 1994. *Making monsters: False memories, psychotherapy, and sexual hysteria.* New York: Charles Scribner's Sons.

Orne, M. T., D. A. Soskis, D. F. Dinges, and E. C. Orne. 1984. "Hypnotically induced testimony." In G. L. Wells and E. F. Loftus (Eds.). *Eyewitness testimony: Psychological perspectives.* New York: Cambridge University Press.

Paris, S. G. and A. Y. Carter. 1973. "Semantic and constructive aspects of sentence memory in children." *Developmental Psychology,* 9: 109–113.

Parkin, A. J., C. Bindschaedler, L. Harsent, and C. Metzler. 1994. "Verification impairment in the generation of memory deficit following ruptured aneurysm of the anterior communicating artery." Submitted for publication.

Pendergrast, M. 1995. *Victims of memory: Incest accusations and shattered lives.* Hinesburg, Vt.: Upper Access.

Penfield, W. 1958. *The excitable cortex in conscious man.* Springfield, Ill.: C. C. Thomas.

Penfield, W. and P. Perot. 1963. "The brain's record of auditory and visual experience." *Brain,* 86: 595–696.

Perkins, F. T. 1932. "Symmetry in visual recall." *American Journal of Psychology,* 44: 473–490.

Perry, C. and J.-R. Laurence. 1984. "Mental processing outside of awareness: The contributions of Freud and Janet." In K. S. Bowers and D. Meichenbaum (Eds.). *The unconscious reconsidered* (pp. 9–48). New York: Wiley.

Pezdek, K. 1994. "The illusion of illusory memory." *Applied Cognitive Psychology,* 8: 339–350.

Pezdek, K. and C. Roe. 1994. "Memory for childhood events: How suggestible is it?" *Consciousness and Cognition,* 3: 374–387.

Pick, A. 1903. "On reduplicative paramnesia." *Brain,* 26: 260–267.

Polster, M. R., L. Nadel, and D. L. Schacter. 1991. "Cognitive neuroscience analysis of memory: A historical perspective." *Journal of Cognitive Neuroscience,* 3: 95–116.

Pope, H. G. J. and J. I. Hudson. 1994a. "Can memories of childhood sexual abuse be repressed?" Submitted for publication.

Pope, H. G. J. and J. I. Hudson. 1994b. " 'Recovered memory' therapy for eating disorders: Implications of the Ramona verdict." Submitted for publication.

Posner, M. I. and S. W. Keele. 1968. "On the genesis of abstract ideas." *Journal of Experimental Psychology,* 353–363.

Read, J. D. Dec. 1993. "From a passing thought to a vivid memory in ten seconds: A demonstration of illusory memories." Clark University Conference on Memories of Trauma, Worcester, Mass.

Read, J. D. and D. S. Lindsay. 1994. "Moving toward a middle ground on the 'False Memory Debate': Reply to commentaries on Lindsay and Read." *Applied Cognitive Psychology,* 8: 407–435.

Register, P. A. and J. F. Kihlstrom. 1988. "Hypnosis and interrogative suggestibility." *Personality and Individual Differences*, 9: 549–558.

Reyna, V. F. and B. Kiernan. 1994. "Development of gist versus verbatim memory in sentence recognition: Effects of lexical familiarity, semantic content, encoding instructions, and retention interval." *Developmental Psychology*, 30: 178–191.

Roediger, H. L., III and K. B. McDermott. 1995. "Creating false memories: Remembering words not presented in lists." *Journal of Experimental Psychology: Learning, Memory, and Cognition*, 21: 803–814.

Roediger, H. L., III, M. A. Wheeler, and S. Rajaram. 1993. "Remembering, knowing and reconstructing the past." In D. L. Medin (Ed.). *The psychology of learning and motivation: Advances in theory and research* (30: 97–134). New York: Academic Press.

Ross, B. M. 1991. *Remembering the personal past.* New York: Oxford University Press.

Ross, M. 1989. "Relation of implicit theories to the construction of personal histories." *Psychological Review*, 96: 341–357.

Rozin, P. 1976. "The psychobiological approach to human memory." In M. R. Rosenzweig and E. L. Bennet (Eds.), *Neural mechanisms of learning and memory* (pp. 3–46). Cambridge, Mass.: MIT Press.

Rubin, D. C. 1986. *Autobiographical memory.* Cambridge: Cambridge University Press.

Saywitz, K. J. and S. Moan-Hardie. 1994. "Reducing the potential for distortion of childhood memories." *Consciousness and Cognition*, 3: 408–425.

Schacter, D. L. 1982. *Stranger behind the engram: Theories of memory and the psychology of science.* Hillsdale, N.J.: Lawrence Erlbaum Associates.

Schacter, D. L. 1987. "Implicit memory: History and current status." *Journal of Experimental Psychology: Learning, Memory, and Cognition*, 13: 501–518.

Schacter, D. L. 1992. "Understanding implicit memory: A cognitive neuroscience approach." *American Psychologist*, 47: 559–569.

Schacter, D. L. 1994. "Priming and multiple memory systems: Perceptual mechanisms of implicit memory." In D. L. Schacter and E. Tulving (Eds.), *Memory systems 1994.* Cambridge, Mass.: MIT Press.

Schacter, D. L. 1995. "Memory wars." *Scientific American*, 272: 135–139.

Schacter, D. L. In press. *Searching for memory.* New York: Basic Books.

Schacter, D. L. and T. Curran. In press. "The cognitive neuroscience of false memories." *Psychiatric Annals*.

Schacter, D. L., J. E. Eich, and E. Tulving. 1978. "Richard Semon's theory of memory." *Journal of Verbal Learning and Verbal Behavior*, 17: 721–743.

Schacter, D. L., J. L. Harbluk, and D. R. McLachlan. 1984. "Retrieval without recollection: An experimental analysis of source amnesia." *Journal of Verbal Learning and Verbal Behavior*, 23: 593–611.

Schacter, D. L., J. Kagan, and M. D. Leichtman. 1995. "True and false memories in children and adults: A cognitive neuroscience perspective." *Psychology, Public Policy, and Law*, 1: 411–428.

Schacter, D. L., A. K. Kaszniak, J. F. Kihlstrom, and M. Valdiserri. 1991. "The relation between source memory and aging." *Psychology and Aging*, 6: 559–568.

Schacter, D. L. and J. F. Kihlstrom. 1989. "Functional Amnesia." In F. Boller and J. Grafman (Eds.), *Handbook of Neuropsychology* (3: 209–231). Amsterdam: Elsevier.

Schacter, D. L., D. M. Osowiecki, A. F. Kas=niak, J. F. Kihlstrom, and M. Valdiserri. 1994. "Source memory: Extending the boundaries of age-related deficits." *Psychology and Aging,* 9: 81–89.

Schacter, D. L. and E. Tulving. 1994. "What are the memory systems of 1994?" In D. L. Schacter and E. Tulving, *Memory systems 1994* (pp. 1–38). Cambridge, Mass.: MIT Press.

Schimek, J. G. 1987. "Fact and fantasy in the seduction theory: A historical review." *Journal of the American Psychoanalytic Association,* 35: 937–965.

Schooler, J. W. 1994. "Seeking the core: The issues and evidence surrounding recovered accounts of sexual trauma." *Consciousness and Cognition,* 3: 452–469.

Schooler, J. W., R. A. Foster, and E. F. Loftus. 1988. "Some deleterious consequences of the act of recollection." *Memory and Cognition,* 16: 243–251.

Schudson, M. 1992. *Watergate in American memory: How we remember, forget, and reconstruct the past.* New York: Basic Books.

Scoville, W. B. and B. Milner. 1957. "Loss of recent memory after bilateral hippocampal lesions." *Journal of Neurology, Neurosurgery and Psychiatry,* 20: 11.

Semon, R. 1904/1921. *The mneme.* London: George Allen and Unwin.

Semon, R. 1909/1923. *Mnemic psychology.* London: George Allen and Unwin.

Shallice, T., P. Fletcher, C. D. Frith, P. Grasby, R. S. J. Frackowiak, and R. J. Dolan. 1994. "Brain regions associated with acquisition and retrieval of verbal episodic memory." *Nature,* 368: 633–635.

Sheehan, P. W. 1988. "Memory distortion in hypnosis." *International Journal of Clinical and Experimental Hypnosis,* 36: 296–311.

Sheehan, P. W., V. Green, and P. Truesdale. 1992. "Influence of rapport on hypnotically induced pseudomemory." *Journal of Abnormal Psychology,* 101: 690–700.

Sherry, D. F. and D. L. Schacter. 1987. "The evolution of multiple memory systems." *Psychological Review,* 94: 439–454.

Shimamura, A. P. and L. R. Squire. 1987. "A neuropsychological study of fact memory and source amnesia." *Journal of Experimental Psychology: Learning, Memory, and Cognition,* 13: 464–473.

Shimamura, A. P. and L. R. Squire. 1991. "The relationship between fact and source memory: Findings from amnesic patients and normal subjects." *Psychobiology,* 19: 1–10.

Smith, M. 1983. "Hypnotic memory enhancement of witnesses: Does it work?" *Psychological Bulletin,* 94: 387–407.

Smith, M. L., M. H. Kates, and E. R. Vriezen. 1992. "The development of frontal-lobe functions." In F. Boller and J. Grafman (Eds.). *Handbook of Neuropsychology* (7: 309–330). Amsterdam: Elsevier.

Snyder, M. and S. W. Uranowitz. 1978. "Reconstructing the past: Some consequences of person perception." *Journal of Personality and Social Psychology,* 36: 941–950.

Sorabji, R. 1972. *Aristotle on memory.* London: Duckworth.

Spanos, N., E. Menary, N. Gabora, S. DuBreuil, and B. Dewhirst. 1991. "Secondary identity enactments during hypnotic past-life regression: A sociocognitive perspective." *Journal of Personality and Social Psychology,* 61: 308–320.

Spence, D. P. 1984. *Narrative truth and historical truth.* New York: Norton.

Spence, D. P. 1994. "Narrative truth and putative child abuse." *The International Journal of Clinical and Experimental Hypnosis,* 42: 289–303.

Squire, L. R. 1987. *Memory and Brain.* New York: Oxford University Press.

Squire, L. R. 1992. "Memory and the hippocampus: A synthesis from findings with rats, monkeys, and humans." *Psychological Review,* 99: 195–231.

Squire, L. R., J. G. Ojemann, F. M. Miezin, S. E. Petersen, T. O. Videen, and M. E. Raichle. 1992. "Activation of the hippocampus in normal humans: A functional anatomical study of memory." *Proceedings of the National Academy of Sciences,* 89: 1837–1841.

Standing, L., J. Conezio, and R. N. Haber. 1970. "Perception and memory for pictures: Single trial learning of 2560 visual stimuli." *Psychonomic Science,* 19: 73–74.

Stern, W. 1910. "Abstracts of lectures on the psychology of testimony and on the study of individuality." *American Journal of Psychology,* 21: 270–282.

Stuss, D. T., M. P. Alexander, A. Lieberman, and H. Levine. 1978. "An extraordinary form of confabulation." *Neurology,* 28: 1166–1172.

Sulin, R. A., and D. J. Dooling. 1974. "Intrusion of a thematic idea in retention of prose." *Journal of Experimental Psychology,* 103: 255–262.

Talland, G. A. 1961. "Confabulation in the Wernike-Korsakoff Syndrome." *Journal of Nervous and Mental Disease,* 132: 361.

Talland, G. A. 1965. *Deranged memory: A psychonomic study of the amnesic syndrome.* New York: Academic Press.

Terr, L. 1994. *Unchained memories.* New York: Basic Books.

Tulving, E. 1983. *Elements of episodic memory.* Oxford: Clarendon Press.

Tulving, E., S. Kapur, F. I. M. Craik, M. Moscovitch, and S. Houle. 1994. "Hemispheric encoding/retrieval asymmetry in episodic memory: Positron emission tomography findings." *Procedures of the National Academy of Science,* 91: 2016–2020.

Underwood, B. J. 1965. "False recognition produced by implicit verbal responses." *Journal of Experimental Psychology,* 70: 122–129.

van der Kolk, B. A. 1994. "The body keeps the score: Memory and the evolving psychobiology of PTSD." *Harvard Review of Psychiatry,* 1: 3.

van der Kolk, B. A. and O. van der Hart. 1991. "The intrusive past: The flexibility of memory and the engraving of trauma." *American Imago,* 48: 425–454.

Vidal-Naquet, P. 1992. *Assassins of memory: Essays on the denial of the Holocaust.* Trans. Jeffrey Mehlman. New York: Columbia University Press.

Weaver, C. A., III. 1993. "Do you need a 'flash' to form a flashbulb memory?" *Journal of Experimental Psychology: General,* 122: 39–46.

Wells, G. L. and E. F. Loftus. 1984. *Eyewitness testimony: Psychological perspectives.* New York: Cambridge University Press.

Whitehouse, W. G., E. C. Orne, M. T. Orne, and D. F. Dinges. 1991. "Distinguishing the source of memories reported during prior waking and hypnotic recall attempts." *Applied Cognitive Psychology,* 5: 51.

Whittlesea, B. W. A. 1993. "Illusions of familiarity." *Journal of Experimental Psychology: Learning, Memory, and Cognition,* 19: 1235–1253.

Whitty, C. W. M. and W. Lewin. 1957. "Vivid day-dreaming: An unusual form of confusion following anterior cingulectomy." *Brain,* 80: 72.

Williams, L. M. 1994. "Recall of childhood trauma: A prospective study of women's memories of child sexual abuse." *Journal of Consulting and Clinical Psychology,* 62: 1167–1176.

Williams, M. W. and C. Rupp. 1938. "Observations on confabulation." *American Journal of Psychiatry,* 95: 395.

Winograd, E. and U. Neisser. 1992. *Affect and accuracy in recall.* New York: Cambridge University Press.

Wright, L. 1994. *Remembering satan.* New York: Alfred A. Knopf.

Wulf, F. 1922. "Über die Veränderung von Vorstellungen." *Psychologische Forschung,* 1: 333–373.

Wyke, M. and E. Warrington. 1960. "An experimental analysis of confabulation in a case of Korsakoff's syndrome using a tachistoscopic method." *Journal of Neurology, Neurosurgery and Psychiatry,* 23: 327.

Yapko, M. 1994. *Suggestions of abuse.* New York: Simon and Schuster.

Zangwill, O. L. 1937. "An investigation of the relationship between the process of reproducing and recognizing simple figures with special reference to Koffka's trace theory." *British Journal of Psychology,* 27: 250–276.

Zaragoza, M. S. and J. W. Koshmider III. 1989. "Misled subjects may know more than their performance implies." *Journal of Experimental Psychology: Learning, Memory, and Cognition,* 15: 246–255.

Zaragoza, M. S. and S. M. Lane. 1994. "Source misattributions and the suggestibility of eyewitness memory." *Journal of Experimental Psychology: Learning, Memory, and Cognition,* 20: 934–945.

Acknowledgments

Preparation of this chapter was supported by National Institute of Mental Health grant RO1 MH45398, National Institute on Aging grant R01 AG08441, and National Institute of Neurological Disorders and Stroke grant PO1 NS27950. I am grateful to Tim Curran, Gerald Fischbach, Eric Kandel, Wilma Koutstaal, Kevin Ochsner, Roddy Roediger, Michael Schudson, and Larry Squire for helpful comments and suggestions concerning an earlier version of this chapter. I am also grateful to Kimberly Nelson and Chrissy Thurmond for help with preparation of the chapter.

Cognitive Perspectives

I

The Reality of Illusory Memories

1

Elizabeth F. Loftus
Julie Feldman
Richard Dashiell

Ten thousand different things that come from your memory or imagination—and you do not know which is
which, which was true, which is false.

Amy Tan (1991)

In the science fiction film *Total Recall,* people can travel to
other planets without leaving home. The lead character, played by Arnold
Schwarzenegger, cannot afford his dream vacation to the planet Mars. So
he contacts the company Rekall Incorporated to have exotic memories of
traveling to Mars implanted into his brain. Rekall Incorporated prides itself
in creating low-cost vacation memories—and besides, there is no chance
that your luggage will be lost. Unfortunately for Arnold, things don't work
out as planned. Arnold discovers that he has already lived on Mars, where
he worked in a corrupt government; he must remove parts of his memory
to keep the corruption secret. In the process, he becomes thoroughly confused about what is real and what is not.

What is particularly intriguing about *Total Recall* is the mere idea that we
might one day possess the technical capability to create artificial memories in
the mind of a person who would then experience those pseudomemories as
indistinguishable from genuine recollections of the past (Garry et al., 1994;
Yapko, 1994). Yet most people don't realize that that day is here. We now
know a great deal about how to "implant" memories, perhaps not of large,
full-blown, exotic adventures in Mars, but certainly ones that are smaller
and less exotic.

The modern work on memory distortion comes from a distinguished heritage in psychology, which can be found under the rubric of interference
theory. The basic idea is that memories do not exist in isolation but rather
in a world of other memories that can interfere with one another (Greene,
1992). In particular, memory has been shown to be especially fragile in the
face of subsequent events, a phenomenon known as retroactive interference.

The fragility of memory in more real-life settings has been simulated in the interference studies of the last two decades. In these studies, subjects first witness a complex event such as a simulated violent crime or an automobile accident. Sometime later, half of the subjects receive misleading information about the event, while the other half do not. During the third phase of the study, all subjects try to recall the original event, and the extent to which the misinformation leads to changes in recollection is assessed. Two decades of research leave little doubt that misleading information can produce errors in what subjects report that they have seen. In some studies, the deficits in memory performance following exposure to misinformation have been dramatic, with performance differences exceeding 30%. With a little help from misinformation, subjects have recalled seeing stop signs when they were actually yield signs, hammers when they were actually screwdrivers, and curly-haired culprits when they actually had straight hair. Subjects have also recalled nonexistent items such as broken glass, tape recorders, and even something as large and conspicuous as a barn in a scene that contained no buildings at all.

Why Do People Make These Memory Mistakes?

Do errors in memory arise because the misinformation causes representations/traces to be partially or completely lost from the memory system, or is it because the misinformation causes those representations to be harder to locate at the time the memory test is given? Wording the issue slightly differently, do the errors arise because misinformation causes a loss of information from the person's prior memory? Or because misinformation causes a loss of access to that prior memory? Brainerd and colleagues (1990) provide an excellent review of the earliest theoretical positions on this issue, beginning with Hoffding in 1891 and continuing with Freud, Kohler, Wulf and others in the early part of the twentieth century. As Brainerd and associates correctly note, Hoffding, Freud, and others believed that representations, once formed, do not get changed by subsequent events. Rather, forgetting is a matter of retrieval failure. Conversely, other prominent early theorists assumed that representations do not remain crystallized, but rather degenerate through decay, reorganization, substitution, or some other mechanism.

This fundamental question about memory has captivated scholars throughout the twentieth century, as noted by Brainerd and Ornstein (1991). Associationists claimed that memory traces remain intact once they get into long-term memory. This idea constituted an important feature of models from a quarter-century ago, like that of Atkinson and Shiffrin (1968), who conceived of long-term memory as a permanent system and attributed forgetting to retrieval failure. Gestalt psychologists, on the other hand, thought the traces were altered with time. Related ideas can be seen in the writings of memory theorists through the century (e.g., Bartlett, 1932; Alba and Hasher, 1983; Brewer and Nakamura, 1984), who felt that forgetting occurs in part because people are continually processing new information through mental structures that are built up from the knowledge and beliefs they already have about the world. A number of recent formal models, even those heavily based on associationistic ideas, seem to favor storage changes. For example, consider CHARM (Composite Holographic Associative Recall Model; Metcalfe, 1990). CHARM demonstrates a formal mechanism by which new inputs can impair ability to remember earlier details. Although the mathematics underlying this model are unique to holographic memory models (Schooler and Tanaka, 1991), the representations that result from the model are similar to those of other distributed memory models such as the ones developed by McClelland and Rumelhart (1986) (see also McClelland, 1988).

In the modern memory distortion/misinformation literature, investigators are now asking questions analogous to those posed fifty years ago. When people are exposed to misinformation about an event, is that original memory impaired at all? After all, people can give erroneous misinformation responses for reasons that have nothing to do with impairment of original memories, such as demand characteristics. If impairment of event memories can be shown to occur, what kind of impairment is it? As Brainerd et al. and Belli et al. (1992) note, two classes of memory impairment hypotheses have been addressed in the literature. The first is "retrieval-based memory impairment," and it holds that the stored representation of an event remains intact, but misinformation renders it more difficult to access. On the other hand, the "storage-based memory impairment" hypothesis holds that misinformation changes the storage of the event information in some way. If evidence is found for storage-based memory impairment, the next question to be answered is how this process should be characterized (Brainerd and Ornstein, 1991). Does it principally involve a mechanism of trace destruction, trace fading, reorganization, or some other mechanism?

Who (other than cognitive psychologists) cares if memories are impaired by subsequent events? One significant group is psychotherapists, many of whom have adopted their own conceptions of forgetting that may need to be revised. Pillemer (1992) provides several examples of psychotherapeutic beliefs in the unchanging nature of memory, at least traumatic memory: "original situational memories are unlikely to be changed" (Brewin, 1989, p. 387); "traumatic events create lasting visual images . . . burned-in visual impressions" (Terr, 1988, p. 103); "memory imprints are indelible, they do not erase—a therapy that tries to alter them will be uneconomical" (Kantor, 1980, p. 163). Others have echoed similar beliefs: "traumatic memory is inflexible and invariable" (van der Kolk and van der Hart, 1991). In fact, data bearing on the fate of once-formed memory traces contradicts these psychotherapeutic conceptions.

Whether event memories are impaired or not, there still remains the issue of the extent to which people in general, and clinical patients more specifically, believe in the accuracy of their false memories. Johnson (1988) has suggested that certain mental dysfunctions (for example, schizophrenia) can be discussed in terms of reality monitoring failures in general, and, more specifically, in terms of patient difficulty in discriminating between internal thoughts and memories, on the one hand, and external information, on the other hand. Put another way, the patients believe in their false memories.

The preceding discussion raises two of the most pressing questions about the impact of misinformation on a person's ability to accurately recall the past. Does misinformation actually impair a person's ability to remember details? And, once misinformation is embraced and reported, do people genuinely believe in their misinformation memories?

The Fate of the Original Memory

Does misinformation alter preexisting memory traces? Some investigators have suggested that even the showing of abundant errors following receipt of misinformation does not provide evidence for impairment of prior traces. Demand characteristics and response biases could readily lead subjects to perform more poorly in the face of misinformation. For example, a subject who does not remember some event detail (say, a hammer) could report a suggested detail (say, a screwdriver) in order to go along with the perceived desires of the experimenter (McCloskey and Zaragoza, 1985). Or they could report a suggested detail because they remember reading something about it, not because they think they saw it. While it is clear that these mechanisms are partially responsible for erroneous reporting, the question remains whether misinformation ever leads to memory impairment. Several procedural innovations have been developed to explore this issue.

One of these procedures involves an adaptation of Jacoby's logic of opposition (Jacoby and Kelley, 1992; Lindsay, 1990, 1993). Subjects saw an event that contained critical details such as a hammer. Then they read an erroneous narrative that mentioned, say, a screwdriver. Finally, they were tested on what they saw. The experimental innovation involved informing subjects when they were tested that the postevent information that they read did not include any correct answers to the test questions. In other words, the subjects were given a strong warning that said, in essence: "If you remember that you read it, it isn't accurate." Half the subjects were exposed to conditions that made it easy to remember the postevent suggestions, and the other half were exposed to conditions that made it difficult. Before taking their test, all subjects were warned to report what they saw, and that anything they remembered reading was not accurate. The results showed that subjects with the easy conditions were quite able to identify the source of their memories of suggested details and refrained from reporting seeing these in the event. Despite this ability, the misleading suggestions still interfered with their ability to correctly report the event details. In other words, they knew it wasn't a screwdriver, but they weren't so sure it was a hammer. Lindsay (1993, p. 88) has argued that this finding constitutes powerful evidence that misleading suggestions can impair the ability to remember event details.

Another important finding from Lindsay occurred in the "difficult" condition. Here, subjects who received misinformation about a critical item were far more likely to claim that they had seen the suggested item than subjects who were not misinformed about that item. Indeed, more than a quarter of the responses on misled items were details that were only suggested. What this finding means is that misinformation effects are not simply due to a blind trusting of the postevent narrative. The finding further implicates poor source memory as a contributor to memory distortion.

Implicit Testing

Most tests to assess memory distortion are explicit tests of memory in which subjects are instructed to remember recent events and try to do so. Implicit measures, on the other hand, are those in which subjects are not told to remember particular events, but rather are asked to perform some other task, such as completing a word fragment. "Memory" exists to the extent that it influences later performance on the implicit task relative to some baseline. Implicit measures have been known to reveal evidence of memory where explicit measures fail to do so (Graf and Schacter, 1987; Roediger, 1990; Schacter, 1987).

Suppose a hypothetical subject, Mary, has seen a hammer and been misled about a screwdriver. On an explicit test, she reports the screwdriver, with high confidence, and insists that she did not see a hammer. In other words, the explicit test produces no evidence of memory for a hammer. What would happen if she were given an implicit test instead? For example, assuming that prior exposure to the hammer in the absence of misinformation "primes" her performance on the implicit test, would performance still be primed in the face of misinformation?

Three attempts to address this issue have appeared in the recent literature—with mixed results. Birch and Brewer (1989) found evidence for impairment of memories with an implicit test, but their materials were somewhat unusual. Dodson and Reisberg (1991) found no evidence for impairment of memories with an implicit memory test, but interpretation of their results is compromised because their subjects were first given an explicit test.

Kilmer and Loftus (cited in Loftus, 1991) found evidence for impairment of memories using an implicit test. In this study subjects saw a complex event containing numerous critical details (e.g., Hammer). Following this, they read a narrative containing some misinformation (e.g., Screwdriver); they took an implicit memory test; and finally they took an explicit test. The particular implicit test, part of a seemingly unrelated experiment, required subjects to produce the names of category members (e.g., Name the first five tools that come to mind). The results were mixed. First, seeing an item in the slides increased its chance of being produced on the category list (seeing a hammer increased the production of "hammer" on the category list). This is a small priming effect, caused by the recent exposure to the item. Did misinformation reduce the priming effect? The answer, overall, was no. Misinformation did not reduce the likelihood that the critical event item was produced. However, when Kilmer and Loftus looked only at the generation of event details (e.g., Hammer) for those subjects who ultimately (on the explicit test) bought the misinformation, the priming effect disappeared. While this result is consistent with the notion that the event memory was impaired, the particular implicit test used makes the results open to other interpretations. Responding to prior criticisms, we explored the memory impairment issue with a new implicit memory test involving picture fragments.

The Picture-Fragment Study

The overall design of the study involved four major phases. Subjects (1) viewed a sequence of slides depicting a complex event, then (2) read a post-event narrative containing misinformation about the event, then (3) completed an implicit (degraded picture) test, and finally (4) took an explicit memory test.

The subjects were 345 undergraduates from the University of Washington who watched a series of 51 slides that depicted a female college senior ("Kristine") visiting a local department store. While shopping, Kristine visited six different departments, picking up various items along the way. Of these items, Kristine put some into her cart, while surreptitiously slipping the more expensive items into her oversized purse. Kristine did not get caught the first time, but did get caught when she returned to the store a second time.

After viewing the event containing a number of critical items, subjects read a narrative that contained some misinformation. For example, subjects may have seen Kristine handle a hammer that was later described in a narrative erroneously as a screwdriver or neutrally as a tool. After the narrative, they were questioned about their attitudes regarding Kristine's actions, a sham activity designed to convince them that the experiment was over. They were debriefed and then asked to take part in a second short experiment. Subjects were taken to a separate testing room and signed a separate consent form to maximize the chance that the "two experiments" were not related in the subject's mind.

The implicit test was a degraded picture task developed by Snodgrass and Vanderwart (1980) and adapted for the Apple Macintosh computer (see Snodgrass, Smith, Feenan, and Corwin, 1987, for a detailed description). Subjects had to "identify pictures of common objects and animals which would appear in fragments on the computer screen." Each picture was presented from level 1 (highly fragmented) to level 8 (complete picture). As soon as they felt they could identify the picture, they typed the picture's name into the computer. After the implicit task, they were tested on their memory for the slide sequence, with a recognition test. For example, a question might be of the form: "What was the tool that you saw Kristine handle? Hammer or Screwdriver?"

The results showed a large misinformation effect on the explicit recognition test. Accuracy was higher for control items than for misled items (72.1% versus 55.4% correct). Misinformation led to a decrease in accuracy for all but one of the 20 critical items as a result of misleading postevent information.

The next question of interest is how performance on the implicit test was influenced by having seen the slides or being exposed to misinformation. Did seeing a critical item in the slides benefit subjects on the implicit test? The answer is yes. For 18 of the 20 critical items, subjects who had seen the item in the slides in the control condition showed more priming than subjects who had not seen any slides at all. In other words, for 18 of 20 items, control items showed priming relative to baseline. In terms of the level at which the picture fragment was recognized, it was 4.32 for control items, which was less than the value of 4.44 for baseline items.

We now turn to the issue of major interest to the present study: Did misinformation affect performance on the implicit test? If subjects had seen a hammer and been given misinformation about a screwdriver, did they still show a benefit in recognizing fragments of a hammer? The impairment hypothesis predicts that misinformation would reduce or eliminate the priming benefit that control items exhibited (producing data similar to those in the top panel of Figure 1.1). If there is no impairment of memory for the event item, one might expect to still see priming (producing data similar to those in the bottom panel of Figure 1.1). The results, in fact, showed a very small reduction in priming of the event item after exposure to misinformation (see Figure 1.2). Of the 18 items that showed priming in control over baseline conditions, only 8 showed a reduction of the priming benefit that

Impairment

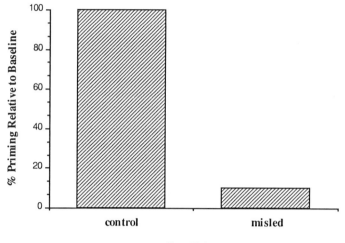

Permanence/Coexistence

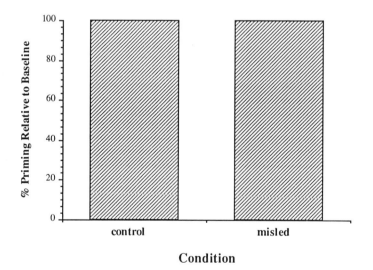

Figure 1.1 Predictions for picture-fragment study.

Our Results

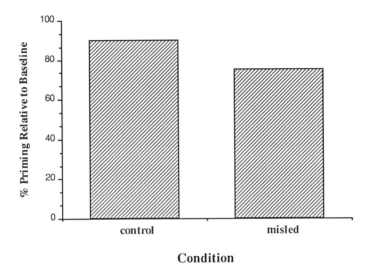

Figure 1.2 Data from picture-fragment study.

control items exhibited. The mean level of fragment identification for 20 items in the misled condition was 4.31, indistinguishable from the mean of 4.32 reported above for the control condition.

These analyses indicate that critical items that were primed by having been seen earlier in the slides remain almost equally primed despite the presence of misinformation. Even when the data were examined separately for misled subjects who were correct on the explicit test as opposed to the misled subjects who were incorrect on the explicit test, the conclusion did not change. The picture-fragment study provides little or no evidence of impairment of event details by misinformation. Misled performance was "better" than baseline performance, but no different from control performance. However, the priming obtained even in the control condition was so unexpectedly small (4.44 versus 4.32) that there was not much room to maneuver. Small priming effects may have been attributed to any one of a number of factors. The original items were presented pictorially in slides quite unlike the computerized picture fragments. Differences in physical features of stimuli from study to test can have large effects on priming. Also, priming does decrease over time, and subjects in this study experienced at least a 30- to 40-minute delay between time of exposure to the series of slides and administration of the implicit test. The next attempt to use picture fragments or any implicit test to search for lost memories should first strive to ensure that priming in the control condition is sufficiently large to detect deviations due to misinformation, should they exist.

One last comment is in order. The finding that misinformation reduces priming of event items would constitute fairly strong support for impairment. However, the finding that misinformation does not reduce priming (as in the picture-fragment study) does not constitute strong support for the intact nature of the event trace. Misinformation might indeed impair episodic information (assessed by explicit measures of memory), but it might simultaneously leave unaffected activation in semantic memory (assessed by implicit tests or priming). Put another way, under an episodic/semantic memory theory, failure to obtain a reduction in priming with misinformation could co-occur with impairment of episodic traces. Perhaps this is one reason why past research shows that explicit memory tests commonly reveal interference effects, while implicit memory tests are not as susceptible to interference (Graf and Schacter, 1987).

The fate of original memories in the face of misinformation remains an issue of continuing interest to scholars of the misinformation effect. Whether the underlying traces remain intact or are modified, what the subject reports is often the misinformation option. Thus a separate issue to explore is the extent to which the overt report reflects a genuine belief on the part of the subject that the misinformation was actually experienced.

Do People Really Believe in Their Misinformation Memories?

It is tempting to claim that people genuinely believe in their misinformation memories because they often report those memories with a great deal of confidence. But some subjects might use high confidence ratings simply because they believe the misinformation is right and assume that they must have seen it (Zaragoza and Lane, 1994). Fortunately, there are other techniques for showing that subjects really believe in their misinformation memories.

One finding that is consistent with the idea that subjects genuinely believe in their misinformation memories is that they will bet money on those memories (Weingardt, Toland, and Loftus, 1994). On the other hand, it could be argued that subjects might be willing to bet money on a particular item even if they don't remember seeing it but for other reasons conclude it is the right answer. These reasons are developed below.

It is clear that there are many reasons why a subject who sees a "hammer" and receives misinformation about a "screwdriver" will subsequently come to report seeing a screwdriver. Some subjects could have failed to encode the hammer in the first place, and could choose the screwdriver on the test because they remember reading about it ("misinformation acceptance"). Other subjects might remember both hammer and screwdriver, and choose the screwdriver on the test because they trust the misinformation more than their own memory ("deliberation"). Some subjects might have a subjective experience of memory for the misinformation ("memory"). Other subjects might simply be guessing. In other words, multiple "process histories" could be responsible for different subjects' report of the same item, screwdriver. Most of the previous research on the misinformation effect simply examines the proportion of subjects who report screwdriver, or the average confidence or speed with which they do so. While such data are often useful, they sometimes mask important results because they are averages from subjects who undoubtedly have different process histories. And even worse, the procedure of averaging performance across subjects and trials can be especially misleading if subjects vary in the strategies they use to perform a given task (Newell, 1973). If one wants to know something about how often the various strategies are used in a typical misinformation study, another method is needed.

One new approach to gaining information about individual strategies relies on a simple but clever methodology used by Siegler (1987, 1989) in a completely different cognitive domain—namely, the study of children engaged in addition and subtraction. In the subtraction study, for example, when the data were averaged from all trials, and over all strategies, the conclusion reached was that children solved subtraction problems mostly by counting down from the larger number or counting up from the smaller one. However, when the data were analyzed separately according to the particular strategy that a child claimed to use, a different picture was suggested. It is no wonder that Siegler (1987) titled his paper with the phrase "the perils of averaging data," and that in his later (1989) paper he referred to the "hazards" of the practice of averaging.

A similar research strategy would yield useful data in the misinformation domain. If data were analyzed separately, according to some retrospective indication of the specific strategy subjects said they used on the trial, more informed conclusions about the impact of misinformation might be reached. Subjects who arrive at a misinformation response via one strategy (e.g., deliberation) versus another (e.g., pure acceptance of the misinformation) might express different levels of confidence in their memories, might describe the memories in different ways, and might be differentially resistant to being convinced that their memory is wrong.

Like Siegler, we asked subjects on each trial the strategy they used to arrive at their response. The technique of asking people immediately after each response how they generated their answers has been successful in a variety of domains (see Ericsson and Simon, 1984). It is particularly useful when the processing episode being asked about is not extremely brief in duration. Although protocol analysts are well aware of the argument that verbal reports can give a misleading picture of what people are doing (Nisbett and Wilson, 1977), Siegler has argued convincingly that indirect methods of cognitive assessment (such as chronometric analyses) can give an equally misleading picture. Moreover, some related work in memory (Gardiner and Java, 1990) points to the potential benefits of gathering post-response verbal reports. In this related work, subjects recognized previously presented words, and then indicated whether they actually "remembered" the previous occurrence or whether they simply "knew" that it had occurred before but without being able to consciously recollect anything about its occurrence. These "remember" versus "know" judgments tapped qualitatively different components of memory. Analogously, we hoped that by simply asking subjects the reason why they reported a particular item, we would discover whether subjects did so because they genuinely believed they had seen those items.

A dilemma arose as to whether we should leave the subject free to describe the reason she reported an item using her own words, or whether we should provide the subject with a list of options to choose from. Obviously providing options would facilitate our analysis; however, we might be forcing subjects to select a reason that did not quite match their real reason. Thus we did the experiment both ways.

A New "Reasons" Study

The subjects, 301 students, watched a series of 67 slides depicting a man visiting a local bookstore. The man interacted with a number of critical items (e.g., a screwdriver or a wrench, a can of Coke or 7-Up). After the event, the subjects read a postevent narrative that contained some misinformation. Finally, subjects answered questions about what they had seen during the event. The questions took this form: Did you see a screwdriver or a wrench? One member of the pair was actually in the slides, and the other had been given as misinformation to half the subjects. The innovation in this study is that after subjects indicated what they had seen, they indicated the reason for their choice.

The results showed a strong misinformation effect. Subjects were correct more often when they had not been given misinformation than when they had (78% versus 51%). Next, we examined the reasons that subjects gave for choosing the misinformation option. The open-ended responses of subjects were classified into categories. Next to each category, in parentheses, is the percentage of items that were classified into each category. Six percent of the time, no reason was given or else the response given was uncodable. The remaining 94% of responses were categorized into one of eight categories (see Figure 1.3).

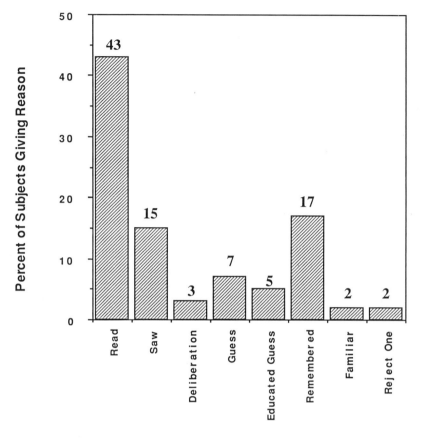

Reason For Choosing Misinformation

Figure 1.3 Data from reasons study: free choice.

1. Read: (The subject remembered reading about the item, e.g., "I read it in the narrative.")

2. Saw: (The subject remembered seeing the item in the slides, e.g., "I saw that the can was red.")

3. Deliberated: (The subject remembered one item in the slides and another in the narrative, and finally opted for the narrative.)

4. Guessed: (The subject indicated a pure guess.)

5. Educated guess: (The subject made a guess based on some piece of apparently relevant information other than the item itself, e.g., "Since I think he was screwing something, it must have been a screwdriver.")

6. Remember: (The subject indicated remembering without stating a source for the memory, e.g., "I remember it" or "I memorized it.")

7. Familiar: (The subject indicated a sense of familiarity about the item, e.g., "I hear it in my mind.")

8. Reject one: (The subject rejected one option and chose the other by default, e.g., "I would have remembered a Mickey Mouse shirt.")

These data reveal that the major reason why subjects choose the misinformation option is that they remember having read it (43%). A smaller, but sizable, minority (19%) chose the misinformation item because they simply remembered it from somewhere (17%) or because it just seemed familiar (2%). But it is also important that 15% of the misled items were selected because the subject explicitly, but incorrectly, remembered "seeing" the item.

One potential concern about the study is that subjects were asked for their strategies about an item immediately after revealing which item they thought they had seen. Thus, they knew at the time they made their choices that they would be pressed for information about their strategy. Perhaps this requirement affected the choices they made. For this reason, in the next study, subjects first indicated for all items which ones they thought they had seen. Later they went back and revealed for each item the reason they had selected it.

The first strategy study gave us some indication of the types of reasons subjects gave when permitted to express those reasons in their own words. In the second strategy study, we gave subjects a list of six possible reasons for selecting the misinformation option, and urged them to select one of the six.

The second "reasons" study used 282 students as subjects. They viewed the same event, read a postevent narrative that contained some misinformation, and finally were tested. They responded by using a black pen. When they were finished, the black pens were collected and blue ones handed out. With the blue pens the subjects indicated the reason for their earlier choices. The change in pens prevented subjects from changing their earlier answers. The "strategy" instructions urged the subjects to choose from the following:

1. Saw—"I remember seeing it in the slides."

2. Saw and Read—"I remember it was in both the slides and the narrative."

3. Read—"I read it in the narrative."

4. Conflict—"I thought I saw one choice in the slides, but I thought that I read the other in the narrative."

5. Guess—"I couldn't remember which it was so I guessed or made an educated guess based on what I did remember."

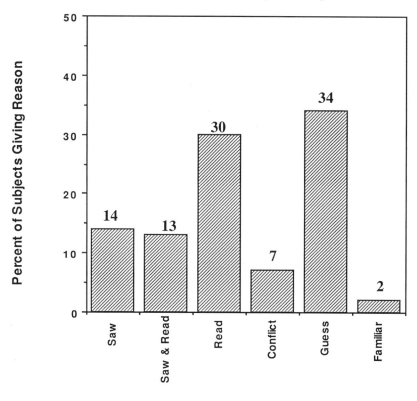

Reason For Choosing Misinformation

Figure 1.4 Data from reasons study: forced choice.

6. Familiar—"I remembered my answer from the experiment, but I don't remember what the source was" (slides or narrative).

Subjects were also told that if they could not classify a strategy using this system, they should try to explain their strategy in their own words.

Again, the results showed a reliable misinformation effect. Misled subjects were more likely to choose the misinformation option, and thus to perform more poorly than control subjects. What reasons did subjects give for picking the misinformation? Figure 1.4 shows the distribution of reasons. This time, the largest percentage of misinformation responses resulted from guesses (34%). Next largest was the option Read (30%). Relatively few subjects indicated that they chose the misinformation after a conflict (7%) or because it just seemed to be familiar (2%). Of greatest interest, however, was the finding that over a quarter of the subjects claimed to have seen the misinformation item, either by checking Saw (14%) or Saw and Read (13%).

Taken together, these studies are consistent with the idea that at least a fraction of the subjects pick the misinformation item because they remember seeing it. Even when given the choice of saying that they remember both seeing and reading the item, one in seven subjects still claim only that they saw it. Of course it must be kept in mind that subjects who saw the items neither in the slides nor in the narrative sometimes still remember "seeing" the item in the slides. In this study, false claims of "seeing" happened nearly as often for control items. Thus, explicit exposure to misinformation is not the only reason why people can come to remember seeing things that they didn't see. But the data do complement those of Zaragoza and Lane (1994), who showed that misled subjects definitely do sometimes come to believe they remember seeing items that were merely suggested to them, a phenomenon they refer to as a "source misattribution effect" (p. 934).

The Creation of False Memories

It is one thing to change memory for a detail about some recently experienced event, and quite another thing to implant an entire memory for something that never happened. To determine whether it is even possible to implant entire memories that come to be believed, Loftus and Coan (1994) suggested to five individuals that they had been lost for an extended time when they were about the age of five. With the help of some prodding from a trusted family member (a mother, an older brother, an aunt), these individuals, ages 8 to 42, were convinced they had been lost. For example, 14-year-old Chris received the suggestion from his older brother that he had been lost in the University City shopping mall in Spokane, Washington. After some time, Chris was supposedly rescued by an elderly man and reunited with his mother and brother. Just two days after receiving the suggestion, Chris could remember the event with feelings: "That day, I was so scared that I would never see my family again. I knew I was in trouble." The next day, he recalled that his mother told him never to do that again. On the fourth day he could remember the old man's flannel shirt. Two weeks later he remembered the balding head and glasses of the man who rescued him. When he was finally debriefed and told that his memory was false, he said, "Really? I thought I remembered being lost . . . and looking around for you guys. I do remember that. And then crying, and Mom coming up and saying 'Where were you? Don't you—don't you ever do that again.'"

More recently, with Jacqueline Pickrell, we have tried to convince 24 individuals, ages 18 to 53, that they had been lost for an extended period of time, that they were crying or scared, and that they were eventually rescued by an elderly person and reunited with their families. The subjects thought they were participating in a study of "the kinds of things you may be able to remember from your childhood." The subjects were given a brief description of four events that supposedly occurred while the subject and family member were together. Three were true events and one was the false "lost" event. Subjects tried to write about these events in detail. Approximately a week later they were interviewed about the events, and about a week after that they were interviewed again.

The four "memories" were described in one paragraph apiece. Thus, for example, the family member of one 20-year-old Vietnamese female subject constructed this "lost" memory: "You, your Mom, Tien and Tuan, all went to the Bremerton K-Mart. You must have been five years old at the time. Your Mom gave each of you some money to get a blueberry ICEE. You ran ahead to get into the line first, and somehow lost your way in the store. Tien found you crying to an elderly Chinese woman. You three then went together to get an ICEE."

The subject embraced much of the information, and expanded upon it: "I vaguely remember walking around K-Mart crying and looking for Tien and Tuan. I thought I was lost forever. I went to the shoe department, because we always spent a lot of time there. I went to the handkerchief place because we were there last. I circled all over the store it seemed 10 times. I just remember walking around crying. I do not remember the Chinese woman, or the ICEE (but it would be raspberry ICEE if I was getting an ICEE) part. I don't even remember being found."

During the first interview, the subject described how horrible she felt: "I felt really lost, I felt like nobody is going to find me, they're going to leave without me for home. They're just going to forget about me. Where is everybody? I just remember thinking that . . . I don't think my mom knew I was lost yet and I was . . . I just remember feeling that nobody was going to find me. I was destined to be lost at K-Mart forever."

Of the 24 subjects to whom we suggested three true events and one false one, 75% said they couldn't remember the false event. The remaining subjects developed a complete false memory or a partial one. The false memories were described in fewer words than the true memories, and they were rated as less clear than the true memories. Despite these statistical differences between true and false memories, it was still the case that sometimes the false memories were described in quite a bit of detail, and embraced with a fair degree of confidence.

Where do their memories of being lost come from? One possibility is that subjects may be combining a genuine experience of being lost, or a stereotyped experience of being lost, with their semantic memories of the location selected by their family member (Bremerton K-Mart in the above example). Retrieval of a fragment of a "lost" memory, with enough source confusion about that memory, could lie at the heart of the ability to use this fragment to construct the kind of memory being sought.

The question arises of whether it would be possible to implant a false memory of something that is far less common in human experience than being lost. Several attempts have been made to create entire autobiographical memories for events that are not so common. One is that of Hyman and colleagues (1993). In one experiment, parents of college students supplied information about a series of personal events that occurred to their child before the age of 10. Subjects were asked to remember some "real" events, and also to remember a false one. One false event was about an overnight hospitalization for a high fever with a possible ear infection. Hyman and associates found that no subjects "recalled" the false events during the first interview. But in the second interview, which occurred from 1 to 7 days later, 20% of the subjects remembered something about the false events. A sample protocol is shown below from one of the misled subjects who was asked if she could remember something about a hospital event that had happened to her about the age of 5.

S: I just, I can remember the doctor always probing my ear and stuff, and I'm just crying all the time and it hurts.
I: Local hospital emergency room.
S: I remember the hospital.
I: The hospital, ok, anything at all you can remember, who might have been around.
S: Uh, I remember the nurse, she was a church friend. That helped.
I: Anything, just whatever you can think of, things like that.
S: The doctor was a male, I think so. That's it.

Hyman's results show again the possibility of being able to implant entire false memories. In current work, Hyman and colleagues are convincing adult subjects that as children they went to a wedding, knocked over the punch bowl, and spilled punch all over the parents of the bride or groom. These empirical demonstrations support the feasibility, with sufficient suggestion, of inducing entire false memories, including memories of relatively uncommon experiences.

Even more startling results were obtained in a study using children as subjects (Ceci, Crotteau, Smith, and Loftus, in press; see Ceci, Chapter 3, for more details). The subjects were 96 children ranging in age from 3 to 6 who completed a minimum of seven interviews about past events in their lives. They were interviewed individually about real (parent-supplied) and fictitious (experimenter-contrived) events, and had to say whether each event had happened to them or not. One "false" event concerned getting one's hand caught in a mousetrap and having to go to the hospital to get it removed; another concerned going on a hot air balloon ride with classmates.

The children were interviewed many times, and by the seventh interview, approximately three months later, about 36% of the younger children and 32% of the older ones now claimed that the events happened.

These children not only said that the events happened, but they greatly embellished their false memories. One 4-year-old boy described his contact with the mousetrap this way: "My brother Colin was trying to get Blowtorch from me, and I wouldn't let him take it from me, so he pushed me into the wood pile where the mousetrap was. And then my finger got caught in it." He remembered the trip to the hospital as a family affair: "And then we went to the hospital, and my mommy, daddy, and Colin drove me there, to the hospital in our van, because it was far away." He even remembered the particular finger that the doctor put the bandage on.

One interesting aspect of the study occurred at the debriefing phase. When the parents tried to explain to their children that the false events hadn't really happened, some of the children insisted that they had. One boy, when told by his mother that he had never had his hand caught in a mousetrap, still claimed that he had: "But it did happen. I remember it!" Another girl argued with her mother, claiming the mother didn't know the truth because the mother wasn't home at the time when the mousetrap was engaged.

This study shows that it is indeed possible to suggest an entire false event to a child that can become part of the child's memory. Although repeated interviews did not significantly increase the false beliefs, in a similar study involving more interviews about different fictitious items (falling off a tricycle and getting stitches in the leg), the rate of "buying" the false memory was greater with more interviews (Ceci et al., 1994).

Taken together, these studies show that one can implant entire false memories into the minds of adults as well as children. One intuitively appealing way to think about these findings is in terms of source confusions. People tend to pick up information from different sources, different times, different parts of their lives. When asked to recall, they use this information to construct memories. The studies of memory malleability provide good support for something that Lindsay and Johnson (1989) suggested some time ago, namely that two memories can become confused because people forget their sources.

Final Remarks

What do we now know as a result of hundreds of studies of misinformation, spanning two decades and most of the world's continents? That misinformation can lead people to have false memories that they appear to believe in as much as some of their genuine memories. That misinformation can lead to small changes in memory (hammers become screwdrivers) or large changes (barns that didn't exist, and hospitals that were never visited).

These findings have some bearing on what Kihlstrom (1994) has called "an epidemic of cases of exhumed memory," referring to people (sometimes patients in psychotherapy) who appear to recover long-forgotten memories of childhood abuse and trauma. While Kihlstrom, we, and almost everyone who writes on this subject acknowledge that childhood trauma is a major problem for our society, it is also true that some of the cases seem to reflect something other than actual experience. A number of clinicians and researchers have worried that false memories about an abusive childhood might sometimes be created in the minds of vulnerable patients (Ganaway, 1989; Lindsay and Read, in press; Loftus and Ketcham, 1994; Ofshe and Watters, 1994; Persinger, 1994; Yapko, 1994). Coons (1994) recently analyzed his patients' memories of childhood satanic ritual abuse and concluded that "pseudomemories may be created by therapists in highly suggestible patients" (p. 1376). Coons and others have worried in particular about false memories of abuse being created by suggestion, hypnosis, social contagion, and regression. His worries are well-founded; if a simple suggestion from a family member can create an entire autobiographical memory for an event that would have been mildly traumatic, how much more powerful would be a combination of techniques, over the course of years of therapy? Understanding how we can become mentally tricked by suggestion can help therapists gather true memories of the past and avoid inadvertently creating false ones. Such an understanding offers a way for all of us to avoid being tricked, and ultimately provides an important window into the malleability of the mind.

References

Alba, J. W. and Hasher, L. (1983) Is memory schematic? *Psychological Bulletin, 93,* 203–231.

Bartlett, F. C. (1932) *Remembering: A study in experimental and social psychology.* Cambridge: Cambridge University Press.

Belli, R. F., Windschitl, P. D., McCarthy, T. T., and Winfrey, S. E. (1992) Detecting memory impairment with a modified test procedure: Manipulating retention interval with centrally presented event items. *Journal of Experimental Psychology: Learning, Memory and Cognition, 18,* 356–367.

Birch, S. L. and Brewer, W. F. (1990) Memory permanence versus memory replacement in sentence recall. Unpublished manuscript, University of Illinois at Urbana-Champaign.

Brainerd, C. and Ornstein, P. A. (1991) Children's memory for witnessed events. In J. Doris (Ed.) *The suggestibility of children's recollections.* Washington D.C.: American Psychological Association.

Brainerd, C. J., Reyna, V. F., Howe, M. L., and Kingma, J. (1990) The development of forgetting and reminiscence. *Monographs of the Society for Research in Child Development, 55* (3, Whole No. 222).

Brewer, W. F. and Nakamura, G. V. (1984) The nature and functions of schemas.

In R. S. Wyer and T. K. Srull (Eds.) *Handbook of Social Cognition* (Vol. 1, pp. 119–160). Hillsdale, N.J.: Erlbaum.

Brewin, C. R. (1989) Cognitive change processes in psychotherapy. *Psychological Review*, 96, 379–394.

Ceci, S. J., Crotteau, M. L., Smith, E., and Loftus, E. F. (in press) Repeatedly thinking about a non-event: Source misattributions among preschoolers. *Consciousness and Cognition.*

Ceci, S. J., Loftus, E. F., Leichtman, M., and Bruck, M. (1994) The role of source misattributions in the creation of false beliefs among preschoolers. *International Journal of Clinical and Experimental Hypnosis.*

Coons, P. M. (1994) Reports of satanic ritual abuse: Further implications about pseudomemories. *Perceptual and Motor Skills*, 78, 1376–1378.

Dodson, C. and Reisberg, D. (1991) Indirect testing of eyewitness memory: The (non)-effect of misinformation. *Bulletin of the Psychonomic Society*, 29, 333–336.

Ganaway, G. K. (1989) Historical truth versus narrative truth: Clarifying the role of exogenous trauma in the etiology of Multiple Personality Disorder and its variants. *Dissociation*, 2, 205–220.

Garry, M., Rader, M., and Loftus, E. F. (in press) Classic and contemporary studies on the impact of misleading information. In Y. Itskushima, S. Hamada, K. Ichinose, and Y. Watanabe (Eds.) *Eyewitness testimony: Interdisciplinary perspectives.* Tokyo: Shakaihyouron Press.

Graf, P. and Schacter, D. L. (1987) Selective effects of interference on implicit and explicit memory for new associations. *Journal of Experimental Psychology: Learning, Memory and Cognition*, 13, 45–53.

Greene, R. L. (1992) *Human memory: Paradigms and paradoxes.* Hillsdale, N.J.: Erlbaum.

Hyman, I. E., Billings, F. J., Husband, S. G., Husband, T. H., and Smith, D. B. (1993) Memories and false memories of childhood experiences. Poster presented at the annual meeting of the Psychonomic Society, Washington D.C. Unpublished manuscript, Western Washington University.

Jacoby, L. L. and Kelley, C. M. (1992) A process-dissociation framework for investigating unconscious influences. *Current Directions in Psychological Science*, 1, 174–179.

Johnson, M. K. (1988) Discriminating the origin of information. In T. F. Ohmanns and B. A. Maher (Eds.) *Delusional beliefs: Interdisciplinary perspectives* (pp. 34–65). New York: Wiley.

Kantor, D. (1980) Critical identity image. In J. K. Pearce and L. J. Friedman (Eds.) *Family therapy: Combining psychodynamic and family systems approaches* (pp. 137–167). New York: Grune and Stratton.

Kihlstrom, J. F. (July 1994) The social construction of memory. Paper presented at the American Psychological Society Annual Meeting, Washington, D.C.

Lindsay, D. S. (1990) Misleading suggestions can impair eyewitnesses' ability to remember event details. *Journal of Experimental Psychology: Learning, Memory and Cognition*, 16, 1077–1083.

Lindsay, D. S. (1993) Eyewitness suggestibility. *Current Directions in Psychological Science*, 2, 86–89.

Lindsay, D. S. and Johnson, M. K. (1989) The eyewitness suggestibility effect and memory for source. *Memory and Cognition*, 17, 349–358.

Lindsay, D. S. and Read, D. (in press) *Applied cognitive psychology.*

Loftus, E. F. (1991) Made in memory: Distortions of recollection after misleading information. In G. Bower (Ed.) *Psychology of learning and motivation* (Vol 27, pp. 187–215). New York: Academic Press.

Loftus, E. F. and Coan, J. (in press) The construction of childhood memories. In D. Peters (Ed.) *The child witness in context: cognitive, social, and legal perspectives.* New York: Kluwer.

Loftus, E. F. and Ketcham, K. (1994) *The myth of repressed memory.* New York: St. Martin's Press.

McClelland, J. L. (1988) Connectionist models and psychological evidence. *Journal of Memory and Language,* 27, 107–123.

McClelland, J. L. and Rumelhart, D. E. (1986) *Parallel distributed processing.* Cambridge, Mass.: MIT Press.

Metcalfe, J. (1990) Composite holographic associative recall model (CHARM) and blended memories in eyewitness testimony. *Journal of Experimental Psychology: General,* 119, 145–160.

Ofshe, R. and Watters, E. (1994) *Making monsters.* New York: Scribner's.

Persinger, M. A. (1994) Elicitation of "childhood memories" in hypnosis-like settings is associated with complex partial epileptic-like signs for women but not for men: Implications for the False Memory Syndrome. *Perceptual and Motor Skills,* 78, 643–651.

Pillemer, D. B. (1992) Remembering personal circumstances: A functional analysis. In E. Winograd and U. Neisser (Eds.) *Affect and accuracy in recall.* New York: Cambridge University Press.

Roediger, H. L. (1990) Implicit memory: Retention without remembering. *American Psychologist,* 45, 1043–1056.

Schacter, D. L. (1987) Implicit memory: History and current status. *Journal of Experimental Psychology: Learning, Memory, and Cognition,* 13, 501–518.

Schooler, J. W. and Tanaka, J. W. (1991) Composites, compromised, and CHARM: What is the evidence for blend memory representations? *Journal of Experimental Psychology: General,* 120, 96–100.

Terr, L. (1988) What happens to early memories of trauma? A study of 20 children under age five at the time of documented traumatic events. *Journal of the American Academy of Child and Adolescent Psychiatry,* 27, 96–104.

Van der Kolk, B. A. and Van der Hart, O. (1991) The intrusive past: The flexibility of memory and the engraving of trauma. *American Imago,* 48, 425–454.

Weingardt, K. R., Toland, H. K., and Loftus, E. F. (1994) Reports of suggested memories: Do people truly believe them? In D. Ross, J. D. Read, and M. P. Toglia (Eds.) *Adult eyewitness testimony: Current trends and developments* (pp. 3–26). New York: Springer-Verlag.

Yapko, M. (1994) *Suggestions of abuse.* New York: Simon and Schuster.

Zaragoza, M. S. and Lane, S. M. (1994) Source misattributions and the suggestibility of eyewitness memory. *Journal of Experimental Psychology: Learning, Memory and Cognition,* 20, 934–945.

Constructive Memory and Memory Distortions: A Parallel-Distributed Processing Approach

2

James L. McClelland

Bartlett (1932) introduced and insisted on the view that memory is a constructive process. His view was essentially that recall is not a retrieval, but a reconstruction, in which aspects of the content of previously presented material are woven into a coherent whole, with the aid of preexisting knowledge. Details may be distorted to increase coherence; rationalizations not present in the original may be introduced; details that are consistent with the synthesized coherent story may be added; and details that are inconsistent may be dropped. Neisser (1967) likened both perception and memory to the constructive activities of a paleontologist, who uses a collection of bone fragments, as well as everything she knows about dinosaurs from previous experience, to reconstruct the skeleton of a particular dinosaur. These ideas are consistent with what we would refer to today as a constraint satisfaction process, in which remembering is simultaneously constrained by traces left in the mind by the event we are remembering itself, by background knowledge of related material, and by constraints and influences imposed by the situation surrounding the act of recollection. Obviously if memory is constructive in this way, this has profound implications for the question of the veridicality of memory and the extent to which it may be influenced by suggestion, preexisting knowledge, and other related experiences.

My interest is in the mechanisms that may implement this constructive, constraint satisfaction process. Remembering, I will argue, takes place in a parallel distributed processing system—a system consisting of a large number of simple but massively interconnected processing units. Processing in such systems takes place through the propagation of activation among the units, based on excitatory and inhibitory connections. Forming a memory trace for something—say, an episode or event—begins with the construction of a pattern of activity over the processing units, with the experience itself strongly influencing the pattern. But the existing connections among the units will also influence the pattern constructed, thereby introducing the possibility of additions, omissions, and distortions. Storage of a trace of the episode or event then occurs through the modification of the strengths of the connections among the units; to a first approximation, the connection from a unit that is active in the representation to another such active unit will tend to increase in strength, while the strength of connections between active and inactive units will tend to decrease.

Remembering may occur when some aspect or aspects of an event arise again as input. This may activate some of the units that previously participated in the representation of the episode or event, and these may in turn activate other units, via the weighted connections. The pattern that is constructed again depends on the connections among the units, and since these were adjusted previously when the episode was first experienced, the pattern that is constructed will tend to correspond to the pattern that was present at the time of storage. But the units that participate in representing one episode or event also participate in representing other episodes, and so the representation that is constructed may be affected by many other experiences. This means that my memory of any one episode or event will tend to reflect the influence of what I have learned from many other episodes or events.

I will describe two models that capture this constructive process in different ways. Both models have their origins in early connectionist papers, one by myself (McClelland, 1981) and one by Hinton (1981). Neither model is fully adequate in itself, but I will propose a synthesis of the two that may capture some of the main features of human memory, including aspects of memory distortions. The synthesis may provide as well one way of thinking about amnesia.

A Trace Synthesis Model

The first model (McClelland, 1981) focuses on distortion processes that can occur during acts of remembering, using a simple, localist connectionist network for the storage and retrieval of information. I used in the example the task of remembering facts about a collection of two somewhat unsavory individuals, belonging to two made-up gangs, the Jets and the Sharks. The Jets tended to be in their twenties, to be single, and to have only a Junior High School education, though no one Jet had all these characteristics; the Sharks tended to be older, to be married, and to have attended High School, though again no one Shark had all these properties. Members of both gangs were equally likely to be pushers, bookies, or burglars.

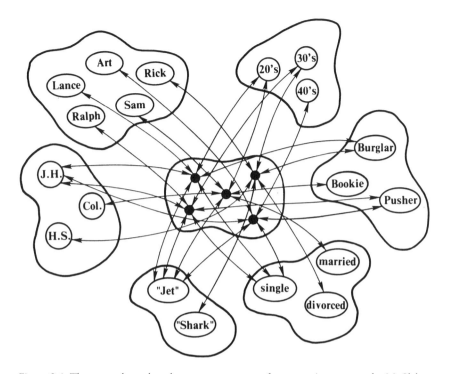

Figure 2.1 The network used to demonstrate aspects of constructive memory by McClelland (1981). The units participating in the representation of a few of the members of the
Jets and Sharks gangs described in the text are shown. Units within the same group are
mutually inhibitory; units connected with bidirectional arrows are mutually excitatory.
From McClelland (1981), fig. 1, p. 171.

In the model, I represented each individual with its own connectionist
processing unit that I will call an instance unit (see Figure 2.1). The model
also contained property units, one for each property an individual might
have. Names were treated as properties, so there were units for names, for
gang membership, for education, for marital status, and for occupation. Bidirectional, excitatory connections between units were used to link instance
units to the units representing their properties, so that if one activated a
name unit, it activated the corresponding instance unit, and the instance
unit activated the other properties of the instance. The instance units formed
a group of units that were mutually inhibitory, so that if one was active it
tended to suppress the others; similarly, the units for each type of property
were grouped into clusters of mutually inhibitory units. The use of single
units to represent whole items is a simplification—I will argue later that it

is more correct to use distributed representations, both for the whole and for the parts. However, even this simple model captures crucial aspects of the kinds of reconstructive processes that take place during remembering.

My focus in the original work reported in McClelland (1981) was on the process of constructing representations of material not explicitly stored in memory. One such case involved constructing a composite recollection of the typical Jet or Shark. In the model this could be done simply by activating the unit for Jet. This unit then sent activation to the instance units for all of the Jets, and these in turn sent activation to the units for each instance's properties. The inhibition among the instance units prevented any of these units from becoming too strongly activated, but they all contributed some activation to their property units. As a result the properties of the typical Jet became active (age in 20's, single, JH education); all of the occupations were partially activated.

This first example shows a desirable property of this sort of memory system—it can spontaneously generalize from examples. Another property—which may often be desirable but which can also be undesirable—is revealed when the model is used to try to retrieve the properties of a single individual by activating the unit for that individual's name. This individual's properties tend to be more strongly activated than the properties of any other individual, but one finds that as the activation process goes on, other, similar individuals become partially activated. This happens because as the properties of the target individual become active, they send activation to the instance units for other individuals, and these, in turn, tend to activate the units for their properties. This effect can be particularly potent—and can lead to strong distortions—when some piece of information about the target individual is missing. To show this, I first deleted the connection between the instance node for Lance and the property node for his occupation—he happened to be a burglar. Then I activated the name unit for Lance. This caused the instance node to become active, and the instance node then activated the property nodes for Jet, 20's, JH education, and married. Now, there happened to be several other Jets who had many of these properties, and they all happened to be burglars. As a result, the model filled in this occupation for Lance. In this instance the result happened to be correct, but the same thing would of course have happened whether Lance had been a burglar or not. Had he been a pusher or a bookie (or, for that matter, someone with an entirely innocuous occupation), the model would have filled in burglar anyway. In that case this would have been a clear example of a memory distortion: Lance would have been guilty by association.

The model illustrates two key points central to the issues raised in this volume. First, it provides an explicit though simple mechanism illustrating how memory distortions can arise from the workings of ordinary memory retrieval processes. These processes are often beneficial—they allow the formation of generalizations over similar instances and the filling in of missing properties based on the properties of other, similar individuals—but they can potentially be harmful in that the information filled in need not be correct.

Second, the model has the same property that human memory has, of often failing to separate information that arises from different sources. Suppose that a new instance node is formed from every experience (a proposal strikingly similar to the memory model of Hintzman, 1988), and suppose one has a number of similar experiences. Then when we try to recall one, pieces of other similar experiences will tend to intrude particularly in those aspects of the original for which the information is weak or missing. In the model, it is unfortunately not possible to inspect each memory trace individually; the information is not stored in the units themselves, but in their connections; like connections among neurons in the brain, we only know what is stored in the connections through the effects these connections have on the outcome of processing. But, since many units and connections contribute to this outcome, full disentangling of the specific cause of each aspect of the outcome is impossible. It will, then, in general not be possible to identify the specific source of any aspect of constructed recollection.

Given the model, then, the memory distortions reported in this volume by Loftus, Ceci, Moscovitch, and others are to be expected. Perhaps the only thing that is unexpected about them is the resistance that often arises to their acceptance. This resistance may come from implicit acceptance of an alternative model of memory, in which memory traces are not so much constructed as retrieved, like books from a library. The metaphor of human memory and human knowledge as a library provides a basis for accounting for the role of organization in memory, but gives no basis for understanding distortion. I believe that as we come to understand memory better and better, it will become increasingly clear that this is a misleading metaphor.

An Experimental Test of the Trace Synthesis Model

To test the model described above, and to extend the empirical data base of evidence of memory distortions, Leigh Nystrom and I developed an experimental paradigm designed to elicit trace synthesis errors in remembering (Nystrom and McClelland, 1992). In this paradigm, subjects study a list of sentences, and then are later cued for complete recall of individual whole sentences when a fragment is presented as a probe. Consider sentences of the form: "The policeman gave the accountant the hammer in the basement." We imagine that the sentence is analyzed into a set of role-filler pairs, which are then represented by the activations of input units in the network shown in Figure 2.2. The network is strictly analogous to the model previously described. There is a pool of instance units, with one unit assigned to

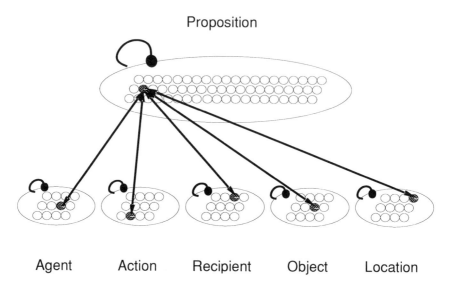

Proposition

Agent   Action   Recipient   Object   Location

Figure 2.2 Sketch of the network architecture used by Nystrom and McClelland (1992). The units participating in the representation of a particular proposition are shown, along with the bidirectional connections that allow this model to perform cued recall of the whole sentence when part of the sentence is represented as a cue.

each proposition. The model also contains several pools of property units, one for each type of role that can occur in one of the sentences. Each pool contains a unit for each word that can appear in that role. We represent the sentence about the policeman as shown in the figure. Another sentence, with a non-overlapping set of words, would involve a different word-in-role unit in each property unit pool, and a different proposition unit.

In a model such as this, cued remembering occurs by simply turning on the units for the words contained in the probe, and asking the network to essentially fill in the rest. This occurs via a gradual constraint satisfaction process. Processing begins with the units for the cue words clamped and continues until a stable pattern of activation is achieved. When the cue uniquely matches one stored sentence, and there are no other very similar sentences, the correct sentence tends to be recalled. However, errors can occur when there are two or more stored items that have the same or a similar degree of match to the probe. In this case the "remembered" pattern is a constructed synthesis of two or more stored traces.

Nystrom and I studied the adequacy of this model to account for memory and memory distortions in a series of four experiments. Here I will discuss only one of these. The subjects studied lists of sentences set up so that some of the sentences shared three content words in common with another paired

Table 2.1 Example overlap and control sentence pairs from Nystrom and McClelland (1992), with corresponding test probes

---

Overlap Pair:
  The policeman gave the accountant the hammer in the dining room.
  The farmer gave the accountant the hammer in the garage.

Control Pair:
  The driver showed the receptionist the toaster in the kitchen.
  The swimmer loaned the salesman the envelope in the basement.

Overlap Probe:
  The . . . gave the accountant the hammer in the . . .

Control Probe:
  The . . . showed the receptionist the toaster in the . . .

---

sentence. One such pair of overlapping sentences is shown in Table 2.1; a pair of control sentences, with no overlap, is also shown. In the model, we assigned a different proposition unit to each sentence, and connected this unit to the input units for each of the corresponding words. In the case of overlap sentences, three of the five role-fillers are the same, so the proposition units in these cases are connected to overlapping sets of input units, as shown in Figure 2.3.

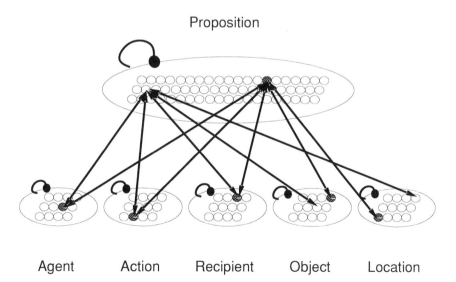

Proposition

Agent   Action   Recipient   Object   Location

Figure 2.3 The units and connections participating in the representation of a second sentence that overlaps with the first one shown previously in Figure 2.2. Presentation of an ambiguous probe tends to activate both sentences and may produce a blend error.

Our focus in this research was on trace synthesis at the time of recall, and we therefore went to some lengths to minimize the possibility that subjects would be reminded of the first member of each overlap pair when given the second member during the exposure phase of the experiment. This was done, first of all, by developing a cover task that focused subjects on analyzing each individual sentence separately from all of the others without any mention of a later memory test: subjects were told their task was to rate each sentence for its overall plausibility and to say how well they thought each word fit with the overall event described by the whole sentence. Other precautions included varying the placement within the sentences of the overlapping words, and separating overlapping sentences as far as possible in the study list of 34 sentences. Although subjects did notice that some words were occasionally repeated, only a few subjects reported that the second member of an overlap pair ever caused them to recall the previous member of the pair, and eliminating these subjects from the analyses did not change the results. Thus we were reasonably confident that reminding and trace synthesis during the study phase was not a major factor in determining the results.

After the subjects completed a filler task for 5 minutes, the cued recall phase of the experiment was administered. This involved presenting 16 sentence fragments, each with blanks for two content words. Eight fragments were from overlap pairs and eight were from control pairs. Thus a subject might see probes like the ones shown in Table 2.1.

In both cases, the subjects were told to complete the probe with the first studied sentence that came to mind. Subjects were alerted to the fact that sometimes the probe matched two studied sentences equally well, and they were told to recall only one of the two sentences and to take care not to mix up the two. After the first recall they were given an opportunity to recall the second sentence. I will be discussing only the results of the first recall here. Suffice it to say that second recalls were generally less accurate than first recalls.

On the first recalls, the probability of correctly recalling a complete sentence did not differ between the overlap and control pairs: two words from the same sentence that matched the probe were recalled 42% of the time in the overlap condition and 41% of the time in the control condition. However, in the overlap condition subjects did sometimes make what we can call synthesis errors—errors in which one word came from one of the sentences that matched the probe and the other came from the other of these two sentences. This occurred on nearly 10% of the error trials (5.4% of all trials with overlap probes, compared to less than 1% of trials with control probes). The rate of synthesis errors may seem relatively low, but they were reliably more frequent than chance. Confidence ratings were obtained on each recall trial; confidence was slightly less on average for synthesis errors than for completely correct responses, but on 40% of the synthesis errors subjects gave the highest confidence rating, corresponding to the statement "I am sure both words recalled came from a single studied sentence that matched the probe." We take the experiment, then, as demonstrating that memory distortions can arise from trace synthesis at the time of recall. We would not want to claim, of course, that trace synthesis does not often occur earlier, when an intervening event reminds us of a previous event; indeed, it may be that this is one common source of memory distortions. We would only suggest that our results support the view that trace synthesis can occur at recall as well as between initial study and recall.

We modeled the data from this and the other three studies we conducted using the model discussed previously. To fit the data it was necessary to make two additional stipulations: first, that processing has an inherently random component; and second, that subjects sometimes failed to encode each sentence completely. We implemented this latter assumption by randomly eliminating a fraction of the connections between the input and prop units. These assumptions do different and important work in accounting for the data.

The first assumption—intrinsic variability—allows the network to select essentially randomly between two equally good responses in cases where two studied sentences fit the probe equally well. Intrinsic variability is implemented simply by incorporating normally distributed random noise into the input to each unit. Each time the unit's state is updated, this noise affects the exact degree of activation. If high levels of noise are used, the model becomes totally random in its behavior; but with small amounts of noise, the variability effectively causes the network to choose randomly among equally good alternatives. Without any noise the network will have a tendency to partially activate both matching sentences most of the time, and will not tend to recall one or the other: with the randomness in place, on the other hand, the network will tend to settle to one of the two answers. The idea of intrinsic variability in processing was introduced into connectionist modeling by several investigators in the mid-1980s (Geman and Geman, 1984; Smolensky, 1986; Hinton and Sejnowski, 1986). I have suggested elsewhere that intrinsic variability is a general property of human cognitive function, and I think it is necessary if we are to model the kinds of results we see in a wide range of tasks, such as free association, stem completion, or perceptual identification, where subjects generally emit one or the other of a set of alternative coherent responses, rather than a blend of many alternatives (McClelland, 1991). Others have established that the outcome of this settling process is optimal from the point of view of maximizing the probability of selecting the correct answer, given that the weights accurately encode information about the domain (Geman and Geman, 1984).

The second assumption—encoding failures—allows the model to account simultaneously for the existence of synthesis errors, together with the fact that the probability of correct recall did not suffer in the overlap condition compared to the control condition. Simplifying a bit, with this assumption in place, correct recall of a single sentence depends on whether it has been completely encoded, and the probability of complete encoding is independent of whether there is an overlap sentence in the study set. Incomplete encoding offers an opportunity for synthesis errors: we obtained an excellent fit to the data by assuming that subjects failed to encode 20% of the words. In cases where there are gaps in the encoding of one of the sentences, the other can contribute, creating a memory distortion. Intrusions from the other sentence rush in when the most active trace provides no information.

Summary of the Trace Synthesis Model

The model I have described has considerable appeal as a simple descriptive account of the process of memory trace synthesis in cued recall and goes some way toward implementing the constructive memory retrieval process of which Bartlett and Neisser wrote. I should note that there are other models that can account for trace synthesis, including the MINERVA model of Hintzman (1988), as well as the models by Metcalfe (1990) and by Humphreys, Bain, and Pike (1989) that use distributed representations (see also McClelland and Rumelhart, 1985). The model of Metcalfe (1990) has been applied to a number of important findings on blend errors and other memory distortions and shows that such models can offer very nice accounts of much of the existing data on blending and memory distortion.

In spite of their success, all of these models lack something. There are other, deeper, more fundamental forces at work shaping memory performance. These processes, I believe, operate gradually over the course of cognitive development to shape the way we represent the constituents of memory traces—for example, the concepts that contribute to propositions. These representations, in turn, provide the basis for more powerful forms of constructive memory effects.

Models of Representation Formation via Gradual Learning

An early model that pointed the way toward this idea was presented by Hinton (1981). This model is sketched in Figure 2.4. It consists of separate sets of units for representing the first noun, relation, and second noun of three-term propositions such as "Fish can swim," "Sammy is a fish," "Elephants are gray," "Clyde is white," and so forth. The model is similar to the previous model, but now each word is a pattern of activation over the appropriate units rather than a single active unit. The whole proposition is represented as a pattern of activity over the three sets of constituent units,

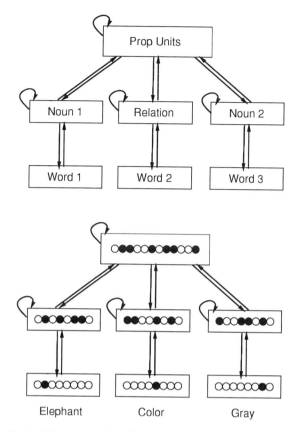

Figure 2.4 A slightly elaborated version of the connectionist network used by Hinton to represent propositions about the concepts. Each rectangle represents a pool of connectionist information processing units, and each arrow represents a full set of connections from each unit on the sending side of the arrow to each unit on the receiving side. Processing occurs by the propagation of activation among the units via the connection weights. Each unit simply sets its activation to a value between 0 and 1 based on the summed input it receives from other units via the weighted connections. For example, the connections from the Word 1 input units to the Noun 1 representation units allow a pattern of activation representing the first word of a proposition to activate the appropriate semantic pattern over the Noun 1 units. The connections between the different pools of constituent units and the Prop units encode the system's knowledge about propositions, and after the weights have been acquired through learning, these connections allow the third constituent of a proposition to be completed given the other two constituents as inputs. Return connections from the constituent units to the word units then provide for output of the pattern filled in by the network. The upper panel shows each pool of units with labels. The lower panel illustrates how a particular proposition would actually be represented.

and over an additional, fourth set of units called "PROP" units. The network contains bidirectional connections from each set of constituent units to the PROP units. There is also another set of connections for input to and output from the network; these allow inputs standing for specific words to activate distributed semantic patterns over the input units. The recurrent connections within each pool of units allow local pattern completion within each pool. The effect of this is to implement a "clean-up" process in which the pattern of activation tends to converge to the representation of a specific word, and has much the same effect as the mutual inhibition within layers in the previous model.

Once again, the knowledge or memory in this system is stored in the connections among the units. We can think of the input/output weights as encoding knowledge about the semantic pattern corresponding to each word of the proposition, and we can think of the connection weights between the constituent and PROP pools as encoding knowledge about the propositions that these constituents enter into with other constituents. Hinton (1981) suggested that this network would be able to generalize what it knows about one concept to other related concepts if similar concepts are represented by similar patterns of activation. Thus, if Clyde is a particular elephant, and Clyde is represented by a pattern that is similar to the pattern for elephant, then what we know about elephants will tend to generalize to Clyde. Such effects do not strictly obey the laws of logic; instead they obey the laws of association.

In Hinton's (1981) work, the representations of the concepts were assigned by hand. Connectionist learning algorithms have evolved considerably since that time, however, and we now have algorithms that can discover how to represent different concepts through repeated exposure to information about the entire semantic domain in which the concept is embedded. I will consider one such domain—the broad domain of living things. I show in Figure 2.5 a representation of a fragment of the knowledge someone might have about living things. This format is typical of the approach to knowledge representation used in classical artificial intelligence approaches to cognition, beginning with Quillian (1968). The knowledge has several characteristics: it is structured, in that it is organized into a hierarchy. Individual types or species are listed at the bottom of the hierarchy, and their organization into broad classes, and the organizations of these into larger classes, is indicated by "isa" links. We can imagine attaching, below the level of the types, specific instances of the types. For example, we could add "Tweety isa canary," and so forth; or if we had an Elephant node, we could add "Clyde isa Elephant." The network is potentially quite economical, in that facts that are true of whole sub-trees of the hierarchy can be attached at the highest level to which they apply. Given this, when some information is not stored on a specific concept, it may be inferred by searching through the tree. The process is equivalent to the standard logical syllogistic reason-

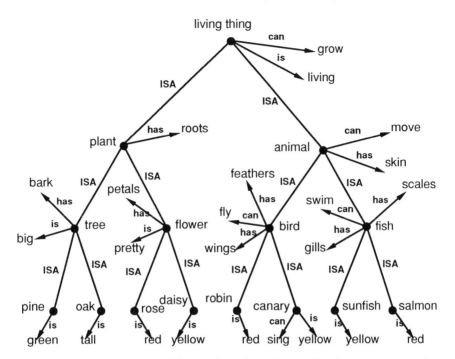

Figure 2.5 A semantic network of the type formerly used in models of the organization of knowledge in memory, containing the concepts and propositions used in the learning experiment of Rumelhart (1990). Adapted from fig. 1.8 of Rumelhart and Todd (1993) by McClelland et al. (1994) as their fig. 3, p. 13.

ing process through which we infer that Socrates is mortal. We know that Socrates is a man, and we know that men are mortal, therefore we can infer that Socrates is mortal too.

When one trains a network like the one shown in the previous figure with example propositions from this domain, it learns two things. It learns connection weights internally that encode the propositions, and that allow completion of a proposition from two of its terms. It also learns connection weights from the word input units to the constituent units that essentially assign useful semantic representations to each word. Hinton (1989) demonstrated this for kinship relationships. Rumelhart (1990; Rumelhart and Todd, 1993) applied the same idea to the domain of living things (the actual simulation model Rumelhart used was slightly simpler than the one shown in Figure 2.5), and I have chosen to use this case as my example. The results on which the following discussion depends come from a repetition of the Rumelhart (1990) simulation reported in McClelland, McNaughton, and O'Reilly (1994).

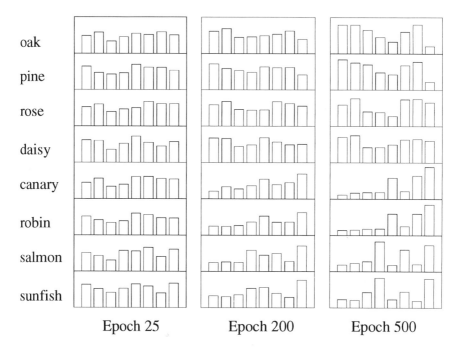

oak

pine

rose

daisy

canary

robin

salmon

sunfish

Epoch 25   Epoch 200   Epoch 500

Figure 2.6 Representations discovered in a replication of Rumelhart's (1990) experiment training a semantic network much like the one shown in Figure 2.5. The figure shows the activation of each of the Noun-1 units for each of the eight specific concepts used. The height of each vertical bar indicates the activation of the unit on a scale from 0 to 1. One can see that initially all the concepts have fairly similar representations. After 200 epochs of training, there is a clear differentiation of the representations of the plants and animals. After 500 epochs, the further differentiation of the plants into trees and flowers and of the animals into fish and birds is apparent. From McClelland et al. (1994), fig. 5, p. 16.

   Through gradual training on examples from the domain of plants and animals, the network learned more than just the propositions. It also learned to assign useful representations to each concept. The representations the network learned to use for the first noun are illustrated in Figures 2.6 and 2.7. These representations are determined by the connection weights from the concept input units to the concept representation units. Through the course of learning, these weights gradually change, so that the representations of the different concepts gradually come to capture how similar the concepts are in terms of the propositions they enter into. Canary and Robin enter into highly overlapping sets of propositions—for example, both are birds, both can fly, both have feathers. As a result of this, the network comes to assign them representations that are very similar; similar representations lead to similar outputs. Most important, once it has learned to use such

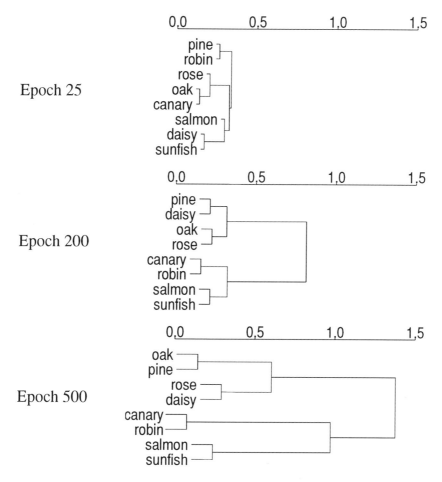

Figure 2.7 Similarity structure discovered in our replication of Rumelhart's (1990) learning experiment, using the representations shown in Figure 2.6. Initially, the patterns are all quite similar, and the weak similarity structure that exists is random. The concepts become progressively differentiated as learning progresses. From McClelland et al. (1994), fig. 6, p. 17.

representations, the network can use the similarity of the representations as the basis for inferences. Thus, once the network has learned how to represent Canary and Robin as similar to each other and distinct from other concepts, it now adds to the training set one proposition about a new type of animal— let's say the proposition that "Sparrow isa bird"—the network learns to assign "Sparrow" a representation similar to the representation it uses for other birds. After this proposition has been learned, we can then ask the network if it knows what a sparrow can do. This can be done by pattern completion—we can test the network to see if it can complete the pattern "Sparrow can . . ." with "fly." Indeed, Rumelhart showed in his simulations that if the network was trained on the full set of propositions concerning canaries and robins, he could teach it only one proposition about sparrows—namely "Sparrow is a bird"—and it was able to correctly complete other propositions about sparrows. The output was quite clear about those things that are generally true of the other birds. For those properties that differed between canary and robin, it produced ambiguous outputs. Thus it applied what it already knows about canaries and robins to sparrows.

Now, taking this model at least as a sketch of a model of our knowledge of facts and events, let us consider the nature of memory as reconstruction again. Individual experiences themselves are not separately represented; instead, they leave what I would call a structured system of knowledge stored in the connection weights. Furthermore, this knowledge is not itself directly accessible to overt responding or direct report. Instead the knowledge provides a mechanism that can construct responses to queries presented to the network, whether the actual proposition was ever actually experienced, as in the case of the actual training examples, or not, as in the case of questions we may ask about, for example, what a sparrow can do after the training described above. The outputs of such a network might then be the basis of performance we take as indicative of remembering, but many times they might reflect generalization based on the accumulated effects of prior experience, rather than the effects of storing anything like the specific item in memory. Such generalization is, I would suggest, central to our ability to act intelligently, and the process of learning the sorts of representations on which such generalizations are based is central to cognitive development (see McClelland, 1994, for discussion). But such generalization gives rise to distortions as an inherent by-product: it becomes impossible to distinguish between what has actually been experienced and what can be constructed based on other related things that have been experienced.

But there is something slightly wrong here. Our ability to isolate particular memories is not as bad as it would appear to be if we assumed that memory consists solely of the gradually acquired residue of a large body of experience. I can tell you a new fact—such as the fact that "Sammy is a Sunfish"—and this can affect your semantic memory right away. We need some mechanism capable of relatively rapid learning of the contents of individual episodes and experiences.

One might think that one could simply add new memories one at a time into a network like the Hinton (1981) network, but in fact this is not so. If one attempts to store additional memories all at once in such systems, it can be done, but at the cost of a phenomenon called "Catastrophic Interference" (McCloskey and Cohen, 1989). The addition of the new material causes a dramatic loss of the ability to perform correctly with other, similar material, particularly when, as is often the case, the new material is not completely consistent with what is already known. Thus if I train the network with the propositions "Sparrow isa bird" and "Sparrow is brown," it will drastically interfere with my ability to recover the color of other birds like canaries and robins (McClelland et al., 1994). The only way to add new information robustly to a structured memory system is to add it through a process called interleaved learning, in which learning occurs very gradually through repeated exposure to the new material, interleaved with ongoing exposure to other examples of the same domain of knowledge. Connection weight adjustments occur during exposure to the new material and the old, thereby gradually allowing the new material to be incorporated into the memory system without at the same time disrupting what is already known.

A Proposed Synthesis of the Models

A natural proposal that arises from this observation, then, is to suggest that the human memory is essentially a synthesis of the two types of models I have described above. One part of the system gradually learns to represent and use concepts as in the Hinton model, while another part is given the task of rapidly learning the specific content of individual events and experiences, storing them in a way that is similar to the method used in the Trace Synthesis model of McClelland (1981). I have presented a visualization of this idea in Figure 2.8.

This proposal may seem at first somewhat unparsimonious, but in fact it provides an account of the pattern of amnesia that results from bilateral lesions to the medial temporal lobes. Individuals with extensive damage to these brain regions show a very striking pattern of memory deficits (for overviews see Squire, Chapter 7 of this volume). These patients appear profoundly deficient in the ability to form new semantic or episodic memories, but the ability to acquire new implicit knowledge such as new cognitive skills or sensitivity to the sequential dependencies among stimuli in implicit learning tasks remains intact, and existing semantic knowledge such as semantic associations can be primed. Semantic and episodic knowledge acquired long before the damage occurred is spared—that is, it is as good in such patients as it is in age-matched controls. In fact, there is a temporally graded retrograde amnesia, which in humans can extend over several years, such that semantic and episodic memories that were acquired shortly before the occurrence of the damage are profoundly affected, and memories that were acquired at progressively earlier times are progressively less and less affected. Crucially, in several studies both in humans and in other animals, memory for the most recent premorbid time periods can actually be much worse than memory for material from slightly more remote time periods.

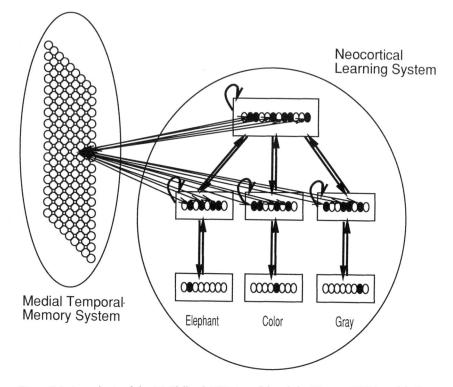

Figure 2.8 A synthesis of the McClelland (1981) model and the Hinton (1981) model. One part, based on the McClelland (1981) model, allows the storage and retrieval of individual traces, subject to trace synthesis, while the other part, more similar to the model of Hinton (1981), makes use of gradual, interleaved learning to acquire a structured system of knowledge gradually from exposures to ensembles of events and experiences. The part of the model based on McClelland (1981) plays a role akin to that played by medial temporal lobe structures in the brain, while the part based on Hinton (1981) plays a role similar to that played by other learning systems in the human neocortex.

We can account for these findings by assuming that older, consolidated memories, as well as cognitive skills and other "implicit" forms of knowledge, are subserved by information processing systems located in the large neocortical information processing system situated outside the medial temporal region. I identify these systems—hereafter labeled collectively the neocortical system—with the systems that acquire knowledge very gradually, through small adjustments to connection weights, represented in Figure 2.8 schematically by the network of the type introduced by Hinton (1981). The connection adjustments in this system, as we have seen, lead to the gradual emergence of structured knowledge systems such as those that are required for adequate generalization in domains that others have tended to treat as implicit—domains such as syntax—and domains that others have tended to treat as explicit—domains such as semantic memory. At the same time we assume that the ability to perform correctly in explicit memory tasks based on rapidly formed memory traces of recent events and experiences arises from learning that takes place within the medial temporal lobes, hereafter called the medial temporal lobe system. Recently, Bruce McNaughton, Randy O'Reilly, and I have proposed an account of the amnesic syndrome based on these ideas (McClelland et al., 1994). On this view, an experience, such as hearing someone say "Sammy is a sunfish," produces a pattern of activation widely distributed throughout the neocortical system; connections from this system into the medial temporal region produce a corresponding pattern of activation over the neurons there. The medial temporal lobe system then plays the role that the proposition units play in the McClelland (1981) model, linking all of the constituents of the event together into a single trace. We do not think this is done by assigning an individual neuron to each episodic memory, as originally proposed by McClelland (1981). However, an explication of the details of our view of the nature of medial temporal lobe representation is beyond the scope of this chapter. Suffice it to say that we think of the representation as sharing many characteristics with the representations used in the trace synthesis model: the representations, though distributed, are relatively sparse (few units active), and each unit that participates in the representation is activated only when a conjunction of elements occurs in the input (for fuller discussion, see O'Reilly and McClelland, in press).

Once a representation has been set up in the medial temporal lobe system, memory can be probed by presenting an incomplete fragment, just as in the trace synthesis model, and reconstruction occurs, via return connections. Each time a trace is synthesized, a small amount of connection adjustment takes place within the neocortical system as well. Consolidation is thought to be the result of this gradual neocortical learning that occurs every time a memory trace is reconstructed. The process is gradual, so that the new information initially stored via the medial temporal system itself can be gradually integrated into the system of representations used in the neocortical system without disrupting existing knowledge stored therein. This sort of dual memory system then allows new information to be rapidly stored in the medial temporal system without producing catastrophic interference with what is known in the neocortex. Information that is repeatedly reinstated, interleaved with ongoing exposure to other information, gradually becomes incorporated into the representations in the neocortex.

Conclusion

I have concurred with those who hold that memory is a constructive process, and I have proposed two rather different types of connectionist mechanisms that can contribute to the synthesis of memory traces; and I have suggested that both models capture aspects of the constructive processes that occur in memory. Indeed, I would suggest that both sorts of constructive processes may contribute to every act of remembering. One contribution to remembering may come from the medial temporal lobe trace of the episode or event itself; if this were the only contribution, we could speak simply of recalling that previous experience, perhaps with gaps arising from forgetting or encoding failure. But remembering involves an activation and synthesis process, in which the representations of other events and experiences stored in the medial temporal lobe can contribute to the reconstructed trace, as they sometimes do in the trace synthesis model. It also involves contributions from background knowledge based on information acquired very gradually over the course of a lifetime of experience directly within the neocortical system. If these ideas have any validity, we cannot see remembering as recall, but as a synthesis of contributions from many different sources of information.

The notion that much of memory may be based on knowledge built up gradually through exposure to large ensembles of experiences has many implications for the likelihood of veridical memory and for our ability to uncover the source of the outputs generated by our memory systems, an issue central to many of the other chapters in this volume. If memory were a propositional network of the Quillian type, then separating real from illusory memories would just be a matter of separating propositions derived from experience from those that were inferred; in principle we might imagine we could train ourselves, like Sherlock Holmes, to avoid making inappropriate inferences and therefore befuddling our memories. If memory is always an active synthesis of traces as in the McClelland (1981) model, there is still hope to somehow minimize the intrusion of inappropriate traces by probing our memory just right, so that activation of inappropriate traces is minimized. But if memories are always constructed with at least a partial reliance on a system of connection weights acquired gradually through extensive experience with a domain of knowledge, our hope of disentangling the individual traces disappears completely, and the likelihood that we can isolate the contribution of a specific experience becomes increasingly remote.

References

Bartlett, F. C. (1932). *Remembering*. Cambridge, Mass.: Cambridge University Press.

Geman, S. and Geman, D. (1984). Stochastic relaxation, Gibbs distributions, and the Bayesian restoration of images. *IEEE: Transactions of Pattern Analysis and Machine Intelligence*, PAMI-6, 721—741.

Hinton, G. E. (1981). Implementing semantic networks in parallel hardware. In

G. E. Hinton and J. A. Anderson (Eds.), *Parallel models of associative memory.* Hillsdale, N.J.: Erlbaum, Chap. 6, 161—187.

Hinton, G. E. (1989). Learning distributed representations of concepts. In R. G. M. Morris (Ed.), *Parallel distributed processing: Implications for psychology and neurobiology.* Oxford: Clarendon Press, Chap. 3, 46—61.

Hinton, G. E. and Sejnowski, T. J. (1986). Learning and relearning in boltzmann machines. In D. E. Rumelhart and J. L. McClelland (Eds.), *Parallel distributed processing: Explorations in the microstructure of cognition,* Vol. 1. Cambridge, Mass.: MIT Press, Chap. 7, 282—317.

Hintzman, D. L. (1988). Judgements of frequency and recognition memory in a multiple-trace model. *Psychological Review, 95,* 528—551.

Humphreys, M. S., Bain, J. D., and Pike, R. (1989). Different ways to cue a coherent memory system: A theory for episodic, semantic, and procedural tasks. *Psychological Review, 96,* 208—233.

McClelland, J. L. (1981). Retrieving general and specific information from stored knowledge of specifics. In *Proceedings of the Third Annual Conference of the Cognitive Science Society.* Berkeley: 170—172.

McClelland, J. L. (1991). Stochastic interactive activation and the effect of context on perception. *Cognitive Psychology, 23,* 1—44.

McClelland, J. L. (1994). The interaction of nature and nurture in development: A parallel distributed processing perspective. In P. Bertelson, P. Eelen, and G. D'Ydewalle (Eds.), *Current advances in psychological science: Ongoing research.* Hillsdale, N.J.: Erlbaum.

McClelland, J. L., McNaughton, B. L., and O'Reilly, R. C. (1994). Why there are complementary learning systems in hippocampus and neocortex: Insights from the successes and failures of connectionist models of learning and memory. Pittsburgh: Department of Psychology, Carnegie Mellon University, Technical Report PDP.CNS.94.1.

McClelland, J. L. and Rumelhart, D. E. (1985). Distributed memory and the representation of general and specific information. *Journal of Experimental Psychology, General, 114,* 159—188.

McCloskey, M. and Cohen, N. J. (1989). Catastrophic interference in connectionist networks: The sequential learning problem. In G. H. Bower (Ed.), *The psychology of learning and motivation.* New York: Academic Press.

Metcalfe, J. (1990). Composite holographic associative recall model (CHARM) and blended memories in eyewitness testimony. *Psychological Review, 119,* 145—160.

Neisser, U. (1967). *Cognitive psychology.* New York: Appleton-Century-Crofts.

Nystrom, L. E. and McClelland, J. L. (1992). Trace synthesis in cued recall. *Journal of Memory and Language, 31,* 591—614.

O'Reilly, R. C. and McClelland, J. L. (in press). Hippocampal conjunctive encoding, storage, and recall: Avoiding a tradeoff. *Hippocampus.*

Quillian, M. R. (1968). Semantic memory. In M. Minsky (Ed.), *Semantic information processing.* Cambridge, Mass.: MIT Press.

Rumelhart, D. E. (1990). Brain style computation: Learning and generalization. In S. F. Zornetzer, J. L. Davis, and C. Lau (Eds.), *An introduction to neural and electronic networks.* San Diego: Academic Press, Chap. 21.

Rumelhart, D. E. and Todd, P. M. (1993). Learning and connectionist representa-
    tions. In D. E. Meyer and S. Kornblum (Eds.), *Attention and performance XIV:
    Synergies in experimental psychology, artificial intelligence, and cognitive neu-
    roscience*. Cambridge, Mass.: MIT Press, 3—30.
Smolensky, P. (1986). Information processing in dynamical systems: Foundations
    of harmony theory. In D. E. Rumelhart and J. L. McClelland (Eds.), *Parallel
    distributed processing: Explorations in the microstructure of cognition*, Vol. 1.
    Cambridge, Mass.: MIT Press, Chap. 6, 194—281.
Squire, L. R. (1992). Memory and the hippocampus: A synthesis from findings with
    rats, monkeys and humans. *Psychological Review*, 99, 195—231.
Squire, L. R. (1995). Biological foundations of accuracy and inaccuracy in memory.
    Chapter 7, this volume.

Acknowledgments

The work reported herein was supported by Grants MH00385 and MH47566. I
would like to thank Craig Stark for contributing to the thinking that led to this
paper.

False Beliefs: Some Developmental and Clinical Considerations

3

Stephen J. Ceci

False reports can be the result of conscious, deliberate decisions on the part of the reporter (e.g., a lie intended to flatter, avoid punishment, gain rewards, protect loved ones), or they can be the result of indeliberate, unconscious processes (e.g., a false belief that arises from a chain of inferential or reconstructive processes that are neither planned nor even accessible to awareness). In this chapter I shall be concerned primarily with the latter form of false belief. It is the one that I believe poses the most troublesome issues for researchers and mental health professionals.

There is a rich history of research dealing with false beliefs, and it is beyond the scope of this chapter to survey it comprehensively, though some of it is so germane to the points I wish to make that some attempt is warranted. Before delving into some of this research, however, it will be useful to describe what I mean by the term "false belief" by way of example. I have culled the following five examples of false beliefs from newspapers, empirical research reports, and historical literature. Each represents a different set of issues, as will be seen. And each entails a different set of cognitive processes and most likely different neuro-architectural underpinnings—issues that I will return to later.

Example 1. The first example comes from a *New York Times* story in 1990, on the occasion of the death of Tony Conigliaro, the one-time slugging sensation with the Boston Red Sox. At age 20, Conigliaro led the American League in homers, with 32, and by age 22 he was the youngest major leaguer to have hit 100 home runs.

Some readers may recall that in 1967 Conigliaro's career was nearly ended when he was hit in the head with a fastball by California Angels pitcher Jack Hamilton. Conigliaro's cheekbone was fractured, his jaw dislocated, and his vision seriously blurred. Although he was to return for two more seasons in which he hit 20 and 36 homers, respectively (after sitting out the 1968 season), eventually his blurred vision returned, forcing him to retire.

On the occasion of Conigliaro's death in 1990, *New York Times* sports writer Dave Anderson interviewed Jack Hamilton, the pitcher whose fastball had nearly killed Conigliaro. Not surprisingly, Hamilton expressed sincere regret over the incident. "I know in my heart I wasn't trying to hit him," Hamilton asserted of the pitch that crushed the right side of Conigliaro's face. After all, Hamilton said, there was no strategic reason for him to have hit Conigliaro. Consider two of Hamilton's recollections of that fateful pitch:

> —"It was like the 6th inning when it happened. I think the score was 2–1, and he [Conigliaro] was the 8th hitter in their batting order . . . I had no reason to throw at him." (Anderson, 1990, p. B-9)

> —"I tried to go see him in the hospital late that afternoon or early that evening but they were just letting his family in." (Anderson, 1990, p. B-10)

Both of these "recollections" are wrong. But they are more than wrong, for they represent a reconstruction that allows Jack Hamilton to maintain his belief that he did not deliberately throw at Conigliaro's head. To begin with, it was only the 4th inning, and there were two outs, and no one on base—the perfect occasion for a brush-back pitch. Second, Conigliaro was batting 6th, and already had amassed 20 homers and 67 RBIs that season, so he represented a real threat. Third, it was an evening game, so Hamilton, who may want to imagine that he tried to visit the hospital immediately after the game, actually did not go until the following afternoon.

Hamilton says that he thinks about that fateful day a lot, and has had to learn to live with it. Yet, for all of his professed ruminations, he seems to have gotten the story wrong, not only in its peripheral details but in its gist, its core truths. He has constructed an account that permits him to view his role in the termination of Conigliaro's career (and nearly his life) as being more benign than it may have been on that summer evening.

Example 2.   The second example of a false belief comes from a letter to the editor of the Gannett television trivia column, *Ask Inman*. The letter comes from a reader inquiring about the details of a show from his youth that he thinks he can remember, yet he appears to have blended memories from three different shows that aired around the same time:

> Dear Inman: Was there ever a TV series called "The Survivors"? I remember it was about some people who'd been stranded on an island in an airplane

crash. I also remember Lily Tomlin appearing on it before she was anybody. Could the time period be around 1969 or 1970? —Rick, Great Falls, Mont.

Dear Rick: Gee, you've managed to remember most of the ABC Monday evening lineup from the Fall of 1969 and mix all of the shows together . . . The show you mention, "The Survivors," was a "Dynasty" style soap opera . . . It starred Lana Turner . . . Her biggest problem was protecting her teenage son Jeffrey (Jan Michael Vincent) from the other sleazy members of her family. The second show about people stranded on an island was called "The New People," and it aired just before "The Survivors." The "New People" were a bunch of teenagers who crash landed on an island where a city had been built for the purposes of atomic testing, so they already had shelter, stoplights, etc. And the third show, the one with Lily Tomlin, was called "The Music Scene."

Example 3.   The third example comes from a laboratory study on auditory memory. Someone calls a subject in the evening and purports to be a pollster. The pollster asks about the respondent's political attitudes, and the conversation lasts 5 minutes. The following morning the respondent comes to the lab to participate in an experiment that had been previously agreed to. When they reach the lab, the experimenter explains that the pollster last night was a confederate, part of the study in which they agreed to participate. They are asked to listen to five voices on tape and decide if any of them are the voice of the pollster from the evening before. None of them are, and respondents typically claim that none of them remind them of the pollster's voice. Two weeks later, respondents return to the lab and are asked to listen to five more voices and decide if any of these are the pollster's voice. Again, none of them are. But this time one of the five voices is one that was included in the earlier voice parade. When this happens, many respondents leap to the conclusion that this is the pollster's voice. In other words, they misattribute the source of the voice's familiarity to the evening telephone call when it was actually part of the voice parade presented the following morning. (Interestingly, more respondents claim that this voice is the pollster's voice than the actual pollster's voice when it is included in the parade!)

Example 4.   The fourth example of a false belief comes from no less than Sigmund Freud himself, on the occasion of learning that he has inadvertently taken credit for an idea of a colleague's that the latter had shared with him several years earlier, an instance of what is now politely referred to as "cryptomnesia." Freud (1901/1960) wrote that while he was developing his theory of original bisexuality, a friend reminded him that he had told Freud of the idea years earlier:

One day in the summer of 1901 I remarked to a friend with whom I used at that time to have a lively exchange of scientific ideas: "These problems of the neuroses are only to be solved if we base ourselves wholly and completely on the assumption of the original bisexuality of the individual." To which he replied: "That's what I told you two and a half years ago at Breslau when we went for that evening walk. But you wouldn't hear of it then." It is painful to be requested in this way to surrender one's originality. (Freud, 1901/1960)

Example 5.   The final example of false belief comes from a highly experienced clinical psychologist, a diplomate of the APA. In 1954, at the age of 14, he was shooting a .22 rifle at a garbage dump. He had no prior hunting experience, and when he saw a large dog wander by, he decided to shoot at it. He shot the dog, and immediately felt remorseful because it would not die; it lay there convulsing. So he shot it again several times to hasten its death and put it out of its misery. Today, he remarks that this was "one of the most shameful moments of my life."

Now fast-forward to 1968 when, at the age of 28, he was in Hawaii, awaiting orders to go to Vietnam. After a week-long wait (because of a delayed briefing), he began to develop a "memory" that he had once murdered a homeless person with a .38 revolver that belonged to a friend's father. He and his friend had often handled his father's revolver, and he recalled exactly what it looked like. He began to recall that after he committed the murder, he buried the revolver in his basement. No one had ever discovered the murder, and he had no prior memory of it until the week in Hawaii. Eventually, he realized that his memory of the murder was a delusion. If he had buried the revolver in his parent's basement his father would surely have noticed the hole in the cement floor (painted gray) and confronted him with it. His friend's father would have noticed the missing weapon, too. In trying to problem-solve the basis of this delusion, he writes:

> "I don't know if killing that dog was the basis for my delusion, but what else could it have been? And isn't it likely that it would arise during a period of anxiety when I was on my way to war? I consider myself fortunate in having a concrete floored basement, and a father who would have called me to account for a hole in the floor—reality factors that no doubt kept me out of psychosis." (clinical psychologist, personal communication, January 20, 1994)

Each of these five examples reveals an aspect of false beliefs, the confusion between real and imagined sources of input into the memory system. The television viewer, the California Angels pitcher, the pseudo-respondent to the fake poll, Sigmund Freud, and the clinical psychologist all forgot one or another type of mental activity that they had invested in thinking about non-existing events, thus setting up the conditions for them to subsequently erroneously believe they had actually experienced those events. For the sake of brevity, I will refer to this as a form of "source amnesia." It deserves to be noted, however, that I am glossing over some important distinctions, such as that between a false memory and a false belief (the latter does not contain the vivid perceptual image required to exceed a threshold needed to judge something as a "memory," yet the individual believes or infers that it nevertheless did happen). For a good example of the concept of false belief in a client trying to recover a presumed lost memory, see Fredrickson (1992).

In the remainder of this chapter, I will consider source amnesia as a factor in developmental differences in suggestibility, focusing on the early stages of development. Although I will have little to say about source amnesia among adults and elderly persons (see Schacter et al., 1993), the relevance of this research to cases of so-called "repressed memory recovery" (or "incest resolution therapy") will be raised. I will briefly review five new studies, all conducted within the past 18 months, that lead to the conclusion that preschoolers' source misattributions are the result of a variety of social and cognitive mechanisms that can eventuate, in some circumstances, in their holding erroneous beliefs that defy our attempts to debrief them. Prior to reporting on these new experiments, however, I will describe the concept of source misattributions, and explain why I think a developmental perspective helps in the search for underlying mechanisms in both false beliefs and so-called "repressed memories."

A Developmental Perspective

> It is all too common for caterpillars to become butter-
> flies and then maintain that in their youth they had been
> little butterflies. Maturation makes liars of us all.
>
> *(Vaillant, 1977, p. 197)*

A developmental perspective is critical to any discussion of false beliefs and repressed memories (e.g., Brainerd, Reyna, Howe, and Kingma, 1990). The reason a developmental perspective is important when discussing the recovery of formerly stored memories is that there are age-related differences in encoding, retention, forgetting, and savings. Put simply, memories cannot be retrieved unless they were adequately processed to begin with, and the retrievability of a memory depends on the status of the operations that occur during each stage of learning, a form of the encoding specificity principle that holds that the effectiveness of a retrieval operation is determined by the degree to which it reinstates operations carried out at the time of the original encoding (Tulving and Thompson, 1973).

What gets retrieved at a later point in time about an event that was encoded at an earlier point in time is a function of the cognitive neuro-architecture at the earlier point in time when the experience was first encoded. It is unlikely that an event that was encoded using an infant's or young child's perceptual-motor schemes can later be retrieved using adult inferential/interpretive schemes unavailable at the time of the original encoding.

Generally, a developmental-cognitive principle states that the cognitive status of the organism at time 1 sets the conditions for memory recovery at time 2. A similar cognitive mechanism must be available at time 2 in order to make contact with the trace as it was originally encoded. While there is some suggestion that original traces can later be recoded using more developmentally advanced architecture that was unavailable at the time of the original experience (Perris, Myers, and Clifton, 1990; Sugar, 1992), such recoding seems to be quite limited—the exception rather than the rule. For example, one child in the Perris et al. study who did not linguistically encode an animal stimulus when it was first presented to him at age 8 months was said to have recoded it linguistically two years later. If the adult mind is organized differently from a 2-year-old's mind, then there is scant evidence that the former can gain access to the cognitive products of the latter. The same schemes used by an immature cognitive system to encode an event are needed to later revisit the encoding of the event. Thus, an event that requires semantic interpretation can only be recalled in adulthood if sufficient perceptual detail was originally encoded and is still recoverable so that it can be recoded and given an adult interpretation. In the absence of a developmental perspective, there is a tendency to think along a retrieval continuum instead of conceptualizing retrieval in terms of qualitatively dissimilar retrieval niches. While it is theoretically possible to retrieve perceptual details from an earlier encoding and reinterpret them in light of the current cognitive awareness, it is probably not the rule because verbatim/perceptual traces fade more quickly than "gistified" traces (Brainerd et al., 1990). Thus, recoding of earlier encodings probably relies on abstractions that are lacking some of the original details. Having said this, there are many clinical case studies that purport to have obtained evidence for recoding. Sugar (1992) claims that a client could retrieve a memory of a red liquid blotch on her floor when she was 18 months old; later, this client's mother informed her that it was probably a miscarriage that she had at that time. If true, then this would indicate that the adult client could still gain access to perceptual details many decades later and reinterpret the meaning of the event using adult interpretive schemes that were unavailable to the young child. Of course, if this is the case, then it can hardly serve as the basis of the symptoms that led the client into therapy in the first place, since the meaning of the event would have been quite different at time 1 than time 2. This becomes particularly important when we consider events that are alleged to be memorable precisely because of their presumed "assaultive" quality—namely, sexual abuse is said to be traumatic because it involves betrayal by a trusted caregiver. Such interpretations require that the young child actually encode the original event as assaultive or betrayal, something that may not be true because many objective abusive experiences may not be perceived as assaultive by the infant or young child (e.g., fellatio, fondling, photography, exhibitionism).

This developmental perspective poses some fascinating clinical questions that I have not seen put forward elsewhere. Suppose that a therapist is convinced that a client has retrieved a so-called repressed memory of childhood abuse, say, from the age of 2 years. (Numerous celebrities have made such claims, such as Roseanne Arnold's claim to have recalled sexual assaults by her mother from the age of 6 months.) How can this happen if there is a mismatch between the original encoding machinery available to the infant and that available to the adult client in therapy? As already noted, one possible means of reconnecting with early experiences would be to retrieve the uninterpreted perceptual details as an adult and reinterpret these perceptions in light of their adult meaning. To do this would require that the original perceptions be vivid and accessible. But if they were not originally interpreted as assaultive by the infant, then how could they be the source of subsequent clinical problems? And if they were simply stored as startling images that created some intrapsychic turmoil for the infant, then why should not the same be true (actually, even more true) of a host of startling nonsexual experiences such as genital catheterizations, circumcisions, insertion of suppositories, repeated enemas, and so forth? In short, as a developmentalist I am struggling with a conception of the encoding-retrieval process that might permit an adult client to gain access to early childhood experiences that were not encoded as sexual abuse when they occurred, and to recode (reinterpret) them as abusive in therapy. I think that this is theoretically possible, but only if we agree that such "memories" could not be the cause of adult psychopathology. For these experiences to be sources of adult psychopathology, they would have had to have been experienced as traumatic (e.g., because of their assaultive nature or their betrayal of trust) when they first occurred; if they were not, then nonsexual events that can claim to be at least as traumatic (e.g., genital catheterizations) would also be a basis for similar psychopathology. But accounts of repressed memories for such procedures are very rare, as are accounts of psychopathology based on early medical procedures, accidents, and the like. In short, while I am struggling to find a developmentally informed framework to explain the clinical case studies that I referred to above, I am not succeeding. Something is wrong, and this has propelled me in the direction of source misattributions as a means of accounting for such phenomena.

Source Monitoring: Distinguishing Reality from Fantasy

Suppose that a child in a laboratory experiment is instructed: (a) to perform certain actions (e.g., touch her ear), and (b) merely to imagine performing other actions (e.g., touch her nose). Later, she is asked to decide which actions she actually performed and which she merely imagined performing. This requires the ability to monitor or keep track of the multiple sources of memory. Sometimes, as in the above example, we must discriminate between an external source (doing something) and an internal source (thinking about or imagining doing something); at other times we must discriminate between two internal sources (e.g., memories resulting from what one said versus what one thought) or between two external sources (e.g., memories of what was said or done by one person versus another). Source monitoring makes use of typical differences between different sources of memories. For example, compared to imagined events, observations of actual events tend to have more perceptual details associated with them and less information about cognitive operations such as inferences (e.g., Schooler, Gerhard, and Loftus, 1986), and they are retrieved more easily than imagined events (see Johnson, Hashtroudi, and Lindsay, 1993). For present purposes, we shall gloss over such distinctions.

The ability to distinguish between various sources of memory is quite important, not only in laboratory tests but also in everyday life. Source monitoring contributes to our ability to exert control over our beliefs, and a failure to attribute the correct source to a memory can result in a false belief.

> If you remember that the source of a "fact" was a supermarket tabloid such as the *National Enquirer* and not *Consumer Reports,* you have information that is important for evaluating the veridicality of the purported fact. Perhaps most important, the subjective experience of autobiographical recollection— the feeling of remembering a specific experience in one's own life—depends on source attributions made on the basis of certain phenomenal qualities of remembered experience. (Johnson et al., 1993, p. 3)

Source Confusions and Suggestibility.   An important though still relatively unexplored cognitive variable is the extent to which suggestibility results from an incapacity to distinguish between the various sources of memory (imagined versus perceived, internal versus external). Freud's seduction theory—postulating that claims of childhood sexual abuse by many of his female adult patients were false, reflecting their inability as children to distinguish reality from fantasy—has never received persuasive empirical support, and many have argued that it is invalid, a reflection of a prior era's refusal to accept the reality of intrafamilial sexual abuse (e.g., Masson, 1984). Freud believed that it was possible, at least in principle, to retrieve original memories, by removal of symbolic/fantasy transformations that "blockaded" them from patients' consciousness (Freud, 1933). Piaget (1926), however, was less optimistic that memories of early experiences could be separated from fantasies, commenting that "the child's mind is full of these 'ludistic' (fantasy play) tendencies up to the age of seven or eight, which means before that age it is very difficult for him to distinguish the truth" (p. 34). Outside of the classical work on animism by Piagetians, the topic of reality monitoring did not receive empirical scrutiny until the 1970s, when a number of studies converged on the view that young children were, in fact, able to reliably distinguish reality and fantasy (Flavell, Flavell, and Green, 1987; Morison and Gardner, 1978; Taylor and Howell, 1973). Morison and Gardner (1978) reported the results of a "triad sorting task" in which 5- to 12-year-olds were instructed to put the two items together that are fantasy figures (e.g., dragon and elf) and exclude the one that is real (e.g., frog). They found that even 5-year-olds were quite aware of this distinction, though accuracy did increase with age, as did explicit fantasy-based explanations (i.e., stating that "they are both fake"). Similarly, the 5-year-old children were quite adept at sorting pictures into piles of real and pretend figures, though they made more errors than the 12-year-old children. Harris, Brown, Marriott, Whittall, and Harmer's results (1991) demonstrated, however, that when situations and questioning become more intense, children appear to easily give up distinctions between what is real and what is only imagined.

In contrast to young children's good ability to distinguish between concrete fantasy and reality figures, there is some evidence that they have difficulty distinguishing between what they experienced through perception and what they only imagined they experienced (see Johnson, 1991 for review; Foley and Johnson, 1985; Lindsay, Johnson, and Kwon, 1991; cf. Roberts and Blades, in press). In Johnson's most embellished model, called MEM, for "Multiple-Entry Modular Memory" system, recollection is based on the interplay of two subsystems, one that is the repository of perceptual processing and the other that contains the contents of reflective processing. The perceptual system records and stores the contents of perceptual processes such as seeing and hearing, while the reflective system records psychologically generated information such as imagining, thinking, and speculating. Without going into the theoretical nuances of the various MEM subsystems, it suffices to say that developmental differences about reality-fantasy monitoring could reflect the earlier functional capability of the perceptual subsystems, and the later development of the reflective systems (there are two of them, R1 and R2, with the latter one concerned with judgment processes). At issue is whether these subsystems are developmentally invariant or whether they unfold over a prolonged period of development (Lindsay et al., 1991).

If subjects are asked to judge whether they had actually said a word, or had imagined saying it, 6-year-olds have more difficulty discriminating between these two possible sources of their memories than do 9-year-olds and adults (e.g., Foley, Johnson, and Raye, 1983). The reason offered for younger children's greater difficulty in distinguishing between memories of their self-generated fantasies and memories of their actual behaviors (so-called realization judgments) is that the cues involved in differentiating between actual versus imagined events are not well developed before late child-hood. However, when asked to judge whether they said (or did) something versus whether it was said (or done) by someone else, it is claimed that children do not have difficulty distinguishing between these different sources, prompting Foley and her colleagues to conclude that young children can differentiate between real and imagined sources of their memories except in the situation where the two sources are both self-generated, as in the case of deciding whether they really touched their nose or just imagined touching it (Foley, Santini, and Sopasakis, in press). Thus, compared with older children and adults, preschoolers are more error-prone at distinguishing between real versus imagined acts or words when they both concern themselves, but they are no worse than adults when it comes to judging whether an act (or words) was performed (or spoken) by themselves versus someone else.

Recently, a more general source monitoring framework has been invoked to account for preschool children's source confusions. According to this more recent account, young children find it especially difficult to separate sources of information that are perceptually and semantically similar. In one experiment, for example (Lindsay et al., 1991, Experiment 3), 7- and 10-year-olds and adults were shown a videotape of a set of actions and were instructed to either perform these actions or watch others perform them, or imagine themselves perform or imagine another perform them (for example, "Please watch the girl touch her nose" versus "Please imagine touching your nose"). Following this procedure, subjects were given a surprise memory test to determine whether they remembered which acts they performed, imagined, or watched. Compared to adults, children found it more difficult to distinguish between imagined and actual actions if the same actor was involved in both kinds of actions (e.g., watching versus imagining the girl touch her nose). In contrast, young children performed as well as adults when the sources of information were relatively discriminable (self versus girl). Thus, while all age groups can reliably distinguish between the actions of two perceptually or semantically distinct actors, a developmental trend can be seen in the discrimination between actual and imagined sources of memories that are perceptually or semantically similar.

Thus, source monitoring studies suggest that children could be susceptible to a wide range of misattributions, some of which involve confusing actual events with suggested events when these are perceptually and semantically similar. Nevertheless, these claims remain speculative because the locus of children's greater misattributions is unclear and there are no data on the interaction of suggestibility and source monitoring difficulties. The experiments described in the following section were intended to begin to provide some developmental data.

Developmental Issues

Study I: The Effect of Visualizations on Children's Narratives
(Ceci, Loftus, Crotteau, and Smith, 1994; Ceci, Loftus,
Leichtman, and Bruck, 1994)

My colleagues and I wondered what would happen if preschoolers were merely asked to think about some event repeatedly, creating mental images each time they did so. We have conducted this experiment in several different ways, but I will describe only one of them here (for details see Ceci, Loftus, Crotteau, and Smith, 1994; Ceci, Loftus, Leichtman, and Bruck, 1994). The events that we asked children to think about were both actual events that they experienced (e.g., an accident that eventuated in stitches) and fictitious events that they never experienced (e.g., getting their hand caught in a mousetrap and having to go to the hospital to get it removed).

As noted in the Introduction, "source misattributions" refer to the problem of separating the various origins of our memories. Occasionally, all of us have experienced these kinds of difficulties. For example, if I showed you a book of mug shots and asked if you recognized someone who staged a mock theft minutes earlier, and if the actual "thief's" photo is not in this mug book, you would probably correctly state that you do not see the thief's photo. But if a week later I ask you to examine a line-up that contains one of the individuals whose photo was in the mug book that you had inspected, you are likely to incorrectly attribute this person's familiarity to actually having observed him commit the mock crime. His face is familiar, but you misattribute the source of the familiarity to the crime context rather than to the mug book context that came later. The question my colleagues and I wished to pursue is whether young children are especially inclined to exhibit source misattributions when they are encouraged to think about events that never occurred. Will they come to think that they actually experienced events that they merely thought about? (Incidentally, although clearly the analogy to therapy is imperfect, I think that such a study has relevance for the testimony of a child who has undergone a certain type of therapy for a long time, engaging in similar imagery inductions and "memory work.")

Each week for ten consecutive weeks, preschool children were individually interviewed by a trained adult. The adult showed the child a set of cards, each containing a different event. The child was invited to pick a card, and then the interviewer would read it to the child and ask if the event ever happened to him or her. For example, when the child selected the card that read: *"Got finger caught in a mousetrap and had to go to the hospital to get the trap off,"* the interviewer would ask: *"Think real hard, and tell me if this ever happened to you. Can you remember going to the hospital with the mousetrap on your finger?"* Each week, the interviewer would ask the child to think "real hard" about each actual and fictitious event, with prompts to visualize the scene.

After ten weeks of thinking about both real and fictitious events, these preschool children were given a forensic interview by a new adult. All of these interviews were videotaped. The interviewer began by establishing a rapport with the child, discussing events that were unrelated to the event in question, and giving the child the expectation that the interviewer wanted elaborated answers, not simple yes/no ones. Initially, the interviewer asked: "Tell me if this ever happened to you: Did you ever get your finger caught in a mousetrap and have to go to the hospital to get the trap off?" Following the child's reply, the interviewer asked for additional details (e.g., "Can you tell me more?" "What did you see/hear?" "Who was with you?" "How did it feel?"). When the child indicated that he or she had no additional details, the interviewer asked a number of follow-up questions that were based on the child's answers. For instance, if the child said that she did go to the hospital to get the mousetrap off, the interviewer asked how she got there, who went with her, and what happened at the hospital.

While we had anticipated that asking children to think about events repeatedly would result in later confusions about whether they actually participated in the events, we had no expectation that this would result in the sort of highly detailed, internally coherent narratives that the children produced. In one study, 58% of the preschool children produced false narratives to one or more of the fictitious events, with 25% of the children producing false narratives to the majority of them. What was so surprising was the elaborateness of the children's narratives. They were very embellished; the children would provide an internally coherent account of the context in which their finger got caught in the mousetrap as well as the affect associated with the event.

We showed these videos to psychologists who specialize in interviewing children at two conferences, and the results were sobering: Professionals were fooled by the children's narratives. They were not reliably different from chance at detecting which events were real, because they did not expect that such plausible, internally coherent narratives could be fabricated by such young children. And I think they are right—if by fabrication we mean "a conscious attempt to mislead a listener about the truth as one understands it" (Ceci and Bruck, 1993). I am of the opinion, though I cannot prove it in any scientifically satisfying manner, that many of the children had come to believe what they were telling the interviewer. This is why they were so believable to the professionals who watched them. The children exhibited none of the telltale signs of duping, teasing, or tricking. They seemed sincere, their facial expressions and affect were appropriate, and their narratives were filled with the kind of low-frequency details that make accounts seem plausible:

e.g., "My brother Colin was trying to get Blowtorch [an action figure] from me, and I wouldn't let him take it from me, so he pushed me into the wood pile where the mousetrap was. And then my finger got caught in it. And then we went to the hospital, and my mommy, daddy, and Colin drove me there, to the hospital in our van, because it was far away. And the doctor put a bandage on this finger [indicating]."

As can be seen, this child supplies a plausible account, not simply yes/no answers. One can imagine how believable such children might be to someone who was shown these children's "disclosures" and asked to judge their authenticity.

One further bit of evidence supports our position that at least some of these children had come to believe that they actually experienced the fictitious events. Twenty-seven percent of the children in this study initially refused to accept debriefing, claiming that they remembered the fictitious events happening. When told by their parents that these events never occurred and they were merely imagined, these children often protested, "But it really did happen. I remember it!" Although such insistence, in the presence of their parents, is not proof that this subset of children believed what they were reporting about fictitious events, it does suggest that they were not duping us for any obvious motive, given that the demand characteristics were all tilted against their making such claims. We are presently pursuing this hypothesis with a new set of experiments, but it is too early to report the results. Thus, repeatedly thinking about a fictitious event can lead some preschool children to produce vivid, detailed reports that professionals are unable to discern from their reports of actual events.

Study II: The Effect of Repeated Suggestions and Stereotypes (Leichtman and Ceci, in press)

In many court cases a constellation of factors co-occurs. Children in these cases are given an expectancy about the defendant (e.g., the defendant might be an estranged parent who is criticized by the custodial parent in the child's presence, and the child comes to accept these criticisms as stable aspects of the parent's character). As an example, in 1990 I was asked to write a *Stay of Execution* brief in a death row case in El Paso, Texas, in which the most important testimony at the original trial had been given by a child who claimed she remembered seeing the defendant with blood on his shirt at his trailer. It was known that the child's mother had told her on numerous occasions that the defendant was a bad man—long before he was accused of murder. From interviews with the child, it was clear that she possessed a stereotype about the defendant, and that her mother had warned her against being friendly with him. Another ingredient that occurred in this case, and in others like it, was the relentless pursuit of the child's memory in a series of highly suggestive interviews, extended over several months.

One wonders whether combining a negative expectancy about a defendant with repeated suggestive interviews will seriously reduce the accuracy of the child's report. In the El Paso case, the child later gave three sworn depositions, at least one of which had the effect of recanting her courtroom testimony. She said that the repeated interviews had confused her, and she had said things that she now thinks were wrong because she wanted to help the adults and because she knew this man was bad. This statement, made 12 days before the defendant's scheduled execution, resulted in a stay of execution. (Ultimately, the defendant was freed.)

To examine this issue experimentally, my colleague Michelle Leichtman and I conducted an experiment called the "Sam Stone Study" (Leichtman and Ceci, in press). A stranger named Sam Stone paid a two-minute visit to preschoolers (ages 3–6 years) in their daycare center. Following Sam Stone's visit, the children were asked for details about the visit on four different occasions over a 10-week period. During these four occasions the interviewer refrained from using suggestive questions. She simply encouraged children to describe Sam Stone's visit in as much detail as possible. One month following the fourth interview, the children were interviewed a fifth time, by a new interviewer, who used forensic procedures (e.g., first acclimating the child, then eliciting a free narrative, then using probes, urging the children to say when they do not recall, taking breaks). This interviewer asked about two "non-events," which involved Sam soiling a teddy bear and ripping a book. In reality, Sam Stone never touched either item.

When asked in the fifth interview: "Did Sam Stone do anything to a book or a teddy bear?" nearly all children correctly replied "No." Only 10% of the youngest (3–4 year old) children's answers contained claims that Sam Stone did anything to a book or teddy bear. When asked if they actually saw him do anything to the book or teddy bear, as opposed to "thinking they saw him do something, or hearing he did something," now only 5% of their answers contained claims that anything occurred. Finally, when these 5% were gently challenged ("You didn't *really* see him do anything to the book/teddy bear, did you?"), only 2.5% still insisted on the reality of the fictional event. None of the older (5–6 year old) children claimed to have actually seen Sam Stone do either of the fictional things. This condition can be considered as a control against which we can assess the effects of the use of repeated suggestive questioning, especially about characters who are the object of children's stereotypes.

A second group of preschoolers were presented a stereotype about Sam Stone before he ever visited their school. We did this to mimic the sort of stereotypes that some child witnesses have acquired about a defendant. Each week, beginning a month prior to the visit, the children were told a new Sam

Stone story, in which he was depicted as very clumsy. (In earlier versions of this study, we also used other stereotypes besides being clumsy, including being a thief. The results were essentially the same as for being clumsy, although we never reported these results because of small sample sizes and their exploratory nature.) For example:

> You'll never guess who visited me last night. [pause] That's right. Sam Stone! And guess what he did this time? He asked to borrow my Barbie and when he was carrying her down the stairs, he tripped and fell and broke her arm. That Sam Stone is always getting into accidents and breaking things!

Following Sam Stone's visit, these children were treated identically to the control group; that is, they were interviewed four times, avoiding all suggestions, and then they were given the same forensic interview by a new interviewer, starting with free narrative, then proceeding to probes about anything happening to the book/teddy bear.

The stereotyping had an effect for the youngest children, 42% of whom claimed that Sam Stone ripped the book or soiled the teddy bear in response to suggestive probes. Of these 42%, 19% claimed they *saw* Sam Stone do these misdeeds (i.e., not just heard that he did these things). But, after being gently challenged, only 11% continued to claim they witnessed him do these things. In contrast, older preschoolers were significantly more resistant to the influence of the stereotype; their error rates were approximately half of those of the younger children.

A third group of children were assigned to a "suggestion-only condition," which involved the provision of suggestive questions during the four interviews following Sam Stone's visit. They were not given the clumsy stereotype, however. Each suggestive interview contained two erroneous suggestions, one having to do with ripping a book and the other with soiling a teddy bear (e.g., "Remember that time Sam Stone visited your classroom and spilled chocolate on that white teddy bear? Did he do it on purpose or was it an accident?" "When Sam Stone ripped that book, was he being silly or was he angry?").

Ten weeks later, when the forensic interviewer probed these children about these events ("Did anything happen to a book?" "Did anything happen to a teddy bear?"), 52% of the younger children's answers and 38% of the older children's answers contained claims that Sam Stone was responsible for one or both misdeeds.

Thirty-five percent of the youngest children's answers contained the claim that they actually witnessed Sam doing these things, as opposed to just being told that he did them. Even after being gently challenged, 12% of these children continued to claim they saw him do one or both misdeeds. Older children were also susceptible to these suggestive interviews, though at a somewhat reduced level.

Finally, a fourth group of children were assigned to a condition that combined the features of the "stereotype" and the "repeated suggestions" conditions. During the fifth (i.e., forensic) interview conducted 10 weeks later, 72% of the youngest preschoolers claimed that Sam Stone did one or both misdeeds, a figure that dropped to 44% when they were asked if they actually saw him do these things.

It is noteworthy that 21% continued to insist that they saw him do these things, even when gently challenged. For the older preschoolers, the situation, though better, was still cause for concern, with 11% insisting they saw him do the misdeeds.

Some researchers have opined that the presence of perceptual details in children's reports (Raskin and Yuille, 1989; Loftus and Hoffman, 1989) is one of the indicators of an accurate memory, as opposed to a confabulated one. In the previous study as well as in this study, however, the presence of perceptual details was no assurance that the report was accurate. In fact, it was surprising to see the number of false perceptual details that children in the combined stereotype *plus* suggestion condition provided to embellish the non-events (e.g, claiming that Sam Stone took the teddy bear into a bathroom and soaked it in hot water before smearing it with a crayon). This may be another difference between this study, which involved repeated erroneous suggestions over a relatively long period of time, coupled with a stereotype that was consistent with these suggestions, and many other studies in the suggestibility literature that are based on single leading questions over brief durations and without stereotypes.

It is one thing to show that children can be induced to make errors and include perceptual details in their reports, but it is quite another matter to show that such faulty reports are convincing to an observer, especially a highly trained one. To examine the believability of the children's reports, we showed videotapes of the children during the final interview to more than a thousand researchers and clinicians who work with children. These researchers and clinicians (including psychiatrists) were simply told that all of the children observed the visit of a man named Sam Stone to their daycare centers. They were asked to watch the tapes carefully, and to decide which of the things that were alleged by the children actually transpired during Sam Stone's visit and which did not. At the conclusion of their viewing the tape, they were asked to rank the children in terms of their overall accuracy, and to rate the accuracy of specific statements the children had made.

Strikingly, the majority of these highly trained professionals were highly inaccurate. Our analyses indicated that experts who conduct research on children's testimonial competence, who provide therapy to children suspected of having been abused, and who carry out law enforcement interviews with children, failed to detect which children were accurate and which were not, despite being confident in their mistaken opinions. The overall credibility ratings they made of individual children were highly inaccurate; the very children who were least accurate were rated as being most accurate. Despite claims from some to the contrary, our data attest to the fact that even extensive training does not always make it possible to detect the validity of young children's reports when they have been subjected to persistent erroneous questioning over long delay intervals.

Study III: Children's Reports of an Inoculation (Bruck, Ceci, Francouer, and Barr, in press)

It could be argued that the Sam Stone Study is not relevant to evaluating the reliability of a child witness who reports personally experienced events that involve her own body, especially when the experience involves some degree of distress or potential embarrassment. Furthermore, some might argue that the Sam Stone data are not germane to testimony about predictable and scripted events. In cases where the event: (a) involves their own body, (b) is somewhat stressful, and (c) is predictable, it is often thought that children may be resistant to suggestion (Goodman, Rudy, Bottoms, and Aman, 1990).

To determine if children could be misled under such circumstances, we examined the influence of postevent suggestions on children's reports about two specific pediatric visits. I will describe these two studies briefly here. The first study had two phases. In the first phase, the subjects were five years old and visited their pediatrician for their annual checkup. The visit was scripted as follows: First, the pediatrician examined the child. Then the child met a research assistant who talked about a poster that was hanging on the wall in the examining room. Next, with the research assistant present, the pediatrician gave the child an oral polio vaccine and a DPT inoculation. Immediately after the inoculation, the pediatrician left the room. The research assistant then gave the child feedback about how she/he had acted when receiving the inoculation. Some children were given pain-affirming feedback: they were told that it seemed as though the shot really hurt them, but that's OK because shots hurt even big kids (hurt condition). Some children were given pain-denying information, that is, they were told that they acted as if the shot did not hurt much, and that they were really brave (no-hurt condition). Finally, some children were merely told that the shot was over (neutral condition). After giving the feedback, the research assistant gave each child a treat, and then read the child a story. One week later, a second research assistant asked each child to indicate through the use of various rating scales how much he or she cried when receiving the shot, and how much the shot hurt.

The children's reports during this interview did not differ as a function of feedback condition. Essentially, children's reports about the stressful, personally significant, and physically invasive checkup procedures were not rendered less accurate by our suggestive questions. These findings resemble those of other researchers who have studied the effects of providing children with suggestions about personally relevant, stressful past experiences in a single interview.

The picture changed, however, when we re-interviewed the children three more times, approximately one year after the shot. During these three interviews, children were provided with repeated suggestions about how they had acted when they received their inoculations. Thus, as in the first phase of the study, some children were told how brave they had been when they got their shot, whereas other children were not given any information about how they had acted. (For ethical reasons, we did not continue with the pain-affirming feedback, in case it had the effect of making children doctor-phobic.) When the children were interviewed for a fourth time and asked to rate how much the shot had hurt and how much they had cried, there were large suggestibility effects. Those who had been repeatedly told that they acted bravely and didn't cry when they received their inoculation one year earlier reported significantly less crying and less hurt than children who were not provided with any information about how they acted. Thus, these data indicate that under certain circumstances children's reports concerning stressful events involving their own bodies can be influenced by erroneous postevent suggestions.

We also provided children with different types of misleading information about the agents of actions that occurred in the pediatrician's office during the original inoculation visit. Some children were falsely reminded (on three occasions) that the research assistant had given them the inoculation and the oral vaccine, whereas the control group children were merely reminded that "someone" did these things. Other children were falsely reminded on three occasions that the pediatrician had shown them the poster, had given them treats, and had read them a story, whereas the control group children were merely reminded that "someone" did these things. According to some researchers, children should not be suggestible about such central and important events, particularly shifting the gender of the person who administered the inoculation. The male pediatrician had never given them treats or read them a story, and the female research assistant had never inoculated them.

Contrary to these predictions, the children *were* misled. In the fourth interview, when asked to tell what happened to them when they visited their doctor one year previously, 45% of the misled subjects and 22% of the control subjects reported that the pediatrician had shown them the poster, given them treats, and read them a story. For children who had been told that the research assistant had given them the shot and the vaccine, nearly 2 out of 5 of their reports, versus only 1 out of 10 of the control children's reports, were consistent with this suggestion. Interestingly, 38% of the misled children and none of the control children said that the research assistant had performed other scripted events that were not accurate (e.g., checked their ears and nose), although these events had not been suggested.

Hence, our suggestions to these children influenced not only their reports of personally experienced, central events, but also their memories for non-suggested scripted events that were related to the suggested events. One final aspect of these data is of interest: Children in this study often produced errors of commission in their free recall, something that is rare to find in the literature (Ceci and Bruck, 1993).

In sum, these data indicate that under certain circumstances preschool children's reports concerning stressful events involving their own bodies can be influenced. As in the Sam Stone study, two important factors included in this study were repeated suggestions over multiple interviews and a long delay interval. These same two factors were independently confirmed as important determinants of suggestibility by Warren and Hagood (in press) and Cassel and Bjorklund (in press), in their respective studies of children's reports of a theft.

The results of this study are therefore consistent with those of the Sam Stone study, even though the events and experiences about which children were misled were different. In the Sam Stone study, repeated suggestions and stereotypes led to convincing claims of witnessing non-occurring events. In the inoculation study, misleading information given in repeated interviews after a long delay influenced children's memories of personally experienced, salient, and predictable events.

Study IV: Using Anatomical Dolls to Symbolically Represent Actions (Bruck, Ceci, Francouer, and Renick, in press)

The next study was an effort to determine whether the report errors that we have observed in these prior studies could be extended to sexualized events. To approach this issue in an ethically permissible manner, we took advantage of 70 naturally occurring pediatric visits to the offices of our colleagues, two of whom are professors of pediatrics. The procedure involved a pediatric exam in which thirty-five 3-year-olds were given a genital exam, and thirty-five were given a non-genital exam. Five minutes following the exam, with the child's mother present, the child was asked to describe in her own words where the doctor had touched her. Following this, the child was presented with anatomical dolls, and asked once more to tell where the pediatrician had touched her. The major finding from this study was that 3-year-olds were generally confused about their bodies when questioned with *or* without dolls. Because of the sizable portion of these children who made errors of commission, they ought not to be interviewed with anatomical dolls. Approximately 60% of the children who were touched in their genital region refused to indicate this with or without the dolls. Thus, they made errors of omission. Dolls did not alleviate this problem. On the other hand, approximately half of the children who were *not* touched in the genital region correctly refrained from saying they were touched when they were interviewed without the dolls. When the dolls were used, nearly 60% of these children indicated genital insertions, and other acts that could be cause for concern. This goes against the common beliefs of most people that children will not indicate sexual events with the dolls. Although research by Goodman and her colleagues did not find that 5-year-olds made errors of commission with the dolls (Saywitz, Goodman, Nicholas, and Moan, 1991), they also did not find that the dolls were beneficial in eliciting information (Goodman and Aman, 1990). Therefore, it seems best not to use the dolls with 3-year-olds until and unless their incremental validity can be demonstrated, which at this point seems unlikely. If anything, it appears that the use of dolls may actually reduce the validity of reports with 3-year-olds when they are added to a predictive equation. Maggie Bruck and I are extending this research with a sample of older children at this time, to determine whether we will replicate the claims of others or whether the story will need to be modified. All of this emphasizes just how out of touch with current research is the APA Council of Representatives' 1991 statement on the benefit of doll use by experienced clinicians:

> Neither the dolls nor their use are standardized or accompanied by normative data . . . We urge continued research in quest of more and better data regarding the stimulus properties of such dolls and normative behavior of abused and nonabused children . . . Nevertheless, doll-centered assessment of children, when used as part of a psychological evaluation and interpreted by experienced and competent examiners, may be the best available practical solution for a pressing and frequent clinical problem. (APA, 1991, p. 1)

Elsewhere, I criticized this statement on the grounds that it is contradictory in noting first that there are no standardized methods for doll interviews or normative data on nonabused or abused children's doll play, but then stating that experienced interviewers may nevertheless find doll-centered assessment the best available method for evaluating children suspected of sexual abuse (Ceci, 1994).

To give an example of how 3-year-olds behave when they are presented with dolls in our study, I am going to describe a child who was given a nongenital exam in which her underpants were never removed and the pediatrician never touched her genital or anal areas.

Five minutes following the exam, the child made two errors: she interdigitated the doll's vagina, and she incorrectly used a measuring tape on her head and on the doll's ankle. Other than these two errors, she responded correctly to all questions about where the doctor touched her, and she correctly demonstrated the other props (stethoscope, light, reflex hammer) on herself and on the doll.

The following day, however, this child made several more errors, including interdigitating the doll's vagina and anus, plus two very interesting uses of the props used during the exam. She inserted a stick that the pediatrician had used to tickle her foot into the doll's vagina, and then hammered it in violently with the reflex hammer. When the interviewer asked: "Eva, did Dr. Emmett really do this to you?" the child replied that he did. A follow-up question by her father elicited a similar claim. Finally, when the father said that her mother didn't see Dr. Emmett do this to her, the child replied that he did it when the mother left the room. A majority of these 3-year-olds used the dolls inappropriately immediately following the non-genital exam.

Study V: Cryptomnesia: Two Oppositely Valenced Developmental Trajectories (Ceci, Masnick, and Hembrooke, in preparation)

In this study we examined developmental factors related to the unconscious plagiarism that was illustrated in the Freud vignette described at the beginning of this chapter. Specifically, we were interested in whether younger children, because of their undeveloped source monitoring skills, and more generally their poor metacognitive ability, would be more likely to fall prey to cryptomnesia than older children.

To study this, we arranged children between 3 and 6 years of age in a circle on the floor to play a game. The game entailed naming an object or performing some act that no one had named or performed before. For instance, if the category was FRUITS, then the first child might name "apple," the next child "orange," and so forth. Whenever a child repeated an item that had been named by a peer, the interviewer corrected him and asked for a novel item. The same procedure was applied to acts that could be performed. For instance, when asked what things could be done with hands, one child might enact "clapping," another might enact "waving," another "touching her peer's nose," and so forth.

Two weeks later the children were asked to recall all of the items they named and acts they performed. Following this, they were asked to name some items and acts that no one had performed or said. Finally, they were presented with a number of acts and items and were asked to identify who contributed them in the game (i.e., themselves or their peers).

Contrary to our prediction, younger preschoolers (3- and 4-year-olds) were not worse than older ones (5- and 6-year-olds) in this task. In fact, the trend was opposite, with older preschoolers plagiarizing more of their peers' contributions than the younger children. In observing children play this game, we realized an important difference between the way the younger and older ones played. Older children would often plan in advance what item or act they would contribute; their advance preparation was palpable. In contrast, younger children waited until it was their turn to think about an act or item. Why is this important? It might be the case that one is most likely to plagiarize an act/item when the mental work for its production has been done. If you intended to say "banana" when it was your turn, and the person immediately before you preempted you, then perhaps this is when you are most likely to claim that you said it. Even though you did not, you did the advance encoding. Later, you may confuse the images of articulated and planned acts. We sought to test this in a follow-up experiment that was identical to the one just described, with one twist. This time the experimenter whispered in each child's ear an item or act that he should say if no one said it before him. This ensured that the youngest preschoolers would engage in advance encoding activities.

As predicted, the youngest preschoolers were now significantly more likely to plagiarize their peers' contributions. And, significantly, their plagiarisms were not random but came disproportionately from the child sitting immediately before them. In other words, the children would not claim to have said something that was contributed by someone following them because such individuals could not have preempted them—only the child sitting before them could do this because of the way the experiment was designed.

If we put together these two subexperiments they tell a nice developmental story: There appear to be two oppositely valenced developmental trends at work. One of them works to the advantage of the youngest children. By not engaging in active encoding, the 3- and 4-year-olds are immune from cryptomnesia because they are never preempted from what they plan to say or do. They do not plan! However, when the children are encouraged to plan, as was done when we whispered in their ear an item or act, the second developmental trend kicks in; younger children make far more source confusions than older preschoolers. They not only claim ownership of their peers' contributions (i.e., claim they said or did things that their peers really said or did), but they also exhibit some implicit memory by naming items that were said by others when they are asked to name only things that were never said by anyone.

Study VI: The Effect of Interviewers' Confirmatory Biases on Children's Reports (Ceci, Leichtman, and White, in press)

So far, I have described a series of manipulations that tilt the odds in the direction of young preschoolers' making more source confusions than older ones. In this final experiment we decided to put children in a situation that might more closely resemble what happens in an actual forensic interview. Characteristic of forensic interviews is their abundant use of leading questions and failure to consider alternative explanations (Lamb et al., 1994; Pettit et al., 1991).

The failure to test alternative hypotheses that are believable (based on our prior knowledge) can pose serious risks to obtaining a scientifically adequate answer (Dawes, 1992). This point is just as true for forensic investigators and therapists as it is for scientists. Failure to test an alternative hypothesis to one's favored hunch can lead to a "confirmatory bias," where inconsistent evidence is ignored and the interview is shaped toward consistent information.

In our analysis of interviews conducted by therapists, police, and social workers, my colleagues and I discovered that interviewers and therapists rarely tested alternative hypotheses (for review of the evidence that therapists rarely test alternatives and fall prey to illusory correlations and confirmatory biases, see Alloy and Tabachnik, 1984; Brehm and Smith, 1986; Kayne and Alloy, 1988). Instead, many interviewers exhibit a confirmatory bias, seeking to elicit support for their hunches about what the child experienced, and engaging in little questioning about disclosures that are inconsistent with their hypotheses. As a particularly telling example of this, consider the interview from a recent court case that is reproduced in Appendix A at the end of this chapter.

In this study preschoolers were exposed to an event, and then interviewed one month later. The interviewer, a trained social worker, was given a one-page report containing information about events that she was told *might* have occurred. She was asked to conduct an interview to determine what the child could, in fact, still recall. The only instruction given to the social worker was that she should begin by asking the child for a free narrative of what had transpired, avoiding all forms of suggestions and leading questions. Following this, she was allowed to use any strategies that she felt necessary to elicit the most factually accurate recall from the child. The one-page report contained both accurate and erroneous information. For example, if the event involved child A touching child B's nose and child B rubbing her own stomach, the interviewer might be told that child A had touched child B's toe (inaccurate), and that child B had in turn rubbed her own stomach (accurate).

The information we provided in the one-page sheet influenced the interviewer's hypothesis about what had transpired and powerfully influenced the dynamics of the interview, with the interviewer eventually shaping some of the children's reports to be consistent with her hypothesis, even when it was inaccurate. When the interviewer was accurately informed, she got children to correctly recall nearly 100% of the events. However, when she was misinformed, 34% of the 3- to 4-year-olds and 18% of the 5- to 6-year-olds corroborated one or more events that the interviewer falsely believed had occurred. Interestingly, the children seemed to become more credible as their interviews unfolded. Many children initially stated details inconsistently or reluctantly, but as the interviewer persisted in asking leading questions about non-events that were consistent with her hypothesis, a significant number of these children abandoned their earlier contradictions and hesitancy, and endorsed the interviewer's erroneous hypothesis.

One month later, we gave the social worker's notes from this interview to another interviewer, and asked her to re-interview the children. Do the original interviewer's notes serve the same function as the one-page information sheet we gave the first social worker, namely, do they help the second interviewer form a hypothesis? The answer is yes. The second interviewer not only got the children to continue to assent to erroneous hypothesis-consistent statements, but many children did so with increasing levels of confidence and in increasing numbers. If we had continued to re-interview the children in this study, each time passing along the notes of the prior interviewer to the new interviewer, there is no telling how far astray the children might have gone. After two such interviews, children gave detailed, but false, accounts of bodily touching (e.g., their knees being licked and marbles inserted into their ears). In criminal investigations, to provide a comparison, children are *formally* interviewed, on average, between 3 and 11 times prior to testifying. It is unknown how many times they are *informally* interviewed, e.g., by parents, therapists, and teachers.

Ideally, scientists try to arrive at truth by ruling out rival hypotheses—particularly, the most reasonable rivals—and by attempting to falsify their favored hypothesis (Ceci and Bronfenbrenner, 1991; Dawes, 1992). Similarly, in order for interviewers to obtain the most reliable information, they should also attempt to rule out rival hypotheses rather than exclusively attempting to confirm their favored hypothesis. Because of the needs of child protective service interviewers, however, it is not feasible or even desirable to insist that they generate and test all conceivable hypotheses or, conversely, be "blinded" from all relevant information that pertains to the prosecutor's main hypothesis. Doing the latter could result in missed opportunities whenever an interviewer did not recognize the relevance of a given piece of information provided by the child. But, as I have just described, the failure to test a rival hypothesis can result in various types of errors (e.g., suggestibility effects, misattributions, source confusions).

Most therapists argue that therapeutic goals are quite different from forensic goals—with some purporting to be less interested in the latter than in their client's feelings and interpretations about what may have happened. Thus, many therapists do not see themselves as conducting law enforcement interviews, and their goal may be to bring to fruition some intrapsychic material that they believe is at the root of their young client's problems. If this is their goal, then many techniques that are potentially suggestive (e.g., visually guided imagery inductions, fantasy play, role playing) may be suitable for bringing this material to fruition. A problem arises, however, when the client or her therapist ends up giving testimony after many months of such therapy. I have made these risks clear in my description of the experiment that was conducted to illuminate the effects of visually guided imagery on young children's reality monitoring. We saw that asking young children repeatedly to visualize a scenario can result in some of them subsequently claiming they experienced it even though they have not.

Summary of Current Literature

The six studies that I briefly described highlight the different techniques that researchers are now employing to examine suggestibility in children. As mentioned earlier, the most recent studies, in contrast to the older literature, are somewhat more equivocal in their conclusions about children's testimonial competence. As a result, it is easy to locate in the recent literature studies claiming that young children are quite resistant to suggestion (e.g., Marin, Holmes, Guth, and Kovac, 1979; Saywitz, Goodman, Nicholas, and Moan, 1991), and it is also easy to find studies claiming the opposite (Ceci, Ross, and Toglia, 1987; Cohen and Harnick, 1980; King and Yuille, 1987). This has resulted in a confusing juxtaposition of claims and counterclaims (as well as newspaper headlines).

However, a careful reading of the scientific literature suggests that there *are* reliable age differences in suggestibility, with preschool children's reports being more readily impeded by the presence of erroneous suggestions by an interviewer than older children's reports. Table 3.1 (adapted from Ceci and Bruck, 1993) shows the basis for this claim; in 14 out of 17 modern studies, suggestibility was greater among preschoolers than among older children or adults. To be sure, there are many caveats that accompany this conclusion. For example, some researchers have claimed that age differences in suggestibility are evident principally with non-participating children (i.e., bystanders as opposed to children who were the recipients of some action), and principally on non-sexual questions (Rudy and Goodman, 1991). Others, however, have demonstrated that pronounced age differences can be obtained for sexual questions, too, as well as when the child is a participant in a stressful event. The safest conclusion is probably that suggestibility effects can be and have been found for all types of events, but perhaps they are somewhat harder to obtain when the event is salient for a child.

In sum, our work leads to the following conclusion: *The majority of children are neither as hypersuggestible and coachable as some pro-defense advocates have alleged, nor are they as resistant to suggestions about their*

Table 3.1 Summary of studies that compared suggestibility of preschoolers to older children or to adults

Study	Reliable age effects for suggestibility
1. Ceci, Leichtman, and White (in press)	+
2. Ceci et al. (1987, Exp. 1)	+
3. Ceci et al. (1987, Exp. 2)	+
4. Gordon et al. (1991)	+
5. Goodman and Aman (1990)	+
6. Goodman et al. (1990, Exp. 4)	+
7. Goodman, Hirschman, et al. (1991, Exp. 3)	+
8. Goodman, Hirschman, et al. (1991, Exp. 2)	+
9. Goodman, Hirschman, et al. (1991, Exp. 4)	+
10. Goodman and Reed (1986)	+
11. Oates and Shrimpton (1991)	+
12. Ornstein et al. (1992)	+
13. Rudy and Goodman (1991)	+
14. Saywitz et al. (1989)	+
15. Marin et al. (1979)	0
16. Howe (1991)	0
17. Delamothe and Taplin (1992)	0

Note: Exp. = Experiment. A plus sign denotes that preschoolers were significantly more impaired by misleading questions than older subjects. A zero denotes no significant age differences in the suggestibility effect. Copyright 1993 by the American Psychological Association. Adapted from Ceci and Bruck (1993) by permission of the publisher and author.

own bodies as some pro-prosecution advocates have claimed. In all of the studies outlined here, some young children were more resistant to suggestions and source confusions than were some older children, though the means were always in the normal direction of greater vulnerability among the youngest children. Children can be led to incorporate false suggestions into their accounts of even intimate bodily touching, if these suggestions are made by powerful adult authority figures and delivered repeatedly over prolonged periods. They also can be amazingly resistant to false suggestions, and able to provide highly detailed and accurate reports of events that transpired weeks or months ago (e.g., Baker-Ward, Ornstein, Larus, and Clubb, 1993). This underscores the need for great care in accepting the claims of those who are eager to put a one-sided "spin" on the data. Unfortunately, some of the better-known figures in this area of research have exhibited a partisanship that prods them to discuss their findings without making clear the limits and alternate interpretations.

On the basis of the six studies that I reviewed here, I now believe that some of the things that we might do in therapy or in repeated interviews *could* taint a young child's understanding of the past. For example, if therapists aim to bring intrapsychic material to fruition, and their methods involve "memory work," imagery inductions, and fantasy play, then this might be incompatible with forensic needs. To the extent that such techniques actually overwrite part of a child's biography, and to the extent that an accurate knowledge of the child's past is important to achieving the therapeutic goals, then the use of potentially suggestive techniques with preschoolers would seem to have costs beyond the forensic ones alluded to. But these are many *ifs*, and I leave it to the reader to judge how great these risks are.

Conclusions

Despite the findings of the six studies I described, it is clear that children—even preschoolers—are capable of recalling much that is forensically relevant. For example, when there was no attempt by the interviewers in the Sam Stone study to mislead them, even 3-year-olds recalled large amounts of information accurately. The same is true when the social-worker interviewer in the last study was not herself misled into misleading the child; in such conditions even very young preschoolers do quite well. In this chapter I have focused on preschoolers' weaknesses rather than on their strengths, which are many, because these weaknesses are real and they may not be obvious, given the recency of the results (they are still "in press" and are not scheduled to appear in print for some time). While it is always true that research findings may be modified by subsequent research, this does not imply that it is safe to gainsay or ignore them. However, the fact that preschool-aged children's reports are more vulnerable to postevent distortion than those of older children, and that they can be induced to make false reports in response to certain practices or motives, is not meant to imply that they are incapable of providing accurate testimony. In many of the studies that have been reported during the past decade, young children have accurately recollected the majority of the information that they observed, even when they have not recalled as much as older children. They may be more likely to succumb to erroneous suggestions than older children and adults, but their vulnerability is a matter of degree only. Even adults are suggestible, as Loftus amply demonstrates in Chapter 1 (see also Belli, 1989; Belli, Windschitl, McCarthy, and Winfrey, in press; Loftus, 1979; Loftus and Hoffman, 1989), and in the absence of persistently misleading suggestions from powerful adults, the effect size for *age* is often modest and, at times, nonexistent.

Finally, the studies described in this chapter take as a starting point a "non-event" rather than an actual experience. Identifying the neuro-architecture for a representation that is not grounded in an actual event may prove challenging. McClelland's framework is my nomination for the best fit with data of the type I described in this chapter, though that framework seems to more easily handle representations that result when an original event is altered by the presence of misleading postevent information (e.g., the aggregations of neurons that are used to encode the original representation may be re-aggregated to encode other representations, including the misleading information), than when there is no original event representation. In many of the studies reported here, the only representation available is the result of the suggestive exercises (self-induced or experimenter-induced), so no neural re-aggregation seems to be involved. According to McClelland's connectionist approach, a given memory is represented by a pattern of activation across neurons and connections, some of which are also part of the representations of other memories. Thus, these aspects of the memory get re-accreted in the process of storing and retrieving other memories, giving rise to conditions of alteration and distortion (i.e., as Schacter points out in the Introduction to this volume, "the memories are superimposed on each other, the output that a connectionist model produces as a 'memory' of a particular event always contains some influence from other memories." The connectionist approach would seem useful to developmentalists working in this area, because it makes contact with a number of issues that are important (e.g., trace strength influences the degree of distortion). Moscovitch's approach also makes clear that some neural systems may be intimately involved in the sorts of misattributions seen in these studies, the most promising of which appears to be the late-developing frontal and prefrontal regions that subserve many time-dependent executive monitoring functions. Even if retrieval functions work well, there is a frontal involvement to evaluate source plausibility, which both very young children and Moscovitch's patients often fail to evidence.

Appendix A

In the following interview an experienced social worker is denoted "I," and he is interviewing a child, denoted "C." Occasionally a police detective (denoted "Police") joins the interview. It illustrates a number of inadvisable practices that I frequently observe in interviews by social workers, law enforcement professionals, and therapists.

> I: We have gotten a lot of other kids to help us since I last saw you.
> C: No. I don't have to.
> I: Oh come on. Did we tell you she is in jail?
> C: Yes. My mother already told me.

Comment: This interviewer is not neutral regarding the defendant's guilt, insinuating that because she is now in jail he need not be afraid of her (if he ever was, which is not clear).

I: Well, we can get out of here real quick if you just tell me what you told me last time.

Comment: There is no desire on the part of this interviewer to test an alternative hypothesis; rather he desires the child to reaffirm on tape what he said in an earlier interview.

C: I forgot.
I: No you didn't, I know you didn't.
C: I did, I did.
I: No, come on.
C: I forgot.
I: I thought we were friends last time.
C: I'm not your friend any more.
I: How come?
C: Because I hate you.
I: Is it because we are talking about stuff you don't want to talk about? What, are you a monster now? Huh? . . .

Comment: This interviewing borders on being coercive. There is little respect for the child's wish not to discuss this matter.

I: We talked to a few more of your buddies—we talked to everybody now. And everyone told me about the nap room, and the bathroom stuff, and the music room stuff, and the choir stuff, and the peanut butter stuff, and nothing surprises me any more.

Comment: Again, further evidence that no alternative hypothesis is being tested. The interviewer essentially tells the child that his friends already told on the defendant, and that he, the child, should do the same.

C: I hate you.
I: No you don't . . . You just don't like talking about this, but you don't hate me.
C: Yes, I do hate you.
I: We can finish this real fast if you just show me real fast what you showed me last time.
C: No.
I: I will let you play my tape recorder . . . Come on, do you want to help us out? Do you want to help us keep her in jail, huh? . . . Tell me what happened to (three other children). Tell me what happened to them. Come on . . . I need your help again, buddy. Come on.
C: No.
I: You told us everything once before. Do you want to undress my dolly?

I: Let's get done with this real quick so we could go to Kings to get popsicles . . . Did (defendant) ever tell you she could get out of jail?

Comment: The interviewer comes close to bribing the child for a disclosure, by implying that the aversive interview can be terminated as soon as the child repeats what he said earlier. Popsicles and playing with a tape recorder are offered as rewards.

Police: She could never get out.
C: I know that.
Police: Cause I got her . . . She is very afraid of me. She is so scared of me.
I: She cries when she sees him (indicating the police detective) because she is so scared . . . What happened to (another child) with the wooden spoon? If you don't remember in words, maybe you can show me.

Comment: There is no attempt to test the hypothesis that the defendant did not do what they believed she did. Instead, we see further attempts to vilify the defendant to make it more likely the child will confirm their hunch about her.

C: I forgot what happened, too.
I: You remember. You told your mommy about everything, about the music room, and the nap room. And all the stuff. You want to help her stay in jail, don't you? So she doesn't bother you any more . . . Your mommy told me that you had a picture of yourself in your room and there was blood on your penis. Who hurt you?
C: (Child names the defendant.)
I: So, your penis was bleeding, oh. Your penis was bleeding. Tell me something else: was your hiney bleeding, too?
C: No.
I: Did (defendant) bleed, too?
C: No.
I: Are you sure she didn't bleed?
C: Yes . . . I saw her penis, too.
I: Show me on the (anatomical) doll . . . you saw that? Oh.
C: She doodied on me . . . She peed on us.
I: And did you have to pee on her at all?
C: Yeah.
I: You did? And who peed on her, you and who else?
C: (Child names a male friend.)
I: Didn't his penis bleed?
C: Yes.
I: It did? What made it bleed? What was she doing?
C: She was bleeding.
I: She was bleeding in her penis? Did you have to put your penis in her penis? Yes or No?
C: Yeah . . . And I peed in her penis.

I: What was that like? What did it feel like?

C: Like a shot.

I: Did (friend) have to put his penis in her penis, too?

C: Yes, at the same time.

I: At the same time? How did you do that?

C: We chopped our penises off.

I: So, she was bleeding in her penis and you had your penis and your friend's inside her penis.

C: At the same time. (pp. 45–50; Superior Court of New Jersey, Appellate Division, from *State of New Jersey v. Margaret Kelly Michaels*, appendix, Vol. 1, Docket No. 199-88T4)

Comment: This type of exchange is very common in the transcripts I am sent: When the child says something that is not part of the interviewer's hypothesis (in this case, that the children chopped off their penises), the interviewer ignores it. There is no attempt to pursue it, probably out of fear that the child may embellish this claim with even more incredible claims.

At this point the child and interviewer began discussing a stream of events in which the child alleged that the defendant urinated in his mouth and he urinated in her mouth; he and others were made to walk in her urine and slide on the classroom floor in her urine. Nowhere in this interview, or in numerous others by this and other social workers and psychologists, is there any evidence that an alternative hypothesis was being tested. Specifically, there is no attempt to get the child to assent to an incompatible hypothesis, e.g., one in which the child's pediatrician put his penis in the child's mouth, or the sheriff made him drink his urine, or that he was just teasing when he allegedly told his mother about the defendant bleeding. As can be seen, there is no attempt to encourage the child to deny that any of this happened. Although it is not possible to know how much of what the child is reporting is factually accurate, there is a certain suspiciousness about his disclosures—and this is even more troubling in the interviews of some of his classmates. Partly, this is due to the heavy-handed use of coercive tactics ("If you tell me real quick, we can go get popsicles"; refusal to believe that the child has forgotten or has a legitimate motive for not wanting to repeat an earlier remark he allegedly made to his mother, e.g., the child may realize the former statement is false). But it is partly due to an absence of incredulity on the part of the interviewer. I think this comes about from a confusion among advocates between taking everything the child says seriously, versus believing everything a child says. To the extent that this type of interviewing is widespread, it raises real concerns, because, as I have shown in this chapter, we are beginning to understand that even mild versions of such interview techniques can increase the risk of eliciting false reports, especially if they are conducted over long delay intervals.

There is a final reason why I am troubled by such interviews. As a parent

I have seen how easily my daughter and her friends lapse into scatological humor with the slightest encouragement from an adult. One wonders if the interviewers realize this about some children. In fact, one wonders why they often tout themselves as specializing in "child-centered" or "developmentally-sensitive" interviewing practices. When used by these interviewers, this phrase seems to mean little more than couching questions in a language structure that the child can understand. Nowhere is there any evidence that the interviewer appreciates the child's "theory of mind," suggestibility, or the salient social factors operative in the child's life. Hence, as a developmentalist, the nomenclature "developmentally-sensitive" strikes me as a somewhat gratuitous presumption.

References

Alloy, L. B., and Tabachnik, N. (1984). Assessment of covariation by humans and animals: The joint influence of prior expectations and current situational information. *Psychological Review, 91,* 112–149.

American Psychological Association. (1991). Statement on the use of anatomically detailed dolls in forensic evaluations. Washington, D.C.: APA Council of Representatives.

Anderson, D. (1990). *New York Times,* p. B-9.

Baker-Ward, L., Gordon, B., Ornstein, P. A., Larus, D., and Clubb, P. (1993). Young children's long-term retention of a pediatric examination. *Child Development, 64,* 1519–1533.

Belli, R. F. (1989). Influences of misleading postevent information: Misinformation interference and acceptance. *Journal of Experimental Psychology, General, 118,* 72–85.

Brainerd, C. J., Reyna, V. F., Howe, M. L., and Kingma, J. (1990). The development of forgetting and reminiscence. *Monographs of the Society for Research in Child Development, 55* (Serial No. 222, 3–4).

Brehm, S. S., and Smith, T. W. (1986). Social psychological approaches to psychotherapy and behavior change. In S. L. Garfield and A. Bergin (Eds.), *Handbook of psychotherapy and behavior change* (3rd ed., pp. 69–116). New York: Wiley.

Bruck, M., Ceci, S. J., Francoeur, E., and Barr, R. (in press). "I hardly cried when I got my shot": Young children's reports of their visit to a pediatrician. *Child Development.*

Bruck, M., Ceci, S. J., Francoeur, E., and Renick, A. (in press). Preschoolers' reports of genital touching. *Journal of Experimental Psychology: Applied.*

Cassel, W. S., and Bjorklund, D. F. (in press). Tell me about . . ., Don't you remember . . .? Isn't it true that . . .? Developmental patterns of eyewitness responses to increasingly suggestive questions. *Law and Human Behavior.*

Ceci, S. J. (1994). Cognitive and social factors in children's testimony. In B. Sales and G. VandenBos (Eds.), *APA master lectures: Psychology and law* (pp. 11–31). Washington, D.C.: American Psychological Association.

Ceci, S. J., and Bronfenbrenner, U. (1991). On the demise of everyday memory: The rumors of my death are greatly exaggerated. *American Psychologist, 46*, 27–31.

Ceci, S. J., and Bruck, M. (1993). The suggestibility of the child witness: A historical review and synthesis. *Psychological Bulletin, 113*, 403–439.

Ceci, S. J., Crotteau, M. L., Smith, E., and Loftus, E. F., (1994). Repeatedly thinking about non-events. *Consciousness and Cognition.*

Ceci, S. J., Leichtman, M., and White, T. (in press). Interviewing preschoolers: Remembrance of things planted. In D. P. Peters (Ed.), *The child witness in context: Cognitive, social, and legal perspectives.* Amsterdam: Kluwer.

Ceci, S. J., Loftus, E. F., Leichtman, M. D., and Bruck, M. (1994). The role of source misattributions in the creation of false beliefs among preschoolers. *International Journal of Clinical and Experimental Hypnosis, 42*, 304–320.

Ceci, S. J., Ross, D., and Toglia, M. (1987). Age differences in suggestibility: Psycholegal implications. *Journal of Experimental Psychology: General, 117*, 38–49.

Cohen, R. L., and Harnick, M. A. (1980). The susceptibility of child witnesses to suggestion. *Law and Human Behavior, 4*, 201–210.

Dawes, R. (Spring 1992). The importance of alternative hypothesis and hypothetical counterfactuals in general social science. *The General Psychologist* (Spring) 2–7.

Flavell, J., Flavell, E., and Green, F. L. (1987). Young children's knowledge about the apparent-real and pretend-real distinctions. *Developmental Psychology, 23*, 816–822.

Foley, M. A., and Johnson, M. K. (1985). Confusions between memories for performed and imagined actions. *Child Development, 56*, 1145–1155.

Foley, M. A., Johnson, M. K., and Raye, C. L. (1983). Age-related confusion between memories for thoughts and memories for speech. *Child Development, 54*, 51–60.

Foley, M. A., Santini, C., and Sopasakis, M. (in press). Discriminating between memories: Evidence for children's spontaneous elaborations. *Journal of Experimental Child Psychology.*

Fredrickson, R. (1992). *Repressed memories: A journey to recovery from sexual abuse.* New York: Parkside Books/Simon and Schuster.

Freud, S. (1901/1960). The psychopathology of everyday life. In J. Strachey (Ed. and Trans.), *The standard edition of the complete psychological works of Sigmund Freud* (vol. 6). London: Hogarth Press.

Freud, S. (1933). New introductory lectures on psychoanalysis. In J. Strachey (Ed.), *The standard edition of the complete psychological works of Sigmund Freud.* London: Hogarth Press.

Goodman, G., and Aman, C. (1990). Children's use of anatomically detailed dolls to recount an event. *Child Development, 61*, 1859–1871.

Goodman, G. S., Rudy, L., Bottoms, B., and Aman, C. (1990). Children's concerns and memory: Issues of ecological validity in the study of children's eyewitness testimony. In R. Fivush and J. Hudson (Eds.), *Knowing and remembering in young children* (pp. 249–284). New York: Cambridge University Press.

Harris, P., Brown, E., Marriott, C., Whittal, S., and Harmer, S. (1991). Monsters, ghosts and witches: Testing the limits of the fantasy-reality distinction in young children. *British Journal of Developmental Psychology, 9*, 105–123.

Johnson, M. K. (1991). Reality monitoring: Evidence from confabulation in organic brain disease patients. In G. Prigatano and D. L. Schacter (Eds.), *Awareness of deficit after brain injury* (pp. 124–140). New York: Oxford University Press.

Johnson, M. K., Hastroudi, S., and Lindsay, D. S. (1993). Source monitoring. *Psychological Bulletin, 114,* 3–28.

Kayne, N. T., and Alloy, L. B. (1988). Clinician and patient as aberrant actuaries: Expectation-based distortions in assessment of covariation. In L. Y. Abramson (Ed.), *Social cognition and clinical psychology: A synthesis.* New York: Guilford.

King, M., and Yuille, J. (1987). Suggestibility and the child witness. In S. J. Ceci, D. Ross, and M. Toglia (Eds.), *Children's eyewitness memory* (pp. 24–356). New York: Springer-Verlag.

Lamb, M., Sternberg, K., and Esplin, P. (in press). Factors influencing the reliability and validity of statements made by young victims of sexual maltreatment. *Journal of Applied Developmental Psychology.*

Leichtman, M. D., and Ceci, S. J. (in press). The effect of stereotypes and suggestions on preschoolers' reports. *Developmental Psychology.*

Lindsay, D. S., Johnson, M. K., and Kwon, P. (1991). Developmental changes in memory source monitoring. *Developmental Psychology, 52,* 297–318.

Loftus, E. F. (1979). *Eyewitness testimony.* Cambridge, Mass.: Harvard University Press.

Loftus, E. F., and Hoffman, H. (1989). Misinformation and memory: The creation of new memories. *Journal of Experimental Psychology: General, 118,* 100–104.

Marin, B. V., Holmes, D. L., Guth, M., and Kovac, P. (1979). The potential of children as eyewitnesses. *Law and Human Behavior, 3,* 295–304.

Masson, J. M. (1984). Freud and the seduction theory. *The Atlantic Monthly,* (February) 33–60.

Milne, A. A. (1957). *The world of Pooh.* New York: E. P. Dutton.

Morison, P., and Gardner, H. (1978). Dragons and dinosaurs: The child's capacity to differentiate fantasy from reality. *Child Development, 49,* 642–648.

Perris, E. E., Myers, N. A., and Clifton, R. K. (1990). Long-term memory for a single infancy experience. *Child Development, 61,* 1796–1807.

Pettit, F., Fegan, M., and Howie, P. (September 1990). Interviewer effects on children's testimony. Paper presented at the International Congress on Child Abuse and Neglect, Hamburg, Germany.

Piaget, J. (1926). *The language and thought of the child.* London: Routledge, Kegan Paul.

Raskin, D., and Yuille, J. (1989). Problems in evaluating interviews of children in sexual abuse cases. In S. J. Ceci, D. Ross, and M. Toglia (Eds.), *Adults' perceptions of children's testimony* (pp. 184–207). New York: Springer-Verlag.

Roberts, K., and Blades, M. (in press). Children's discriminations of memories for actual and pretend actions in a hiding task. *British Journal of Developmental Psychology.*

Ross, D. F., Dunning, D., Toglia, M., and Ceci, S. J. (1990). The child in the eyes of the jury. *Law and Human Behavior, 14,* 5–23.

Rudy, L., and Goodman, G. S. (1991). Effects of participation on children's reports: Implications for children's testimony. *Developmental Psychology, 27,* 527–538.

Saywitz, K. J., Goodman, G. S., Nicholas, E., and Moan, S. F. (1991). Children's memories of a physical examination involving genital touch: Implications for reports of child sexual abuse. *Journal of Consulting and Clinical Psychology, 59,* 682–691.

Schacter, D. L., Osowiecki, D. M., Kasniak, A., Kihlstrom, J. F., and Valdiserri, M. (1994). Source Memory: Extending the boundary of age-related deficits. *Psychology and Aging, 9,* 81–89.

Schooler, J. W., Gerhard, D., and Loftus, E. F. (1986). Qualities of the unreal. *Journal of Experimental Psychology: Learning, Memory, and Cognition, 12,* 171–181.

Sugar, M. (1992). Toddlers' traumatic memories. *Infant Mental Health Journal, 13,* 245–251.

Taylor, D., and Howell, W. (1973). The ability of 3-, 4-, and 5-year-olds to distinguish fantasy from reality. *Journal of Genetic Psychology, 122,* 315–318.

Tulving, E. E., and Thompson, D. M. (1973). Encoding specificity. *Psychological Review.*

Vaillant, G. E. (1977). *Adaptation to life.* Boston: Little, Brown.

Warren, A., and Hagood, P. (in press). Effects of timing and type of questioning in eyewitness accuracy and identification. In M. Zaragoza (Ed.), *Memory, Suggestibility, and Eyewitness Testimony.* New York: Hemisphere.

Acknowledgments

Portions of the research reported in this chapter were supported by grants from NIH RO1 HD25775 and NSF No. 1R01 MH50786–01.

Psychiatric and Psychopathological Perspectives

Hypnosis and Suggestion

4

David Spiegel

Hypnosis has been viewed as both the cause of and the cure for memory distortion. The special characteristics of the hypnotic state and the unusual attributes of those high in the trait of hypnotizability provide opportunities for exploration of memory distortion and retrieval. In one way or another, hypnosis and the related phenomenon of dissociation have been linked in clinical experience to trauma for more than a century. Trauma seems to elicit dissociation, with accompanying distortions in memory, and hypnosis has repeatedly been used to reverse dissociative amnesia and treat other aftereffects of trauma. Yet hypnosis and the enhanced suggestibility associated with it have been linked in the laboratory with increased productivity of memory retrieval at the expense of accuracy, often with a false sense of certainty that the memories produced are correct. This chapter will examine hypnosis and suggestion, their relationship to specific types of memory distortion, and their interaction with clinical phenomena such as dissociation.

Hypnosis

Hypnosis is a state of aroused, attentive, focused concentration with a relative constriction of peripheral awareness (Spiegel, 1988; Spiegel and Spiegel, 1987). It involves attentional processes (Hilgard, 1965; Tellegen and Atkinson, 1974), including imaginative involvement (J. Hilgard, 1970), and heightened responsiveness to social cues (Orne, 1959). Individuals capable of entering a hypnotic state can do so in seconds, utilizing a variety of induction procedures. Indeed, such individuals are prone to spontaneous entry into such states, even without formal induction (Lynn and Nash, 1994; Sheehan et al., 1991; McConkey et al., 1990). On the other hand, individuals with little or no hypnotic capacity are unable to utilize this type of consciousness, even after a formal induction (Hilgard, 1965). Hypnotizability is quite a stable trait throughout the adult life cycle. Piccione and colleagues (1992) recently reported a test-retest reliability of .70 on the Stanford Hypnotic Susceptibility Scale over a 25-year interval.

There are three main components to hypnotic experience: absorption, dissociation, and suggestibility.

Absorption

Absorption is an immersion in a central experience at the expense of contextual orientation (J. Hilgard, 1970; Tellegen and Atkinson, 1974; Tellegen, 1981; Spiegel, 1994). Tellegen, the originator of the term, describes it as " 'total' attention, involving a full commitment of available perceptual, motoric, imaginative, and ideational resources to a unified representation of the attentional object" (Tellegen and Atkinson, 1974, p. 276). The natural tendency to such self-altering experiences has been shown to be positively correlated with measured hypnotizability (Tellegen and Atkinson, 1974; Frischholz et al., 1987), meaning not only that the two constructs are linked, but that aspects of hypnotic experience occur spontaneously among those with the requisite hypnotizability.

Dissociation

In order to become so intensely involved in a central object of consciousness, one must restrict conscious processing of perceptions, thoughts, memories, or motor activities at the periphery (Posner and Petersen, 1990). These experiences may range from the simple, such as a hand feeling not as much a part of the body as usual, to the complex. Even rather complex emotional states or sensory experiences may be dissociated (Spiegel, 1990). Some may involve memory alterations, such as dissociative amnesia for a traumatic event, and others identity and motor function, as in a fugue episode in which for a period of hours to months an individual functions as though he or she had a different name and residence (American Psychiatric Association, 1994). Such experiences can be both induced and reversed with the structured use of hypnosis (Spiegel, 1988).

Dissociated information is temporarily and reversibly unavailable to consciousness, but may nonetheless influence conscious (or other unconscious) experience, analogous to priming effects (Schacter, 1992; Kihlstrom et al., 1980). Out of sight does not mean out of mind. A rape victim may have no conscious memory of the crime, yet become anxious when exposed to stimuli reminiscent of the event (Spiegel, 1990). Absorption and dissociation are thus complementary constructs. Intensifying focal attention facilitates putting other information outside of conscious awareness, but not outside the possibility of influencing consciousness.

Suggestibility

Because of their intense absorption in the trance experience, hypnotized individuals usually accept instructions relatively uncritically; hence the term "suggestibility." Hypnotized individuals are more prone to accept directions, no matter how irrational. This phenomenon has been observed in highly hypnotizable individuals outside of formal hypnosis as well (H. Spiegel, 1974). They are also less likely to distinguish an instruction as coming from another rather than themselves, a phenomenon known as hypnotic source amnesia (Evans and Thorn, 1966; Evans, 1988), and so will tend to act on another person's ideas as though they were their own. This aspect of hypnosis implies that a hypnotized individual is especially vulnerable to the nature of an inquiry, meaning that the trance state can enhance responsiveness, either for good or ill. There is evidence, for example, that under hypnosis utilized for memory retrieval, subjects produce more information, both correct and incorrect, and overestimate the accuracy of their retrieval (Dywan and Bowers, 1983). Some may even be led to produce false memories (Laurence and Perry, 1983; Lynn and Nash, 1994; Stevenson, 1994).

Effects of Hypnosis and Suggestion on Memory Processes

One can conceptualize these components of hypnotic experience as having specific corresponding effects on the three main components of memory processing: encoding, storage, and retrieval. Absorption, narrowing of the focus of attention, can have particular effects on encoding problems, dissociation on storage, and suggestibility on the process of retrieval.

Consider absorption and its effect on encoding of memory. Hypnotic attention involves an intense focus at the expense of peripheral awareness (Spiegel and Spiegel, 1987; Tellegen and Atkinson, 1974). To the extent that individuals enter a hypnotic or hypnotic-like state, they may restrict the range of encoding of new information. An example is the "weapon focus" of mugging victims (Loftus, 1979), who can give a detailed description of the gun pointed at them, but little or no information about the assailant's appearance. Such a constricted fund of information is at least consistent with if not caused by a narrowed attentional focus at the time of the memory encoding. While under normal circumstances it would be surprising to have contact with someone who proved memorable and yet recall little about his facial features, this is less surprising if attentional focus is narrowed and drawn to a threatening object.

Perceptions may be distorted, mislabeled, or omitted, especially when they occur in a stressful or traumatic context. For example, Loftus and Burns (1982) found that subjects shown a shocking film of a boy being shot in the face had poorer recall and recognition memory for other events depicted in the film. They found that this effect occurred not merely because the event was unexpected, but because it was "mentally upsetting." Natural absorption in the intense emotional experience may be intensified by entry into hypnotic-like states during such events, and this in turn can reduce encoding of information outside the boundary of focal attention.

Dissociation

Dissociation is both a normal component of a normal phenomenon (hypnosis) and may occur spontaneously by itself to a degree which may reach pathological proportions. Hypnosis has been defined as formally induced dissociation (Nemiah, 1985). Dissociative effects on memory will be examined from the perspective of dissociation as a continuum from normal to pathological segregation of mental contents (H. Spiegel and Shainess, 1963). Memory storage processes may be particularly influenced by dissociative phenomena. The nature of memory storage and potential for retrievability are profoundly influenced by the associative matrix in which the memories are laid down. The distinction between explicit versus implicit (Schacter, 1987), episodic versus semantic (Tulving, 1983), or declarative versus procedural memory (Squire and Cohen, 1984) illustrates the importance of associational networks in memory retrieval. For example, activation of associations about what a neighbor was like is crucial to recollection of the episode in which this neighbor taught one to ride a bicycle, but is unnecessary to activate the memory schemas required to ride the bicycle. Different networks of association about the same episode yield quite different types of memory retrieval.

Consider, for example, dissociative amnesia, an extreme form of functional memory loss in which there is "inability to recall important personal information, usually of a traumatic or stressful nature, which is too extensive to be explained by ordinary forgetfulness" (American Psychiatric Association, 1994). Such individuals lose access to explicit memories of salient autobiographical information which they consciously acquired and ordinarily would be able to retrieve as explicit memories. A rape victim who had no conscious recollection of the assault became "extremely upset" when taken back to the scene (Schacter and Kihlstrom, 1989). A situation which would ordinarily trigger an association of the scene to conscious recollection instead stimulated uncomfortable affect without explicit content. Indeed, the recollection takes the form of an implicit rather than an explicit memory (Schacter and Kihlstrom, 1989). Lyon (1985, cited in Schacter and Kihlstrom, 1989) reported that a woman with dissociative fugue, a loss of personal identifying information (American Psychiatric Association, 1994), who was asked to randomly dial numbers on the telephone managed without conscious recollection to dial the correct number of her mother, who identified her. Thus, what would ordinarily be considered explicit recollection was retrieved implicitly.

Associative networks, the co-occurrence of related activated associations, are at the heart of connectionist models of memory (McClelland and Rumelhart, 1986). It thus makes sense that mental processes which segregate one set of associations from another might well impair memory storage or retrieval (Kihlstrom, 1980, 1987). Dissociative barriers separating the contents of various aspects of memory or identity from one another cause specific difficulties in retrieval, and may instigate a shift in retrieval model from explicit to implicit.

Functional disorders of memory have been traditionally conceptualized as deficits in memory retrieval (Evans and Kihlstrom, 1979; Schacter and Kihlstrom, 1989). Amnesia has been described as occurring when information which is potentially "available" is currently not "accessible" for recollection as a result of some kind of retrieval problem (Tulving and Pearlstone, 1966). However, some kinds of functional memory disorders may be related to organizational and storage deficits as well. This is likely since the type of memories most commonly rendered inaccessible in dissociative amnesia, "usually of a traumatic and stressful nature" (American Psychiatric Association, 1994), are likely to be stored in a network designed to separate strong affective salience from content. A victim of homosexual rape with dissociative amnesia produced images from his past in hypnosis which he did not initially (but later did) identify as such. However, when shown a TAT card depicting one person being attacked by another from behind, he became quite upset and attempted to commit suicide (Kaszniak et al., 1988, cited in Schacter and Kihlstrom, 1989). His memories were stored in such a manner that the content was dissociated from the affect.

The dissociative disorders represent a disturbance in the integrated organization of identity, memory, perception, or consciousness (American Psychiatric Association, 1994). Events normally experienced on a smooth continuum become isolated from the other mental processes with which they would ordinarily be contiguous. Clinically, this can result in specific deficits. When the dissociation specifically involves memory, it produces dissociative amnesia. When it involves identity, dissociative fugue or dissociative identity (formerly multiple personality) disorder occurs. Dissociation of perception yields depersonalization disorder, while that of consciousness results in acute stress disorder or dissociative trance disorder, which includes various trance and possession states. They are in this sense a disturbance in the organization or structure of mental contents rather than in the contents themselves. Memories in dissociative amnesia are not so much distorted as they are segregated one from another. The problem is the failure of integration rather than the contents of the fragments (Evans, 1988).

Such disorders of memory usually follow some form of acute trauma or traumatic stress and may be gradual or sudden in onset (Spiegel and Cardena, 1990; Spiegel, 1990; Spiegel et al., 1988). They are usually reversible with psychotherapeutic techniques including hypnosis, which may be used to access memory that is otherwise unavailable to consciousness. In contrast to repressed memories, dissociated ones are isolated into discrete periods of time lost from consciousness (Loewenstein, 1991). Thus, the patient may complain of "losing time," not being aware of what happened between one specific time and another. Occasionally, however, such patients may not present with such a complaint. That is, they may not be aware of or remember their failure to remember. Instead, the complaint may come from others that the patient apparently was unaware of certain events, had no memory for a given period of time, or could not recognize certain people or places usually familiar to him.

> A Vietnam combat veteran described a period of complete memory loss covering several weeks which commenced immediately after he learned that a Vietnamese child he had informally "adopted" had been killed in the Tet Offensive. Although he had three previous years of uninterrupted service in Vietnam, and fifteen prior years of good to excellent conduct ratings in the Army, he became unable to function, and was evacuated and eventually discharged for psychiatric reasons. Initial diagnoses included antisocial personality disorder, schizophrenia, and bipolar disorder, and he spent four years in various Army and Veterans Administration Hospitals, becoming increasingly depressed and suicidal. Using hypnosis, he was able to recall consciously for the first time the events subsequent to the boy's death. He relived with intense affect discovering the body, commandeering an ambulance, and setting booby traps for Vietcong. He tearfully relived burying the child and began grieving the loss, with an improvement in his chronic suicidal depression (Spiegel, 1981). Phone calls to people identified in his recollected memories indicated that some of the events were correct but others were not. A soldier he thought had been killed during the Offensive was alive, for example.

When dissociative amnesia occurs it is usually in the aftermath of trauma (APA, 1994), is discrete, and covers an emotionally salient set of events (Loewenstein, 1990, 1991), although other forms have been described. The information kept out of consciousness nonetheless has effects on it, consistent with the suicidal depression observed in the case described above. Experimental evidence from the careful study of an individual with dissociative amnesia indicates a relatively selective deficit in episodic as compared with semantic memory (Schacter et al., 1982) in dissociative amnesia. However, in this case there was some leakage of episodic information from the amnesic period, and some lack of general but personal information not tied to a specific episode, such as the patient's memory of his name. Schacter and colleagues hypothesized that self-information may constitute control elements in the organization of episodic memory. The leakage of information from the amnesic period seemed to be organized affectively rather than temporally, as is the case in organic amnesia. The patient remembered a nickname he had been given during an unusually positive period in his life. This observation is consistent with the idea that dissociation may serve the purpose of affective regulation, especially in coping with the emotional effects of traumatic stress.

Another form of classical dissociative memory loss is dissociative fugue, involving the loss of memory for personal identity. The disorder sometimes involves unplanned and unexpected travel. It may also involve the assumption of a new identity, although this occurs in only a minority of cases (Riether and Stoudemire, 1988).

Dissociation and Trauma

One of the important developments in the modern understanding of dissociative disorders is the exploration of the link between trauma and dissociation. Trauma can be understood as the experience of being made into an object, a thing, the victim of someone else's rage, of nature's indifference. It is the ultimate experience of helplessness and loss of control over one's own body. There is growing clinical and some empirical evidence that dissociation may occur especially as a defense during trauma, an attempt to maintain mental control, just as physical control is lost (Spiegel, 1984; Kluft, 1984; Putnam, 1985; Spiegel, Hunt, and Dondershine, 1988; Spiegel and Cardena, 1993; Koopman et al., 1994; Marmar et al., 1994; Bremner et al., 1992). One Dissociative Identity Disorder patient reported "going to a mountain meadow full of wildflowers" when she was being sexually assaulted by her drunken father. She would concentrate on how pleasant and beautiful this imaginary scene was as a way of detaching herself from the immediate experience of terror, pain, and helplessness. Such individuals often report seeking comfort from imaginary playmates or imagined protectors, or absorbing themselves in the pattern of the wallpaper. Many rape victims report floating above their body, feeling sorry for the person being assaulted below them. According to research on hostage-taking situations, studies of survivors of life-threatening events indicate that more than half have experienced feelings of unreality, automatic movements, lack of emotion, and a sense of detachment (Noyes and Kletti, 1977; Madakasira and O'Brien, 1987; Sloan, 1988). Depersonalization and hyperalertness are prominent experiences during trauma (Noyes and Slyman, 1978, 1979). Numbing, loss of interest, and an inability to feel deeply about anything were reported in about a third of the survivors of the Hyatt Regency skywalk collapse (Wilkinson, 1983), and in a similar proportion of survivors of the North Sea oil rig collapse (Holen, 1991). This is consistent with our studies of survivors of the Loma Prieta earthquake (Cardena and Spiegel, 1993). A quarter of a sample of normal students reported marked depersonalization during and immediately after the earthquake, and 40% described derealization, the surroundings seeming unreal or dreamlike. While the most common reported memory disturbance was intrusive recollection, 29% of the sample reported difficulties with everyday memory. One survivor of the Oakland/Berkeley firestorm who had lost his house reported a strange sense of detachment during the fire:

> It was as though I was watching myself on television. I had this image of myself talking to a policeman, asking if I could go to my home, and whether he had any information about where my son was. I thought that I seemed rather unemotional, and decided that I had better stay that way in order not to upset my wife. It felt like I was watching the experience rather than having it.

Dissociative symptoms have been retrospectively reported as occurring during combat as well (Bremner et al., 1992). Veterans with Post Traumatic Stress Disorder have been found to obtain higher scores on measures of hypnotizability (Stutman and Bliss, 1985; Spiegel et al., 1988) and dissociation (Bremner et al., 1992). Dissociative symptoms, especially numbing, have been found to be rather strong predictors of later PTSD (MacFarlane, 1986; Solomon et al., 1989; Koopman et al., 1994). Thus, physical trauma seems to elicit dissociation or compartmentalization of experience, and may often become the matrix for later post-traumatic symptomatology, such as dissociative amnesia for the traumatic episode. Indeed, more extreme dissociative disorders, such as Dissociative Identity Disorder, have been conceptualized as chronic Post Traumatic Stress Disorders (Spiegel, 1984; Kluft, 1984; Spiegel, 1986). There is recent evidence (Terr, 1991) that children exposed to multiple trauma are more likely to use dissociative mechanisms which include spontaneous trance episodes. Recollection of trauma tends to have an "off/on" quality involving either intrusion or omission (Horowitz, 1986), in which victims either intensively relive the trauma as though it were recurring, or have difficulty remembering it (Madakasira and O'Brien, 1987; Cardena and Spiegel, 1991; Christianson and Loftus, 1987). Thus, physical trauma seems to elicit dissociative responses.

Why consider this a storage problem? If the state of mind occurring at the time of the trauma is altered or hypnotic-like, the way the memories are stored may be influenced by this narrowness of focus. The range of associations may be more limited and therefore those that exist more intense. Strong affect, for example, which is usually associated with traumatic memories, may influence both storage and retrieval. There is evidence that mood congruence between the state in which memories were stored and that in which they are retrieved improves recall (Bower, 1981). Similarly, another form of salient state dependency involves the dissociative state itself. To the extent that individuals do enter a spontaneous dissociated state during trauma, the memories may be stored in a manner that reflects this state (e.g., narrower range of associations to context). There may be fewer cross-connections to other related memories (Evans and Kihlstrom, 1973; Hilgard, 1986). Furthermore, retrieval should be facilitated by being in a similar dissociative state (e.g., hypnosis).

Trauma can be conceptualized as a sudden discontinuity in experience. This may lead to a process of memory storage which is similarly discontinuous with the usual range of associated memories. This may explain the "off/on" quality of dissociative amnesia, and its reversibility with techniques such as hypnosis (Loewenstein, 1990, 1991; Spiegel and Spiegel, 1987). Indeed, there is recent evidence that dissociative symptoms occur frequently in the immediate aftermath of physical trauma such as earthquakes (Cardena and Spiegel, 1993). Half of a normal sample tested within one week of the Loma Prieta earthquake reported memory disturbances, involving either intrusions of traumatic memory or difficulties with everyday memory. The development of dissociative symptoms in the immediate aftermath of a traumatic stressor predicts the development of later Post Traumatic Stress Disorder (Koopman, Classen, and Spiegel, 1994).

Evidence for the phenomenon of dissociation of early life traumatic memory comes from a study by Williams (1994), who studied a sample of women who had been brought to a hospital emergency room for treatment of sexual abuse and collection of forensic evidence. One hundred thirty-six (two-thirds of the sample) were located an average of 17 years later, and interviewed in detail about their histories for an average of three hours by raters blind to their hospital records. Thirty-eight percent of this sample did not report the incident of sexual abuse documented in their medical records, although only 12% reported no memory of any abuse. The author concluded that this failure to report represented lack of accessible memory rather than reluctance because many of these women did report other embarrassing or painful experiences. While some of this lack of recollection may be attributed to normal early childhood amnesia, the study does provide evidence that at least single incidents of documented abuse may not be subsequently available to conscious recollection attempts.

Dissociative symptoms are more frequent in individuals who report histories of trauma in childhood (Chu and Dill, 1990; Herman et al., 1990). Several studies have shown a relationship between a diagnosis of Dissociative Identity Disorder, characterized by the presence of more than one identity or personality state and amnesia (American Psychiatric Association, 1994), and a history of severe and multiple traumas in childhood (Spiegel,

1984; Kluft, 1985). Putnam and colleagues (1986) found that out of 100 DID patients 97% reported experiencing severe trauma in childhood, typically involving a combination of sexual and physical abuse. Coons and Milstein (1986) found that 85% of 20 DID cases reported sexual or physical abuse. Likewise, Ross and colleagues found that 95% of 97 individuals with DID reported they had experienced childhood sexual or physical abuse (Ross et al., 1990). There is some debate as to the accuracy of these reports, particularly given the high hypnotizability of this population (Frankel, 1990). However, Coons and Milstein (1986) were able to find independent corroboration for 17 of the 20 patients' reports of abuse. In another retrospective study involving 19 children with DID and Dissociative Disorder Not Otherwise Specified, Coons (1994) found that all but one reported physical or sexual abuse, and these histories were confirmed through a review of medical records and interviews with parents and other family members, welfare case workers, and pediatricians. A recent survey study demonstrated a relationship between a history of sexual abuse and higher general levels of psychopathology (Mullen et al., 1993). Thus the limited available literature indicates that individuals who have undergone physical trauma are at increased risk for dissociative symptoms, often transient and mild, such as depersonalization. Those who have experienced childhood trauma are at increased risk for subsequent dissociative symptoms (Spiegel, 1984; Kluft, 1985; Terr, 1992), which may include dissociative amnesia for one or more traumatic episodes or the development of Dissociative Identity Disorder.

Suggestibility

It is clear that suggestion independent of hypnosis may exert a powerful influence on memory retrieval. The insertion of a different article in a question ("Did you see a stop sign?" versus "Did you see the stop sign?") will influence the nature of the memory product (Loftus, 1975, 1979, 1991, 1993; Loftus and Loftus, 1980; Loftus et al., 1978). This literature is often cited as grounds for attacking the veracity of the phenomenon of repressed or dissociated memory. Yet the very existence of such a suggestion effect provides evidence of that phenomenon. Proving that memory is malleable and that retrieval can be influenced by suggestion says little about the type of possible distortion. Logically, it should be equally easy to insert false information, as in many of these studies, or to suppress true information by suggesting that something else (or nothing) happened. Evidence for this possibility comes from Ceci's work (see Chapter 3 in this volume) in which children's recollections of the experience of having an injection in the doctor's office were strongly influenced by retrieval cues. Those told a year after the shot that they had "acted brave and didn't cry when they received their inoculation one year earlier, reported significantly less crying and less hurt than children who were not provided with any information about how they acted." In other words, this "false memory" involved suppression of real (if minor) trauma that is recalled by other children not given the positive suggestion.

Furthermore, the provision of a suggestion regarding a memory can produce retroactive interference, the inhibition of a memory through competition with closely associated material placed in consciousness. Depending on the nature of the suggestion and its relationship to memory, it may be necessary to suppress, repress, or dissociate the true memory that it supplants. To falsely remember a stop sign in an automobile accident, it is necessary to suppress veridical recollection of the yield sign that was there. To present themselves as brave when receiving their inoculation, Ceci's children had to repress recollection that they were not so brave and did indeed cry. Thus, suggestion is consistent with rather than contradictory to dissociative amnesia and other forms of "repressed memory." Indeed, several recent studies have shown that hypnotic suggestions exert as much distorting influence on recall of true as of false memories (McConkey, 1992; Lynn et al., 1991).

The formal use of hypnosis can amplify suggestion effects (H. Spiegel, 1980; Hilgard, 1991; Cardena and Spiegel, 1991; Orne et al., 1985; McConkey, 1992; Spanos, Gwynn et al., 1989). The experience of involuntariness is an important component of hypnosis (Weitzenhoffer, 1989; Spiegel and Spiegel, 1987), often coupled with the dissociative experience of observing oneself performing as if one were an outsider (depersonalization). Thus hypnotized individuals may be led to confabulate far more elaborately than is typical of the literature on misguided memory (Putnam, 1979; Zelig and Beidleman, 1981; Timm, 1981; Loftus, 1993).

In the most extreme situation, highly hypnotizable and hypnotized individuals may become what have been called "honest liars," believing strongly in implanted or imagined "recollections" (H. Spiegel, 1974, 1980).

> A highly hypnotizable businessman was instructed in hypnosis that there was a Communist plot to take over the television media, and that he would see three names on a sheet of paper. He was then interviewed on camera by a well-known television reporter. He elaborated a tale of intrigue regarding such a plot, replete with names and dates of meetings. He hallucinated three names when confronted with a blank sheet of paper, saying: "I know him and him, but not that one in the middle." When pushed harder by the interviewer, he stated: "He is a terrible man—maybe he has gotten to you already," thereby elaborating a paranoid defense of his position. As soon as the hypnosis was ended, he recanted the story, viewing it as an amusing experiment.

These clinical examples are consistent with laboratory studies. Laurence and Perry (1983) showed that a substantial minority of hypnotized individuals who had been instructed that they had heard an accident while they were sleeping reported such suggestions as real memories seven days later. Some persisted in this false belief even after they were told that the memory had been the product of a hypnotic suggestion. Such studies underscore the extremes to which hypnosis may influence retrieval processes in certain circumstances. Hypnotic subjects may experience themselves as retrieving information, when they are in fact creating it. Hypnotic age "progression" can appear as compelling as hypnotic age regression. It has been commonly observed that assessment of the validity of recall is out of proportion to its accuracy after hypnotic refreshing of recollection.

More common but mundane effects of hypnosis on memory retrieval involve enhancement of confidence more than accuracy. The memory enhancement literature with hypnosis makes it clear that when individuals use hypnotic techniques to retrieve information they tend to produce more information, both accurate and inaccurate (Dywan and Bowers, 1983; McConkey, 1992; McConkey and Kinoshita, 1988; Nogrady et al., 1985). Indeed, a relationship has been observed between hypnotizability and increased productivity, with or without the formal use of hypnosis (Zelig and Beidleman, 1981). However, the price of these efforts at detecting new information is often a greater willingness to report fantasies as memories—an alteration in response bias, in signal detection terms. The ratio of correct to incorrect information may actually decline, but subjects' conviction that their memories are correct tends to increase (Dywan and Bowers, 1983; Sheehan and Tilden, 1983). Thus, individuals exposed to hypnotic-like techniques of memory retrieval may have a falsely elevated estimate of the veracity of their recollection. However, a similar potential for distortion accompanies nonhypnotic memory retrieval techniques (Scheflin, 1994).

Increasing retrieval productivity is likely to help an individual unearth additional correct information since, as noted before, repeated recall efforts improve true recollection (Erdelyi and Kleinbard, 1978). However, the confounding of productivity with hypnotic product stalks the research literature. Some retrieval attributed to hypnosis may only reflect additional retrieval efforts. In the study which most carefully controlled for productivity, there was no increase in correct or incorrect recollection facilitated by hypnosis (Sheehan and Tilden, 1983). Crawford and Allen (1983) have shown that hypnotizable subjects do better in a visual memory task with hypnosis. The price of this product, however, is a greater likelihood of "confident errors" (McConkey, 1992), if not confabulation.

While it must be borne in mind that most of these studies were conducted in a laboratory setting in which subjects, usually students, watched films, or in one case, watched a staged mock assassination at a university (Timm, 1981), the follow-up time is usually brief and the consequences of a mistake are minimal, certainly far less than they would be in a court of law. Nonetheless, these studies do raise the concern that unduly suggestive efforts at memory retrieval may produce more false than true new information and may exaggerate an individual's conviction that what is recalled is accurate.

If the only goal is the production of more correct information, for example details of a crime scene, hypnosis may be genuinely helpful. For instance, the driver of the school bus hijacked in the Chowchilla kidnapping recalled under hypnosis all the numbers and letters on the license plate of the car that overtook the bus, which led to the arrest of the perpetrators (Kroger and Douce, 1979).

One reason for this disjunction between accuracy and evaluation in memory may come from the dichotomy between episodic and semantic memory (Tulving, 1983; Rosch, 1977), declarative and procedural memory (Shimamura and Squire, 1987; Squire and Zola-Morgan, 1991), or explicit and implicit memory (Schacter, 1987, 1992). This fundamental distinction can be thought of as involving the difference between subjectivity and automaticity in memory, recollection of personal participation in an event versus knowing how to talk, walk, type, or recognize a word as familiar without knowing that one has learned it (Schacter et al., 1982). Implicit or semantic or procedural memory is rarely subjected to much critical scrutiny or even much conscious awareness. Indeed, if we consciously try to "improve" upon our performance of such routine activities as riding a bicycle, we often worsen performance.

Clearly, the task of recalling such information as a long dissociated trauma involves episodic, declarative, or explicit memory. Ironically, hypnosis may involve selectively tapping the implicit memory domain (Spiegel et al., 1993). The involuntariness associated with hypnosis (Weitzenhoffer, 1981; Spiegel and Spiegel, 1987) is very much reminiscent of the automaticity of implicit or procedural memory. Typically, hypnotic tasks involve a subjective sense of automaticity: the instruction that your left hand will "float upward like a balloon" results in a feeling that the hand is moving upward "on its own," a sense of involuntariness (Hilgard, 1965; Spiegel and Spiegel, 1987). Often there is amnesia for such an instruction as well, so the subject experiences the post-hypnotic instruction as an acquired and automatic procedural memory, rather than a declarative one. Furthermore, hypnotized individuals apply little in the way of critical scrutiny to these memories which result in hypnotic compliance: they rationalize rather than question the basis for the often unusual performances (H. Spiegel, 1980; Hilgard, 1986). Thus the attempt to retrieve explicit information in hypnosis may tap a kind of uncritical and automatic retrieval process more typical of implicit memory. For implicit memories, their mere unfolding generally provides evidence of their correctness. That is, they work: you remain upright on the bicycle, you type efficiently, and so forth. This is not the case with explicit memories, which require evaluation: "Was I really there?" "Did he say that?" However, an implicit-like retrieval process could lead a subject to a falsely positive opinion of the quality of explicit information retrieved: it is there so it must be true. Indeed, long dissociated memories may seem more implicit than explicit—there and available but not readily accessible. By definition, we can act on the basis of implicit memory without having any conscious or explicit recollection of how those memories were acquired. We can ride a bicycle even if we cannot recall who taught us and how or where we learned. Thus we can seem to know something without knowing how we know it. Hypnosis may couch "explicit" information in an implicit context. Indeed, a leading theory of the mechanism of hypnotic amnesia is that such memories are decontextualized (Kihlstrom and Evans, 1979), thereby depriving them of networks of association which can enrich explicit recollection and facilitate critical judgment of them. Implicit memories are decontextualized as well: the content is mobilized devoid of its source or historical context (Schacter, 1987, 1992).

Social psychological theorists take the more behavioral orientation of viewing hypnotic amnesia as an output rather than a storage or retrieval problem—the memories are available but simply not reported (Spanos, 1986; Schuyler and Coe, 1989). These theorists emphasize input (social pressure) and output (performance) rather than the mediating psychological and brain processes and individual differences in them (Spiegel, 1986). They assume that it is important to individuals in such experiments to behave like a hypnotized person, and therefore subjective reports and behaviors are distorted in the direction of the task-motivated instruction. In amnesia research, they emphasize the fact that hypnotic amnesia can be breached (although not entirely: see Spanos, 1986; Schuyler and Coe, 1989). Indeed, for hypnotic amnesia to be such and not forgetting, it must be reversible, so the question is the mechanism of its reversibility rather than the possibility of doing so with social pressure instructions. These experiments are similar to crude suggestion, emphasizing strong expectation and minimizing discovery of inner experience—tell me or do not tell me what you remember, versus the hypnotic experience of suddenly discovering or being unable to retrieve recollections. The emphasis on the nature of the social instruction tends to divert useful attention from the subjective phenomenology of hypnotic amnesia. Yet there is substantial evidence that hypnosis may have specific and enhancing effects on memory retrieval (McConkey, 1992).

Conclusion

Hypnosis and suggestion may have important influences on the memory processes of encoding, storage and retrieval, shaping information perceived, the way in which it is stored, and how it is retrieved. Hypnosis is one useful technique for bridging amnesia, especially that resulting from traumatic experience. It may also be used to produce amnesia, and it may influence both the content and assessment of the accuracy of memory retrieval. Hypnosis is neither simply a solution nor a contaminant of memory processes, but rather an interesting if complicating factor in the understanding of memory, especially in relation to traumatic events.

References

American Psychiatric Association. 1994. *Diagnostic and Statistical Manual of Mental Disorders, Fourth Edition.* Washington, D.C.: American Psychiatric Press.

Bower, G. H. 1981. Mood and memory. *American Psychologist* 36(2):129–148.

Bremner, J. D., Southwick, S., Brett, E., Fontana, A., Rosenheck, R., and Charney, D. S. 1992. Dissociation and posttraumatic stress disorder in Vietnam combat veterans. *American Journal of Psychiatry* 149:328–332.

Cardena, E., and Spiegel, D. Dissociative reactions to the Bay Area earthquake. *American Journal of Psychiatry* 150(3):474–478.

Ceci, S. False beliefs: Some developmental and clinical considerations. Chapter 3, this volume.

Christianson, S. A., and Loftus, E. F. 1987. Memory for traumatic events. *Applied Cognitive Psychology* 1:225–239.

Chu, J., and Dill, D. 1990. Dissociative symptoms in relation to childhood physical and sexual abuse. *American Journal of Psychiatry* 147:887–892.

Coons, P. M. 1994. Confirmation of childhood abuse in child and adolescent cases of multiple personality disorder and dissociative disorder not otherwise specified. *Journal of Nervous and Mental Disease* 182:461–464.

Coons, P. M., and Milstein, V. 1986. Psychosexual disturbances in multiple personality: Characteristics, etiology, and treatment. *Journal of Clinical Psychiatry,* 47:106–110.

Crawford, H. J., and Allen, S. N. Enhanced visual memory during hypnosis as mediated by hypnotic responsiveness and cognitive strategies. *Journal of Experimental Psychology: General* 112:662–685.

Diamond, B. L. 1980. Inherent problems in the use of pretrial hypnosis on a prospective witness. *California Law Review* 68:313–349.

Dywan, S., and Bowers, K. S. 1983. The use of hypnosis to enhance recall. *Science* 222:184–185.

Erdelyi, M. H., and Kleinbard, J. 1978. Has Ebbinghaus decayed with time? The growth of recall (hypermnesia) over days. *Journal of Experimental Psychology: Human Learning and Memory* 4:275–289.

Evans, F. J., and Thorn, W. A. 1966. Two types of posthypnotic amnesia: Recall amnesia and source amnesia. *International Journal of Clinical and Experimental Hypnosis* 14:162–179.

Evans, F. J. 1988. Posthypnotic amnesia: Dissociation of context and content. In H. M. Pettinati (ed.) *Hypnosis and Memory.* New York: Guilford, pp. 157–192.

Evans, F. J., and Kihlstrom, J. F. 1973. Posthypnotic amnesia as disrupted retrieval. *Journal of Abnormal Psychology* 82:317–323.

Frankel, R. H. 1990. Hypnotizability and dissociation. *American Journal of Psychiatry* 147(7):823–829.

Frischholz, E. J., Spiegel, D., Trentalange, M. J., and Spiegel, H. 1987. The hypnotic induction profile and absorption. *American Journal of Clinical Hypnosis* 30:87–93.

Herman, J. L., Perry, J. C., and van der Kolk, B. A. 1990. Childhood trauma in borderline personality disorder. *American Journal of Psychiatry* 146:490–495.

Hilgard, E. R. 1986. *Divided Consciousness: Multiple Controls in Human Thought and Action* (rev. ed.). New York: Wiley.

Hilgard, E. R. 1991. Suggestibility and suggestions as related to hypnosis. In J. F. Schumaker (ed.) *Human Suggestibility: Advances in Theory, Research, and Application.* New York: Routledge, pp. 37–58.

Hilgard, E. R. 1965. *Hypnotic Susceptibility.* New York: Harcourt, Brace and World.

Hilgard, J. R. 1970. *Personality and Hypnosis: A Study of Imaginative Involvement.* Chicago: University of Chicago Press.

Holen, A. 1991. Unpublished data.

Horowitz, M. 1986. *Stress Response Syndromes.* Northvale, N.J.: Jason Aronson.

Kaszniak, A. W., Nussbaum, P. D., Berren, M. R., and Santiago, J. 1988. Amnesia as a consequence of male rape: A case report. *Journal of Abnormal Psychology* 97:100–104.

Kihlstrom, J. F., and Evans, F. J. 1979. Memory retrieval processes during posthypnotic amnesia. In J. F. Kihlstrom and F. J. Evans (eds.) *Functional Disorders of Memory.* Hillsdale, N.J.: Erlbaum.

Kihlstrom, J. F., Evans, F. J., Orne, E. C., and Orne, M. T. 1980. Attempting to breach posthypnotic amnesia. *Journal of Abnormal Psychology* 89:603–616.

Kihlstrom, J. R. 1980. Posthypnotic "amnesia" and "semantic" memory. *Cognitive Psychology* 12:227–251.

Kihlstrom, J. R. 1987. The cognitive unconscious. *Science* 237:1445–1452.

Klatzky, R. L., and Erdelyi, M. H. 1985. The response criterion problem in tests of hypnosis and memory. *International Journal of Clinical and Experimental Hypnosis* 33:246–257.

Kluft, R. P. 1984. Treatment of multiple personality disorder. *Psychiatric Clinics of North America* 7:9–29.

Kluft, R. P. 1985. Childhood multiple personality disorder: Predictors, clinical findings, and treatment results. In R. P. Kluft (ed.) *Childhood Antecedents of Multiple Personality Disorder.* Washington, D.C.: American Psychiatric Press, pp. 65–97.

Koopman, C., Classen, C., and Spiegel, D. 1994. Predictors of posttraumatic stress symptoms among survivors of the Oakland/Berkeley, Calif., firestorm. *American Journal of Psychiatry* 151:888–894.

Koopman, C., Classen, C., Cardena, E., and Spiegel, D. 1994. When disaster strikes, acute stress disorders may follow. *Journal of Traumatic Stress.*

Kroger, W. S., and Douce, R. G. 1979. Hypnosis in criminal investigation. *International Journal of Clinical and Experimental Hypnosis* 27:358–374.

Laurence, J. R., and Perry, C. 1983. Hypnotically created memory among highly hypnotizable subjects. *Science* 222:523–524.

Loewenstein, R. L. 1991. Dissociative amnesia and fugue. In A. Tasman and S. M.

Goldfinger (eds.) *American Psychiatric Press Review of Psychiatry, Volume 10.* Washington, D.C.: American Psychiatric Press.

Loewenstein, R. J. 1990. Somatoform disorders in victims of incest and child abuse. In R. P. Kluft (ed.) *Incest-Related Disorders of Adult Psychopathology.* Washington, D.C.: American Psychiatric Press, pp. 75–111.

Loewenstein, R. J. 1991. Psychogenic amnesia and psychogenic fugue: A comprehensive review. In A. Tasman and S. M. Goldfinger (eds.) *American Psychiatric Press Review of Psychiatry, Volume 10.* Washington, D.C.: American Psychiatric Press.

Loftus, E. F. 1993. The reality of repressed memories. *American Psychologist* 48:518–537.

Loftus, E. F., and Burns, T. E. 1982. Mental shock can produce retrograde amnesia. *Memory and Cognition* 10:318–323.

Loftus, E. F., and Loftus, G. R. 1980. On the permanence of stored information in the human brain. *American Psychologist* 35:409–420.

Loftus, E. F., Miller, D. G., and Burns, H. J. 1978. Semantic integration of verbal information into a visual memory. *Journal of Experimental Psychology: Human Learning and Memory* 4:19–31.

Loftus, E. F. 1979. *Eyewitness Testimony.* Cambridge, Mass.: Harvard University Press.

Loftus, E. F. 1975. Leading questions and the eyewitness report. *Cognitive Psychology* 7:560–572.

Lynn, S. J., Milano, M., and Weekes, J. R. 1991. Hypnosis and pseudomemories: The effects of prehypnotic expectancies. *Journal of Abnormal Psychology* 60:318–326.

Lynn, S. J., and Nash, M. R. 1994. Truth in memory: Ramifications for psychotherapy and hypnotherapy. *American Journal of Clinical Hypnosis* 36:194–208.

Lyon, L. S. 1985. Facilitating telephone number recall in a case of psychogenic amnesia. *Journal of Behavior Therapy and Experimental Psychiatry:* 16:147–149.

MacFarlane, A. C. 1986. Posttraumatic morbidity of a disaster: A study of cases presenting for psychiatric treatment. *Journal of Nervous and Mental Disease* 174:4–13.

Madakasira, S., and O'Brien, K. 1987. Acute posttraumatic stress disorder in victims of a natural disaster. *Journal of Nervous and Mental Disease* 175:286–290.

Marmar, C., Weiss, D., Schelenger, W., and Fairbank, J. October 1992. Peritraumatic dissociation and posttraumatic stress disorder. Presentation at the International Society of Traumatic Stress Studies.

McClelland, J. L., and Rumelhart, D. E. 1986. *Parallel Distributed Processing: Explorations in the Microstructure of Cognition, Vol. 1: Foundations; Vol. 2: Psychological and Biological Models.* Cambridge, Mass.: MIT Press.

McConkey, K. M., Lagbelle, L., Bibb, B. C., and Bryant, R. A. 1990. Hypnosis and suggested pseudomemory: The relevance of test context. *Australian Journal of Psychology* 42:197–206.

McConkey, K. M. 1992. The effects of hypnotic procedures on remembering. In E. Fromm and M. R. Nash (eds.) *Contemporary Hypnosis Research.* New York: Guilford, pp. 405–426.

McConkey, K. M., and Kinoshita, S. The influence of hypnosis on memory after one day and one week. *Journal of Abnormal Psychology* 97:48–53.

Mullen, P. E., Martin, J. L., Anderson, J. C., Romans, S. E., and Herbison, G. P. 1993. Childhood sexual abuse and mental health in adult life. *British Journal of Psychiatry* 163:721–732.

Nemiah, J. C. 1985. Dissociative disorders. In H. Kaplan and B. Sadock (eds.) *Comprehensive Textbook of Psychiatry, Fourth Edition*. Baltimore: Williams and Wilkins, pp. 942–957.

Nogrady, H., McConkey, K. M., and Perry, C. 1985. Enhancing visual memory: Trying hypnosis, trying imagination, and trying again. *Journal of Abnormal Psychology* 94:195–204.

Noyes, R., and Slyman, D. J. 1978–1979. The subjective response to life-threatening danger. *Omega* 9: 313–321.

Noyes, R., and Kletti, R. Depersonalization in response to life-threatening danger. *Comprehensive Psychiatry* 18:375–384.

Orne, M. T. 1959. The nature of hypnosis: artifact and essence. *Journal of Abnormal and Social Psychology* 58:277–299.

Orne, M. T., Axelrad, D., Diamond, B. L., Gravitz, M. A., Heller, A., Mutter, C. B., Spiegel, D., and Spiegel, H. 1987. Scientific status of refreshing recollection by the use of hypnosis. *Journal of Experimental Psychology [Learning, Memory and Cognition]* 13:501–518, 1987.

Piccione, C., Hilgard, E. R., and Zimbardo, P. G. 1989. On the degree of stability of measured hypnotizability over a 25-year period. *Journal of Personality and Social Psychology* 56:289–295.

Posner, M. L., and Peterson, S. E. 1990. The attention system of the human brain. *Annual Review of Neuroscience* 13:25–42.

Putnam, F. 1985. Dissociation as a response to extreme trauma. In R. P. Kluft (ed.) *Childhood Antecedents of Multiple Personality Disorder*. Washington, D.C.: American Psychiatric Press, pp. 65–97.

Putnam, F. W., Guroff, J. J., Silberman, E. K., Barban, L., and Post, R. M. 1986. The clinical phenomenology of multiple personality disorder: Review of 100 recent cases. *Journal of Clinical Psychiatry* 47:285–293.

Putnam, W. H. Hypnosis and distortion of eyewitness testimony. *International Journal of Clinical and Experimental Hypnosis* 28:37–448.

Register, P. A., and Kihlstrom, J. F. 1988. Hypnosis and interrogative suggestibility. *Personality and Individual Differences* 9:549–558.

Riether, A. M., and Stoudemire, A. 1988. Psychogenic fugue states: a review. *Southern Medical Journal* 81:568–571.

Rosch, E. 1977. Linguistic relativity. In *Thinking: Readings in Cognitive Science*. P. Johnson-Laird and O. Wason (eds.) New York: Cambridge University Press, pp. 501–522a.

Ross, C. A., Miller, S. D., Reagor, P., Bjornson, L., Fraser, G. A., and Anderson, G. 1990. Structured interview data on 102 cases of multiple personality disorder from four centers. *American Journal of Psychiatry* 147:596–601.

Sanders, G. S., and Simmons, W. L. 1983. Use of hypnosis to enhance eyewitness accuracy: Does it work? *Journal of Applied Psychology* 68:70–77.

Schacter, D. L. 1992. Understanding implicit memory: A cognitive neuroscience approach. *American Psychologist* 47:559–569.

Schacter, D. L. 1987. Implicit memory: History and current status. *Journal of Experimental Psychology [Learning, Memory and Cognition]* 13:501–518.

Schacter, D. L., and Kihlstrom, J. F. 1989. Functional amnesia. In F. Boller and J. Grafman (eds.) *Handbook of Neuropsychology, Volume 3*. Elsevier, pp. 209–231.

Schacter, D. L., Wang, P. L., Tulving, E., and Freedman, M. 1982. Functional retrograde amnesia: A quantitative case study. *Neuropsychologia* 20:523–532.

Scheflin, A. W. 1994. Forensic hypnosis: Unanswered questions. *Australian Journal of Clinical and Experimental Hypnosis* 22:23–34.

Schuyler, B. A., and Coe, W. C. 1989. More on volitional experiences and breaching posthypnotic amnesia. *International Journal of Clinical and Experimental Hypnosis* 37:320–331.

Sheehan, P. W., and Tilden, J. 1983. Effects of suggestibility and hypnosis on accurate and distorted retrieval from memory. *Journal of Experimental Psychology [Learning, Memory, Cognition]* 9:283–293.

Sheehan, P. W., Statham, D., and Jamieson, G. A. 1991. Pseudomemory effects and their relationship to level of susceptibility to hypnosis and state instruction. *Journal of Personality and Social Psychology* 60:130–137.

Shields, I. W., and Knox, V. J. 1986. Level of processing as a determinant of hypnotic hypermnesia. *Journal of Abnormal Psychology* 95:350–357.

Shimamura, A. P., and Squire, L. R. 1987. A neuropsychological study of fact memory and source amnesia. *Journal of Experimental Psychology: Learning, Memory and Cognition* 13:464–473.

Sloan, T. B. July 1988. Neurologic Monitoring. *Critical Care Clinics* 4(3):543–557.

Solomon, Z., Mikulincer, M., and Benbenishty, R. 1989. Combat stress reaction: Clinical manifestations and correlates. *Military Psychology* 1:35–47.

Spanos, N. P. 1986. Hypnotic behavior: A social-psychological interpretation of amnesia, analgesia, and "trance logic." *Behavioral and Brain Sciences* 9:449–502.

Spanos, N. P., Gwynn, M. I., Comer, S. L., and Terrade, K. 1989. Effects on mock jurors of experts favorable and unfavorable toward hypnotically elicited eyewitness testimony. *Journal of Applied Psychology* 74:922–926.

Spiegel, D. 1994. Hypnosis. In R. E. Hales, S. C. Yudofsy, and J. A. Talbott (eds.) *American Psychiatric Press Textbook of Psychiatry*. Washington, D.C.: American Psychiatric Press.

Spiegel, D. 1981. Vietnam grief work using hypnosis. *American Journal of Clinical Hypnosis* 24:33–40.

Spiegel, D. 1986. Dissociating damage. *American Journal of Clinical Hypnosis* 29:123–131.

Spiegel, D., and Spiegel, H. 1986. Hypnosis. In A. K. Hess and I. B. Weiner (eds.) *Handbook of Forensic Psychology*. New York: Wiley.

Spiegel, D. 1990. Hypnosis, dissociation, and trauma: Hidden and overt observers. In J. L. Singer (ed.) *Repression and Dissociation: Implications for Personality Theory, Psychopathology, and Health*. Chicago: University of Chicago Press.

Spiegel, D., and Cardena, E. 1990. New uses for hypnosis in the treatment of posttraumatic stress disorder. *Journal of Clinical Psychiatry* 51:10 (suppl.):39–43.

Spiegel, D., Hunt, T., and Dondershine, H. 1988. Dissociation and hypnotizability in post traumatic stress disorder. *American Journal of Psychiatry* 145:301–305.

Spiegel, D., and Cardena, E. 1991. Disintegrated experience: The dissociative disorders revisited. *Journal of Abnormal Psychology* 100:366–378.

Spiegel, D. 1991. Dissociation and trauma. In A. Tasman and S. M. Goldfinger (eds.)

American Psychiatric Press Review of Psychiatry, Volume 10. Washington, D.C.: American Psychiatric Press.

Spiegel, D. 1984. Multiple personality as a post-traumatic stress disorder. *Psychiatric Clinics of North America* 7:101–110.

Spiegel, D., Frischholz, E. J., and Spira, J. 1993. Functional disorders of memory. In A. Tasman, M. B. Riba, and J. M. Oldham (eds.) *American Psychiatric Press Review of Psychiatry, Volume 12.* Washington, D.C.: American Psychiatric Press.

Spiegel, H. 1974. The grade 5 syndrome: The highly hypnotizable person. *International Journal of Clinical and Experimental Hypnosis* 22:303–319.

Spiegel, H. 1980. Hypnosis and evidence: Help or hindrance? *Annals of the New York Academy of Sciences* 47:73–85.

Spiegel, H. 1963. Current perspectives on hypnosis in obstetrics. *Acta Psychotherapeutica, Psychosomatica et Orthopaedagogica.* 2:412–429.

Spiegel, H., and Spiegel, D. 1978/1987. Trance and treatment: Clinical uses of hypnosis. New York: Basic Books. Reprinted by American Psychiatric Press, Washington, D.C.

Squire, L. R., and Zola-Morgan, S. 1991. The medial temporal lobe memory system. *Science* 253:1380–1386.

Squire, L. R., and Cohen, N. J. 1984. Human memory and amnesia. In N. M. Weinberger, J. L. McGaugh, and G. Lynch (eds.) *Neurobiology of Learning and Memory.* New York: Guilford, pp. 3–64.

Stager, G. L., and Lundy, R. M. 1985. Hypnosis and the learning and recall of visually presented material. *International Journal of Clinical and Experimental Hypnosis* 33:27–39.

Stevenson, I. 1994. A case of the psychotherapist's fallacy: Hypnotic regression to "previous lives." *American Journal of Clinical Hypnosis* 36:188–193.

Stutman, R. K., and Bliss, E. L. June 1985. Posttraumatic stress disorder, hypnotizability, and imagery. *American Journal of Psychiatry* 142(6):741–743.

Tellegen, A., and Atkinson, G. 1974. Openness to absorbing and self-altering experiences ("absorption"), a trait related to hypnotic susceptibility. *Journal of Abnormal Psychology* 83:268–277.

Tellegen, A. 1981. Practicing the two disciplines for relaxation and enlightenment: Comment on "Role of the feedback signal in electromyograph biofeedback: The relevance of attention" by Qualls and Sheehan. *Journal of Experimental Psychology General* 110(2):217–231.

Terr, L. C. January 1991. Childhood traumas: An outline and overview. *American Journal of Psychiatry* 148(1): 10–20.

Timm, H. W. 1981. The effect of forensic hypnosis techniques on eyewitness recall and recognition. *Journal of Police Science and Administration* 9:188–194.

Toland, K., Hoffman, H., and Loftus, E. 1991. How suggestion plays tricks with memory. In J. F. Schumaker (ed.) *Human Suggestibility: Advances in Theory, Research, and Application.* New York: Routledge, pp. 235–252.

Tulving, E., and Pearlstone, Z. 1966. Availability vs. accessibility of information in memory for words. *Journal of Verbal Learning and Verbal Behavior* 5:381–391.

Tulving, E. 1983. *Elements of Episodic Memory.* Oxford: Clarendon Press.

Wagstaff, G. F. 1984. The enhancement of witness memory by 'hypnosis': A review and methodological critique of the experimental literature. *British Journal of Experimental and Clinical Hypnosis* 2:3–12.

Weitzenhoffer, A. M. 1989. *The Practice of Hypnotism: Volume 1: Traditional and Semi-traditional Techniques and Phenomenology.* New York: Wiley.

Weitzenhoffer, A. M. 1980. Hypnotic susceptibility revisited. *American Journal of Clinical Hypnosis* 22:130–146.

Wilkinson, C. B. 1983. Aftermath of a disaster: The collapse of the Hyatt Regency Hotel skywalks. *American Journal of Psychiatry* 140:1134–1139.

Yullie, J. C., and Kim, C. K. 1987. A field study of the forensic use of hypnosis. *Canadian Journal of Behavioural Science* 19:41429.

Zelig, M., and Beidleman, W. B. The investigative use of hypnosis: A word of caution. *International Journal of Clinical and Experimental Hypnosis* 29:401–412.

Post Traumatic Stress Disorder: Psychobiological Mechanisms of Traumatic Remembrance

5

John H. Krystal
Steven M. Southwick
Dennis S. Charney

The most predominant feature of Post Traumatic Stress Disorder (PTSD) is that the memories of traumatic experiences remain indelible for decades and are easily reawakened by all sorts of stimuli and stressors. Despite this fact, there has been relatively little research on the accuracy of traumatic memories in patients with PTSD. In this chapter, we attempt to synthesize the findings from preclinical investigations of learning and memory processes and the neurochemical effects of stress with clinical studies of PTSD to develop a set of hypotheses related to the role of traumatic remembrance in the pathogenesis and treatment of PTSD. In this context, we will discuss the possible mechanisms underlying memory distortion that occurs in PTSD patients.

Neural Mechanisms of Learning and Memory: Relevance to the Reexperiencing Symptoms of PTSD
Fear Conditioning

In many patients with Post Traumatic Stress Disorder, vivid memories of a traumatic event, autonomic arousal, and even flashbacks can be elicited by diverse sensory and cognitive stimuli that have been associated with the original trauma (Litz and Keane, 1989; McNally et al., 1987). Consequently, patients begin to avoid these stimuli in their everyday life, or a numbing of general emotional responsiveness occurs. Modality specific and contextual fear conditioning, which is easily demonstrated in the laboratory, may explain some of these observations. Animals exposed to an emotionally neutral, visual or auditory conditioned stimulus (CS) in conjunction with an aversive unconditioned stimulus (UCS) will subsequently exhibit a conditioned emotional response (CER) to the CS in the absence of the UCS. CERs are also produced when an animal is placed in an environment in which an aversive UCS has previously been experienced. In this circumstance the CERs are not elicited by a modality specific stimulus that was paired with a UCS, but instead by complex, polymodal contextual stimuli that were present in the environment when the UCS originally occurred and are present upon reexposure to the environment (Phillips and LeDoux, 1992). CERs can last for years in laboratory animals (Hoffman et al., 1966) and are used to infer that a state of fear has been produced (Davis, 1990). Therefore, a neural analysis of fear conditioning in animals may be useful in identifying the neurochemicals and brain structures involved in the learning and remembering associations of stimuli with traumatic events, which may form the basis of many of the symptoms associated with PTSD.

Fear conditioning to sensory modality specific stimuli (i.e., auditory, visual) can be mediated by subcortical mechanisms, involving sensory pathways which project to the thalamus and amygdala and modality specific sensory processing areas of the cortex (LeDoux et al., 1990). It has been suggested that emotional memories established via thalamo-amygdala pathways may be relatively indelible (LeDoux et al., 1989).

Contextual fear conditioning, which involves more complex stimuli from multiple sensory modalities, may require projections to the amygdala from higher-order cortical areas that integrate inputs from many sources and the hippocampus (Kim and Fanselow, 1992; Phillips and LeDoux, 1992). It is noteworthy that lesions of the hippocampus one day after fear conditioning abolish contextual fear. Lesions seven days or longer after fear conditioning have no effect. These findings suggest that the hippocampus may have a time-limited role in associative fear memories evoked by contextual sensory (polymodal), but not unimodal sensory stimuli (Kim and Fanselow, 1992). Contextual fear conditioning appears to require exposure to more aversive UCS than modality specific fear conditioning. Apparently, as the intensity of the UCS increases, the organism becomes more sensitive to a wider range of stimulus factors in the environment.

Several behavioral paradigms indicate an important role for noradrenergic neuronal systems in the processes involved in fear conditioning. Neutral stimuli paired with shock produce increases in brain norepinephrine metabolism and behavioral deficits similar to that elicited by the shock (Cassens et al., 1981; Tanaka et al., 1986). In the freely moving cat, the firing rate of cells in the locus ceruleus can be increased by presenting a neutral acoustic stimulus previously paired with an air puff to the whiskers, which also increases firing and is aversive to the cat (Rasmussen et al., 1986). There is also a body of evidence indicating that an intact noradrenergic system may be necessary for the acquisition of fear-conditioned responses (Tsaltas et al., 1987; Cole and Robbins, 1987).

These preclinical investigations are consistent with clinical studies of the pathophysiology of PTSD which have identified a relationship between severe stress exposure and conditioned physiologic and emotional responses. Since the early 1980s, a series of well-designed psychophysiologic studies have been conducted that have further documented heightened autonomic or sympathetic nervous system arousal in combat veterans with chronic PTSD. Combat veterans with PTSD have been shown to have higher resting mean heart rate and systolic blood pressure, as well as greater increases in heart rate, when exposed to visual and auditory combat-related stimuli compared with combat veterans without PTSD, patients with generalized anxiety disorder, or healthy subjects (Blanchard et al., 1982, 1986; Malloy et al., 1983; Orr, 1990; Pallmeyer et al., 1986; Pitman et al., 1987). Furthermore, several psychophysiologic studies have found hyperactive responses to combat-associated stimuli but not to other stressful non-combat-related stimuli (McFall et al., 1990). Because central noradrenergic (LC) and peripheral sympathetic systems may function in concert (Aston-Jones et al., 1991), these data are also consistent with the hypothesis that noradrenergic hyperactivity in patients with PTSD may be associated with the conditioned or sensitized responses to specific traumatic stimuli (Southwick et al., 1993). Studies evaluating the efficacy of psychotherapeutic techniques emphasizing desensitization to reduce hyperarousal responses to stimuli associated with the psychological trauma represent a current focus of investigation (Boudewyns and Hyer, 1990; Keane et al., 1989).

A Possible Failure of Extinction in PTSD

It is possible that the continued ability of conditioned stimuli to elicit traumatic memories and flashbacks in PTSD stems from a deficit in the neural mechanisms involved in response reduction or extinction. Experimental extinction is defined as a loss of previously learned conditioned emotional response following repeated presentations of a conditioned fear stimulus in the absence of a contiguous traumatic event. Extinction has been explained in terms of either an "erasure" of the original associations that led to the production of the conditioned response or the acquisition of new associations that compete with or "mask" the expression of the still intact, response-producing associations. The "erasure" hypothesis predicts that following non-reinforcement, the response-producing associations no longer exist and, therefore, the conditioned response would no longer be present. The "masking" hypothesis predicts that the response-producing associations remain after non-reinforcement, and, therefore, if it were possible to temporarily remove the masking associations, the conditioned response could be elicited.

Several lines of evidence suggest that the original associations are intact following extinction. Expression of extinction may be specific to the stimulus context in which non-reinforcement occurred (Bouton and Bolles, 1985; Bouton and King 1983, 1986). Re-presentation of the conditioned stimulus even up to one year after extinction is sufficient for reinstating extinguished responding to a pre-extinction level (Bouton and Bolles, 1979; McAllister and McAllister, 1988; Pavlov, 1927; Rescola and Heth, 1975). These data indicate the essentially permanent nature of conditioned fear and the apparent fragility of extinction. This phenomenon may help to explain the common clinical observation that traumatic memories may remain dormant for many years, only to be elicited by a subsequent stressor or unexpectedly by a stimulus long ago associated with the original trauma (Solomen et al., 1987; VanDyke et al., 1985).

These studies indicate that extinction does not erase the original aversive memory, but instead involves the learning of a new memory which masks or inhibits the original one. It is important to emphasize, however, that although extinction can be overcome, in normal animals extinction does result in a reduction of the conditioned fear response. Using traditional measures of conditioned fear such as freezing, potentiated startle, or autonomic indices, non-reinforcement leads to a reduction in all these measures. In healthy humans, many childhood fears become extinguished and do not intrude daily in adulthood. In contrast, patients with PTSD describe persistent traumatic memories that do not extinguish. Thus, it is conceivable that PTSD patients have deficits in brain systems that mediate extinction.

The amygdala is not only involved in the acquisition and expression of conditioned fear responses, but may also be necessary for extinction. NMDA antagonists infused into the amygdala prevent the extinction of fear potentiated startle (Falls et al., 1990). Thus, activity in the amygdala during non-reinforced stimuli presentations may be essential for extinction of conditioned fear stimuli. This may result from processes within the amygdala itself, or via structures which project to the amygdala (e.g., hippocampus, prefrontal cortex, septal area) and have been implicated in extinction in several experimental paradigms. Extinction of conditioned fear responses may represent an active suppression by the cortex of subcortical neural circuits (thalamus, amygdala) that maintain learned associations over long time periods (Teich et al., 1989).

Behavioral Sensitization and Stress Sensitivity in PTSD

Sensitization generally refers to the increase in behavioral or physiological responsiveness that occurs following repeated exposure to a stimulus. Behavioral sensitization can be generally context-dependent or conditioned, such that animals will not demonstrate sensitization if the stimulus is presented in a different environment (Post, 1992). However, if the intensity of the stimulus or drug dose is high enough, behavioral sensitization will occur even if the environment is changed. It has been suggested that different mechanisms are called into play with environment-independent sensitization (Weiss et al., 1989).

The neurochemical and neuroanatomical systems mediating environment-dependent and environment-independent behavioral sensitization have begun to be investigated. The mechanisms of the development and maintenance of stress-induced sensitization in mammals have been most extensively studied in catecholaminergic systems.

Single or repeated exposure to a stressor potentiates the capacity of a subsequent stressor to increase dopamine function in the forebrain (Caggiula et al., 1989; Kalivas and Duffy, 1989) without apparently altering basal dopamine turnover (Criswell et al., 1990; Kalivas et al., 1990, 1992). Recently, it has been shown that the conditioned component of sensitization is related to increased dopamine release in the nucleus accumbens (Fontana et al., in press). Behavioral sensitization to stress may also involve alterations in noradrenergic function. Animals previously exposed to a stressor exhibit increased norepinephrine release in the hippocampus (Nisenbaum et al., 1991), hypothalamus (Nisenbaum et al., 1991), and prefrontal cortex (Finlay and Abercrombie, 1991), upon stressor reexposure.

Dopamine D_2 receptor antagonists block the development, but not the maintenance, of sensitization. Conversely, alpha$_2$ receptor agonists, and benzodiazepine agonists, block the maintenance, but not the development, of sensitization (Weiss et al., 1989). In addition, lesions of the amygdala or the nucleus accumbens block the development of cocaine-induced behavioral sensitization. In contrast, lesions of the hippocampus and frontal cortex have no effect (S. R. B. Weiss, Part A, unpublished observations).

There is recent evidence that both the environment-dependent and independent forms of sensitization may be associated with changes in gene expression. Immediate early genes (such as c-fos) act as transcription factors influencing the expression of intermediate substances or late effector genes which could modulate neurotransmitter or peptide receptors in a long-lasting fashion. Conditioned increases in c-fos have been shown to occur (Campean et al., 1991; Smith et al., 1992).

The characteristics of behavioral sensitization suggest that it may be involved in the signs and symptoms of PTSD. In traumatized humans, the magnitude of combat exposure is positively correlated with the development of PTSD (Kulka et al., 1990; Southwick et al., 1993) and prior exposure to childhood trauma. Trauma that is repetitive in nature increases the likelihood of developing PTSD. A study of Israeli combat soldiers who fought in two successive wars reported that soldiers were more likely to develop symptoms during the second war if they had suffered acute combat stress during the first war (Solomen et al., 1987). Further, for many patients the PTSD symptoms do not diminish over time but instead increase in magnitude. In a study of World War II veterans twenty years after the war, Archibald and Tuddenham (1962) reported an increase in symptoms among patients with PTSD with the passage of time.

Altered Memory Functions in PTSD
Dissociation

Dissociative states are an integral component of the response to psychological trauma. The term "dissociation" has been employed to describe a spectrum of subjective states in which perceptual, affective, memory, and identity functions are altered. Particular symptoms associated with dissociative states include distorted sensory perceptions, altered time perception, amnesia, analgesia, derealization, depersonalization, conversion symptoms, fugue states, and multiple personality (Bremner et al., 1992; Freud and Breuer, 1953; Hilgard, 1977; Mayer-Gross, 1935; Spiegel and Cardena, 1991). Dissociation occurs in the context of both civilian and combat-related traumatization (Bremner et al., 1992, 1993; Carlson and Rosser-Hogan, 1991; Fisher, 1945; Janet, 1889; Krystal, 1968, 1988; Spiegel and Cardena, 1991).

Dissociative symptoms and increased hypnotizability also occur as sequelae of adult psychological traumatization (Bernstein and Putnam, 1986; Bremner et al., 1992, 1993; Lowenstein and Putnam, 1988; Spiegel et al., 1988). For example, while recalling their traumatic experiences, individuals may experience time as being slowed, have altered sensory perceptions, and have feelings of unreality (Bremner et al., in review). Less frequently, adult traumatization may produce fugue states, conversion reactions, or multiple personality (Grinker and Spiegel, 1945; McDougle and Southwick, 1990). Childhood psychological traumatization is also associated with dissociative symptoms. In one study, approximately 60% of 450 adults traumatized as children had periods in their lives when they had no memory of their abuse (Briere and Conte, 1993). Dissociative symptoms arising from childhood traumatization continue in adulthood (Hermann et al., 1989; Putnam et al., 1986). For example, psychiatric inpatients with histories of childhood trauma have higher levels of dissociative symptoms than non-traumatized inpatients (Chu et al., 1992).

One common symptom, the flashback, links dissociative and memory-related symptoms of PTSD. During flashbacks, patients vividly reexperience aspects of the traumatic response while feeling detached from their surrounding environment. Ongoing sensory processing may be altered or disrupted, and patients may report that they are "in a fog" or "blacked out" (Bremner et al., 1993). Flashbacks involving the recollection of traumatic experiences are frequently associated with intense emotional responses and panic-like states (Mellman and Davis, 1985). Flashbacks may be brief, lasting only a few minutes, or much longer in duration, lasting from hours to days. While some flashbacks are accurate depictions of a traumatic situation, others have unreal or distorted qualities, similar to dreams. Out-of-body experiences are one type of perspective distortion frequently associated with dissociative states (Rainey et al., 1987; Spiegel and Cardena, 1991).

Dissociative states are comprised of a heterogeneous spectrum of behavioral states involving multiple brain mechanisms. They are associated with alterations in sensory processing and attention, emotional functions, self-monitoring and identity functions, and learning and memory disturbances. Thus, networks within the brain that mediate these functions are involved by implication. Little research has been conducted to identify brain mechanisms associated with dissociative states. Neural circuits involving the thalamus, amygdala, and several cortical areas have been hypothesized (Krystal et al., in press).

Recent clinical studies have suggested the involvement of noradrenergic systems in dissociative symptomatology. Yohimbine, a drug that activates central noradrenergic neurons through blockade of alpha$_2$ receptors located on noradrenergic neurons, produced flashbacks and panic attacks in 40% and 70% of PTSD patients, respectively (Southwick et al., 1993). No panic attacks or flashbacks emerged following placebo administration. Although 45% of the patients in this study also met DSM-III-R criteria for panic disorder, 43% of the yohimbine-induced panic attacks occurred in individuals without panic disorder. However, the risk of a yohimbine-induced panic attack was increased in patients with panic disorder relative to those without comorbid panic disorder (89% versus 43%). A history of panic disorder did not appear to influence the likelihood of experiencing a yohimbine-induced flashback.

Patients experienced varying degrees of derealization and depersonalization that were often accompanied by other dissociative symptoms. Yohimbine elicited a range of altered perceptual experiences, some of which were fragmentary or vague. For example, one patient perceived the shadow produced by a sink in the testing facility to be the shadow made by a tank turret. In addition to stimulating flashbacks, yohimbine significantly increased the recall of traumatic memories. Some patients vividly recalled combat during yohimbine administration, but did not reexperience the actual traumatic events in the form of sensory experiences.

Declarative Memory Function in PTSD

Declarative memory for material unrelated to the trauma appears to be impaired in PTSD patients, whereas recall of trauma-related material is relatively enhanced. Memory and concentration impairments have been reported in Nazi concentration camp survivors (Thygesen et al., 1970) and in prisoners of war from World War II and the Korean War (Goldstein et al., 1987; Sutker et al., 1991). Also, combat veterans from the Vietnam War with chronic PTSD exhibited immediate and delayed recall impairments on the Wechsler Adult Intelligence Scale (WAIS) and the Buschke Selective Reminding Task (Bremner et al., 1993). Zeitlin and McNally (1991) found that veterans with combat-related PTSD performed worse than veterans without PTSD in learning lists of words unrelated to their traumas. However, PTSD patients exhibited a relative facilitation of recall, compared to the non-traumatized veterans, when words were combat-related. Factors involved in post-traumatic learning impairments might include altered allocation of attention, functional alterations in monoamine and neuroendocrine systems that modulate memory function (Krystal et al., 1989), and possible long-term neurotoxic effects of severe stress on neurons within the hippocampus implicated in the encoding of memory (Sapolsky, 1992). It is noteworthy that declarative memory impairments in PTSD patients have been identified in groups with significant exposure to drugs or abuse, such as the combat veterans with chronic PTSD, or groups who survived nutritional deprivation and physical torture, such as the concentration camp survivors or prisoners of war. Future studies will be needed to determine whether declarative memory deficits in PTSD patients are found in groups without other potential medical causes of memory impairment.

Encoding of Traumatic Memories in PTSD

Traumatization appears to alter patterns of memory encoding, leading to the formation of memories with reduced contextual information. Extreme environmental stimulation has been assumed to affect the ability to process and synthesize information by overloading cognitive capacity and attention resources (Easterbrook, 1959). Accumulated research suggests that the impact of stress upon memory formation may depend upon the features of the stressful environment and their relationship to the information to be recalled (Christianson, 1992). Stress enhances the recall of salient stimuli in the environment, but impairs recall of peripheral details (Brown and Kulik, 1977; Burke et al., 1992; Christianson, 1984, 1992; Wagenaar and Groeneweg, 1990; Yuille and Cutshall, 1986). This recall bias is not explained by increased novelty or complexity of traumatic situations (Christianson and Loftus, 1991).

Stress and dissociative states may also alter the predominant mode of memory encoding. For example, memories may be encoded using detail-focused strategies in which components of a memory are encoded and rehearsed separately or holistic strategies where memories are stored and rehearsed as composite images, essentially "snapshots" (Crawford and Allen, 1983). Under usual conditions, detail strategies predominate over holistic strategies. However, during hypnosis, highly hypnotizable individuals tend to utilize holistic rather than detail-focused encoding strategies (Crawford and Allen, 1983). The photographic or cinematographic nature of traumatic memories may suggest that shifts between detail and holistic strategies occur during encoding and rehearsal of traumatic memories. Further, declarative memories may be encoded in verbal, pictorial, and other forms. Encoding in these domains appears to take place concurrently and to be regulated similarly under most conditions (Paivio, 1971; Heil et al., 1994). However, it is possible that during traumatization, there is a shift away from verbal encoding toward encoding in emotional, pictorial, auditory, and other sensory-based memory systems. This shift would help to explain the common experience that verbal descriptions fail to convey an accurate representation of the magnitude of the horror and distress of traumatic experience and the post-traumatic development of alexithymia (Krystal, 1988).

Dissociative states at the time of the trauma may also result in the encoding of bizarre or distorted traumatic memories that reflect altered perceptual states occurring at the time that traumatic memories were formed. For example, one veteran in the yohimbine study (Southwick et al., 1993) had vivid recollections of a "Cheshire cat-like grin" of a dead combat victim, although other features of this victim's face could not be recalled. Alteration in other sensory domains also appears evident in traumatic memories (van der Kolk and Ducey, 1989). Similarly, critical features of the traumatic context may be disturbed, such as the capacity to place events in time (Terr, 1983) and space (Pynoos et al., 1987).

Beyond the selectivity of the information that is encoded at the time of the trauma, repetitive rehearsal of traumatic memories can alter the meaning (Kardiner, 1941) or the content of encoded memories (Craik and Jacoby, 1979; Pynoos et al., 1987). Upon reviewing stress-related memories, individuals think about emotional events in more personalized and concrete ways relative to neutral events (Heuer and Reisberg, 1990). The focus on central details at the expense of contextual information present in the initial encoding process becomes even more pronounced in rehearsal of traumatic memories (Christianson, 1992). These distortions in memory introduced during traumatic memory rehearsal may help to explain why people in a stressful situation show good recall of the central event, but confabulate about motives and reactions of participants in the event (Christianson, 1992).

Traumatic learning cannot entirely be explained by the mechanisms of declarative memory. This point is highlighted by a case in which PTSD developed in the absence of declarative memories of the traumatic event (MacMillan, 1991). This case involved a patient who developed PTSD following a motor vehicle accident associated with a three-day loss of consciousness. Although this patient's traumatic brain injury resulted in a permanent loss of conscious recall of the accident, she suffered from frequent, intrusive thoughts about a friend killed in the accident and avoided reminders of the hospital, a rehabilitation center, the grave of her friend, and a second friend disabled in the accident. She showed increased autonomic symptoms, fear of driving, and a feeling that her career potential was foreshortened. Thus, total disruption of encoding of declarative information did not preclude development of PTSD symptoms, suggesting that traumatic learning was independently encoded by non-declarative mechanisms.

In studies of non-declarative memory function, PTSD patients showed trauma-related alterations in priming and conditioning. In order to study priming, individuals were presented with incomplete words (word stems) that were completed by research subjects. Combat veterans with PTSD, but not those without PTSD, showed a bias in favor of completing combat-related words (Zeitlin and McNally, 1991). This bias was greater for words that they had previously seen compared to completely novel words, suggesting that PTSD patients had an implicit memory facilitation rather than a pure response bias. Since priming generally occurs outside of awareness, this study provided an example of unconscious mechanisms that promoted the recall of traumatic memories in PTSD patients.

Neurobiological studies suggest that the strength of traumatic memories relates, in part, to the degree to which certain neuromodulatory systems are activated by the traumatic experience (McGaugh, 1989, 1990; Pitman, 1989). Evidence from experimental and clinical investigations suggests that memory processes remain susceptible to modulating influences after information has been acquired (Squire, 1986). Locus ceruleus activation by electrical stimulation or alpha$_2$ adrenergic receptor antagonists enhance memory retrieval (Devanges and Sara, 1991; Sara and Devanges, 1989). The memory-enhancing effects of increased noradrenergic activity may be mediated by beta-noradrenergic receptors within the amygdaloid complex (McGaugh, 1989, 109; Devanges and Sara, 1991). Thus, some of the acute neurobiologic responses to trauma may facilitate the encoding of traumatic memories (van der Kolk et al., 1985).

Factors Related to Traumatic Memory Recall

The previous section suggested that traumatization alters the nature of the material which is encoded into declarative and non-declarative memory at the time of the trauma. Further, associative learning might result in the creation of conditioned emotional states. However, a vulnerability toward the involuntary recall of traumatic memories could occur at levels of information processing that are more fundamental than emotional processing or memory retrieval.

Recent research suggests that traumatized individuals preferentially process trauma-related cues and are more distracted by these cues than non-traumatized people. Patients with PTSD appear to have enhanced ability to identify trauma-related words from lists presented binaurally (see Litz and

Keane, 1989). Also, individuals with both rape-related (Foa et al., 1991) and combat-related (McNally et al., 1990) traumas are more easily distracted by trauma-associated words than by other emotionally charged, positively balanced, or neutral words on modified versions of the Stroop task. The heightened distractibility of PTSD patients to trauma reminders may have a physiological parallel in impairments in pre-pulse inhibition of the startle response (C. A. Morgan, C. Grillon, D. Charney, unpublished data). The attention bias toward detection and processing of trauma-related environmental sites in PTSD patients may promote retrieval of traumatic memories through associative mechanisms (Tulving and Thomson, 1973; Craik and Tulving, 1975).

Traumatic memories may intrude into awareness through state- and cue-dependent mechanisms even when they cannot be voluntarily recalled. Traumatic memory retrieval appears to be promoted by environmental cues associated with the trauma (Kline and Rausch, 1985). Also, internal cues, such as emotional state, may provoke retrieval of traumatic memories (Horowitz, 1975). Traumatized individuals who are not troubled by recollections of their trauma when euthymic appear to more readily recall aspects of their trauma when distressed (Krystal, 1968; Solomen et al., 1987). Further, yohimbine and MCPP stimulate autonomic arousal, fear states, and the recall of traumatic memories independent of environmental cues associated with the trauma (Southwick et al., 1991, 1993). Internal or external cues may promote traumatic memory recall in the absence of awareness of these cues (McGee, 1984).

Inaccessibility of traumatic memories may also be state-dependent and may be associated with emotional numbing in PTSD patients. Traumatization produces a suppression of emotional responsivity in many individuals that is reported as emotional numbness, feeling machine-like, and feeling apathetic (Litz, 1992). Reduced emotional responsivity in PTSD patients has been documented in both cognitive and electrophysiological spheres of function. Inpatients with PTSD exhibit a reduction in the expression of affect words in describing emotion-laden situations (Krystal et al., 1986). Similarly, using the Rorschach test, van der Kolk and Ducey (1989) found that, while emotionally numbed, combat veterans with PTSD provided concrete interpretations with a paucity of emotional detail. In contrast, when patients were highly stimulated by Rorschach cards, trauma-related interpretations appeared associated with intense, primitive, and disorganized emotion-laden responses interpreted as "undigested, unsymbolized reliving of traumatic experience." Electrophysiological studies also support the view that many PTSD patients tonically suppress reactivity. Paige and colleagues (1990) found that PTSD patients were in a state of "protective inhibition" of sensory processing relative to healthy subjects on the basis of a study of P200 event-related potentials.

Interpreted together, these findings suggest that when euthymic, patients with PTSD suppress arousal and cognitive associations related to the trauma. Thus, recall impairments in PTSD may arise, in part, from a process that suppresses the retrieval of autobiographical memories. Retrieval disruption has been previously documented in association with hypnosis and may contribute to the inability to recall experiences associated with PTSD (Geiselman et al., 1983; Kihlstrom, 1983). Retrieval impairments may be overcome through associative processes within declarative memory (Tulving and Thomson, 1973) or by inducing trauma-related mood states (Bower, 1981; Lang, 1977; Weingartner et al., 1977). Once trauma-related material intrudes upon consciousness, intense emotions, associations to the trauma, and vivid reexperiencing of the trauma may occur. This relatively dichotomous shift between suppression and reexperiencing has been characterized as the "all-or-none" response pattern in individuals with PTSD (van der Kolk and Ducey, 1989). Aspects of the shifts between suppression and reexperiencing appear to be beyond conscious modulation (Litz and Keane, 1989). However, the common observation that individuals with PTSD actively avoid situations in which they might be exposed to reminders of the trauma suggests that voluntary factors also play a modulatory role.

Assessment and Treatment of PTSD-Related Memory Disturbances

Treatments for dissociative states and traumatic memories cannot delete traumatic memories from the mental record of the victim/survivor. Traumatic experiences are frequently focal experiences shaping the identity of traumatized individuals. Despite their associated distress, traumatic memories guide some traumatized individuals to constructive action, such as working to prevent genocide. Yet patients are frequently concerned that treatment will erase memories. Perhaps some of this concern reflects the degree to which traumatic memories are inaccessible to voluntary recall, so that memories are experienced as either intrusive or nonexistent. Reasonable therapeutic goals include reducing the frequency and severity of dissociative states, enhancing control over the recall of traumatic memories, and reducing distress associated with memory retrieval.

Dissociative phenomena, traumatic memories, and affective regulation are highly interrelated phenomena in PTSD patients. As reviewed earlier, traumatic memories and intense emotions may trigger dissociative phenomena in these patients. Similarly, dissociative states and particular emotional states make the recall of traumatic memories more accessible. Completing the triangle, traumatic memories and dissociative phenomena may precipitate strong emotional responses. Thus, reducing the incidence of flashbacks and the intrusiveness and distress related to traumatic memories must be understood in the context of treating each of the three interactive processes.

The first step in treating dissociative states in traumatized individuals is to alleviate the marked depersonalization, derealization, and extreme emotional arousal. On the World War II battlefield, some psychiatrists employed a technique called narcotherapy, where barbiturates were employed to produce a sustained sleep state for up to three days (Bartemeier et al., 1946). This approach is consistent with, but more extreme than, the current use of benzodiazepines to reduce dissociation (Kluft, 1987). The long-term benefits of acute use of antianxiety drugs are currently unclear. However, Kardiner (1941) emphasized the importance of the peri-traumatic period in creating a long-lasting appraisal of traumatic events. Antianxiety drugs may be helpful in reducing negatively balanced cognitive distortions. In the context of supportive therapy, benzodiazepine treatment may facilitate the development of a more adaptive appraisal of the traumatic stress. This might alter the pairing of emotions and memories and facilitate processing of the traumatic event by reducing dissociative states.

Once hyperarousal symptoms are controlled, a second challenge faced by clinicians is to reduce amnesia for traumatic events. Almost every psychotherapeutic strategy involved in treating acute psychological trauma has, as a goal, the integration of the traumatic experience within the conscious life of patients (Freud and Breuer, 1953; Horowitz, 1976; Krystal, 1988). This task is quite difficult if the patient is amnestic for the trauma. Several guided recollection strategies have been employed to facilitate patients' access to traumatic memories, including relaxation training, free association, dream interpretation, hypnosis, and narcosynthesis (Bartemeier et al., 1946; Grinker and Spiegel, 1943; Krystal, 1988; Keane et al., 1989). Each of these processes takes advantage of an altered state of consciousness associated with increased suggestibility in which there is a reduction in functions usually associated with the frontal cortex, such as reflection, self-monitoring, and editing of thought (Stuss, 1992). A potential risk associated with conducting guided recollection in such a state is that ideas introduced by the clinician may be more readily incorporated into the memories of the patient. In such cases, the patient may not be able to distinguish real memories from those created by the therapist, as may occur under hypnosis (Laurence and Perry, 1983). This concern is particularly relevant to techniques in which the therapist recreates the roles of people within the patient's traumatic memory in order to facilitate memory retrieval (Grinker and Spiegel, 1943, 1945). The use of pharmacologic agents such as amytal may produce drug-induced amnesia (Ghoneim et al., 1984). Because patients may not fully recall information produced during barbiturate narcosynthesis at later times (Grinker, 1944), narcosynthesis may best be viewed as an information-gathering procedure.

Once an individual has access to memories of the trauma, what can the clinician do to help the patient? Freud and Breuer (1953) initially suggested two strategies for reducing dissociative or conversion symptoms associated with hysteria, abreaction and the formation of new associations to the traumatic memories. By abreaction, Freud and Breuer meant the discharge, during therapy, of stored feelings that could not be adequately expressed at the time of the trauma. This "hydraulic" view of emotions has largely been abandoned (Krystal, 1978). Alternatively, modern cognitive, behavioral, and insight-oriented therapies focus on altering cognitive, affective, and identity-related associations to the trauma (Foa et al., 1989; Keane et al., 1989; Krystal, 1988). Psychotherapy may help to reduce the intrusiveness and distress related to traumatic memories by altering associations to the traumatic events.

Clinicians may also promote the linguistic encoding of post-traumatic emotions and memories with the aim of enhancing voluntary control over both domains of symptoms. Traumatic memories may not be encoded or retrieved linguistically. Krystal (1988) has highlighted the difficulty that many individuals with PTSD have in linguistically interpreting their emotional states. He employs cognitive-affective remediation strategies in the psychotherapy of PTSD patients with these difficulties that focus on helping them to learn to label their emotional states, a practice he likens to teaching color-blind individuals to interpret shades of gray. Since sensory processing and emotional reactivity are largely involuntary (LeDoux, 1987), as long as traumatic memories are sensorially encoded and emotionally gated they will intrude unwanted upon consciousness. Perhaps, by linguistically encoding information and emotional responses associated with the trauma, the voluntary control of linguistic function can be brought to bear to achieve the regulation of previously uncontrollable feelings and memories. It is unclear whether the linguistic functions serve primarily an executive function, similar to an operating system on a computer, or whether parallel linguistic memories are created that provide access to the traumatic information in a form that is less distressing. Both processes could be involved in the therapeutic process. However, the latter view is more consistent with the manner in which some patients have a capacity to comfortably review "self-edited" versions of their traumatic memories, while experiencing a great deal of distress when exploring their memories in depth.

The tripartite model highlights challenges facing the clinician treating PTSD. Guided reexperiencing of the trauma could evoke dissociative states that interfere with associative learning and interfere with generalizing therapeutic gains beyond the clinical setting. Intense emotions evoked during such recollections could reinforce the association between traumatic memories and intolerable intense emotions, promoting a sense of helplessness or other negative appraisals of the trauma and making the individual more reluctant or unable to review traumatic material in subsequent therapy sessions (Pitman et al., 1991). Further, by stimulating intense emotional responses and negative association in some individuals, flooding may exacerbate depression or provoke impulsive behavior, including substance abuse (Pitman et al., 1991). These potential problems help explain the need for extensive relaxation training prior to the initiation of guided reexposure therapies, such as flooding (Keane et al., 1989). This step is probably a useful adjunct to all psychotherapies for PTSD patients (Hickling et al., 1986). In addition, one might predict that care must be taken to titrate the level of arousal associated with guided recollection of traumatic memories to the patient's capacity to process information. When, in the course of a therapy session, patients provide clinical data consistent with the induction of dissociative states, further efforts to encourage them to process traumatic material seem less likely to be fruitful. The concern that interference with higher cognitive functions limits the clinical utility of altered states of consciousness applies equally to proposed pharmacologic adjuvants to psychotherapy such as the serotonergic hallucinogens (see Freedman, 1968) and NMDA antagonists (see Krystal et al., 1994). Particularly in patients with chronic PTSD who have been in many years of treatment, there seems to be little benefit in guiding them to reexperience the trauma at the expense of repeated dissociative episodes. Carefully conducted flooding therapy, preceded by relaxation training, may reduce intrusive symptoms of PTSD, but may have no beneficial impact on numbing or avoidance (Keane et al., 1989). These authors highlight significant psychological and social deficits that impair treatment response in patients with chronic PTSD. Thus, treatments aimed at reevaluating traumatic memories may have an important, but carefully delineated, role in therapy.

If, analogous to relaxation training, pharmacologic strategies were developed that preserved cognitive functions in the face of strong affects and traumatic memories, the formation of new associations to traumatic memories might proceed more effectively and rapidly. Benzodiazepines, reportedly useful in some PTSD symptoms in patients with dissociative disorders (Lowenstein et al., 1988), might be helpful by reducing the affective distress, although their amnestic properties might be counterproductive at high doses. Research is needed to develop pharmacologic approaches to enhancing the cognitive processing. In this regard, drugs that facilitate NMDA receptor function via enhancement of the glycine excitatory amino acid site, such as cycloserine or milacemide (Schwartz et al., 1991; Saletu et al., 1986), should be evaluated for antidissociative and other cognitive enhancing properties in PTSD patients.

Antidepressants are the best studied pharmacotherapy for PTSD, and research suggests that they provide only a moderate degree of relief from flashbacks and intrusive memories. The limited efficacy of these agents for many patients with PTSD raises the possibility that other pharmacologic approaches more directly addressing the neurobiology of dissociative states, perhaps via the pharmacology of excitatory amino acid neurotransmission, may have greater efficacy for treating these symptoms in patients with PTSD.

To conclude, in this chapter we have adopted a cognitive neuroscience perspective that assumed that the features of traumatic memories and dissociative states in PTSD are properties of the underlying neural and psychodynamic networks mediating these functions. The process of further identifying and characterizing the regulation of these networks should lead to a better understanding of the pathophysiological consequences of traumatic stress and the discovery of novel and more effective psychotherapy and pharmacotherapy of PTSD.

References

Archibald, H. C., Long, D. M., Miller, C., Tuddenham, R. D. (1962). Gross stress reaction in combat—a 15-year followup. *American Journal of Psychiatry* 119:317–322.

Aston-Jones, G., Shipley, M. T., Chouvet, G., Ennis, M., VanBockstaele, E. J., Pieribone, V., Shiekhattar, R. (1991). Afferent regulation of locus coeruleus neurons: anatomy, physiology and pharmacology. *Progress in Brain Research* 88:47–75.

Bartemeier, L. H., Kubie, L. S., Menninger, K. A., Romano, J., Whitehorn, J. C. (1946). Combat exhaustion. *Journal of Nervous and Mental Disease* 104:489–525.

Bernstein, E., Putnam, T. (1986). Development, reliability, and validity of a dissociation scale. *Journal of Nervous and Mental Disease* 174:727–735.

Blanchard, E. B., Kolb, L. C., Gerardi, R. J., Ryan, P., Pallmeyer, T. P. (1986). Cardiac response to relevant stimuli as an adjunctive tool for diagnosing post-traumatic stress disorder in Vietnam veterans. *Behavioral Therapeutics* 17:592–606.

Blanchard, E. B., Kolb, L. C., Pallmeyer, T. P., Gerardi, R. J. (1982). A psychophysiological study of post-traumatic stress disorder in Vietnam veterans. *Psychiatric Quarterly* 54:220–229.

Boudewyns, P. A., Hyer, L. (1990). Psychophysiological response to combat memories and preliminary treatment outcome in Vietnam veteran PTSD patients treated with direct therapeutic exposure. *Behavioral Therapeutics* 21:63–87.

Bouton, M. E., Bolles, R. C. (1979). Role of contextual stimuli in reinstatement of extinguished fear. *Journal of Experimental Psychology: Animal Behavior Processes* 5:368–378.

Bouton, M. E., Bolles, R. C. (1985). Contexts, event memories, and extinction. In: Balsam, P. D. D., Tomic, K. A., eds. *Context and Learning*. Hillsdale, N.J., Lawrence Erlbaum Associates, pp. 133–166.

Bouton, M. E., King, D. A. (1983). Contextual control of conditioned fear: Tests for the associative value of the context. *Journal of Experimental Psychology: Animal Behavior Processes* 9:248–256.

Bouton, M. E., King, D. A. (1986). Effect of context with mixed histories of reinforcement and nonreinforcement. *Journal of Experimental Psychology: Animal Behavior Processes* 12:4–15.

Bower, G. H. (1981). Mood and memory. *American Psychologist* 36:129–148.

Bremner, J. D., Southwick, S., Brett, E., Fontana, A., Rosenheck, R., Charney, D. S. (1992). Dissociation and posttraumatic stress disorder in Vietnam combat veterans. *American Journal of Psychiatry* 149:328–332.

Bremner, J. D., Steinberg, M., Southwick, S. M., Johnson, D. R., Charney, D. S. (1993). Use of the structured clinical interview for DSM-IV dissociative disorders for systematic assessment of dissociative symptoms in posttraumatic stress disorder. *American Journal of Psychiatry* 150:1011–1014.

Briere, J., Conte, J. (1993). Self-reported amnesia for abuse in adults molested as children. *Journal of Traumatic Stress* 6:21–31.

Brown, R., Kulik, J. (1977). Flashbulb memories. *Cognition* 5:73–99.

Burke, A., Heuer, F., Reisberg, D. (1992). Remembering emotional events. *Memory and Cognition* 20:277–290.

Caggiula, A. R., Antelman, S. M., Aul, E., Knopf, S., Edwards, D. J. (1989). Prior stress attenuates the analgesic response but sensitizes the corticosterone and cortical dopamine responses to stress 10 days later. *Psychopharmacology* 99:233–237.

Campean, S., Hayward, M. D., Hope, B. T., Rosen, J. B., Nestler, E. J., Davis, M. (1991). Induction of the c-fos proto-oncogene in rat amygdala during unconditioned and conditioned fear. *Brain Research* 565:349–352.

Carlson, E. B., Rosser-Hogan, R. (1991). Trauma experiences, posttraumatic stress, dissociation, and depression in Cambodian refugees. *American Journal of Psychiatry* 148:1548–1552.

Cassens, G., Kuruc, A., Roffman, M., Orsulak, P., Schildkraut, J. J. (1981). Alterations in brain norepinephrine metabolism and behavior induced by environmental stimuli previously paired with inescapable shock. *Behavioural Brain Research* 2:387–407.

Christianson, S.-Å. (1984). The relationship between induced emotional arousal and amnesia. *Scandinavian Journal of Psychology* 25:147–160.

———. (1992). Emotional stress and eyewitness memory: A critical review. *Psychological Bulletin* 112:284–309.

Christianson, S.-Å., Loftus, E. F. (1991). Remembering emotional events: The fate of detailed information. *Cognition and Emotion* 5:81–108.

Chu, J. A., Dill, D. L. (1990). Dissociative symptoms in relation to childhood physical and sexual abuse. *American Journal of Psychiatry* 147:887–892.

Cole, B. J., Robbins, T. W. (1987). Dissociable effects of lesions to dorsal and ventral noradrenergic bundle on the acquisition performance, and extinction of aversive conditioning. *Behavioral Neuroscience* 101:476–488.

Craik, F. I. M., Tulving, E. (1975). Depth of processing and the retention of words in episodic memory. *Journal of Experimental Psychology: General* 104:268–294.

Craik, F. I. M., Jacoby, L. L. (1979). Elaboration and distinctiveness in episodic memory. In: Nilsson, L.-G., ed. *Perspectives on Memory Research*. Hillsdale, N.J., Lawrence Erlbaum Associates.

Crawford, H. J., Allen, S. N. (1983). Enhanced visual memory during hypnosis as mediated by hypnotic responsiveness and cognitive strategies. *Journal of Experimental Psychology: General* 112:662–685.

Criswell, H. E., Mueller, R. A., Breese, G. R. (1990). Long-term D₁-dopamine receptor sensitization in neonatal 6-OHD-lesioned rats is blocked by an NMDA antagonist. *Brain Research* 512:284–290.

Davis, M. (1990). Animal models of anxiety based upon classical conditioning: The conditioned emotional response and fear potentiated startle effect. *Pharmacology and Therapeutics* 47:147–165.

Easterbrook, J. A. (1959). The effect of emotion on cue utilization and the organization of behavior. *Psychological Review* 66:183–201.

Falls, W. A., Miserendino, M. J. D., Davis, M. (1990). Excitatory amino acid antagonists infused into the amygdala block extinction of fear-potentiated startle. *Society of Neuroscience Abstracts* 16:767.

Finlay, J. M., Abercrombie, E. D. (1991). Stress induced sensitization of norepinephrine release in the medial prefrontal cortex. *Society of Neuroscience Abstracts* 17:151.

Fisher, C. (1945). Amnesic states in war neurosis: The psychogenesis of fugues. *Psychoanalytic Quarterly* 14:437–458.

Foa, E. B., Feske, U., Murdoc, T. B., Kozak, M. J., McCarthy, P. R. (1991). Processing of threat-related information in rape victims. *Journal of Abnormal Psychology* 100:156–162.

Foa, E. B., Steketee, G., Rothbaum, B. O. (1989). Behavioral/cognitive conceptualizations of post-traumatic stress disorder. *Behavioral Therapeutics* 20:155–176.

Fontana, D. J., Post, R. M., Pert, A. (in press). Conditioned increase in mesolimbic dopamine overflow by stimuli associated with cocaine. *Brain Research*.

Freedman, D. X. (1968). On the use and abuse of LSD. *Archives of General Psychiatry* 18:330–347.

Freud, S., Breuer, J. (1953). On the psychological mechanism of hysterical phenomena. In: Jones, E., ed. *Sigmund Freud, M.D., LLD Collected Papers, Vol. 1*. London, Hogarth Press, pp. 24–41.

Geiselman, R. E., Bjork, R. A., Fishman, D. L. (1983). Disrupted retrieval in directed forgetting: A link with posthypnotic amnesia. *Journal of Experimental Psychology: General* 112:58–72.

Ghoneim, M. M., Hinrichs, J. V., Mewaldt, S. P. (1984). Dose-response analysis of the behavioral effects of diazepam: I. Learning and memory. *Psychopharmacology* 82:291–295.

Goldstein, G., vanKammen, W., Shelly, C., Miller, D. J., vanKammen, D. P. (1987). Survivors of imprisonment in the Pacific theater during World War II. *American Journal of Psychiatry* 144:1210–1213.

Grinker, R. R. (1944). Treatment of war neuroses. *JAMA* 126:142–145.

Grinker, R. R., Spiegel, J. P. (1943). *War Neuroses in North Africa*. New York, Josiah Macy, Jr., Foundation.

Grinker, R. R., Spiegel, J. P. (1945). *War Neuroses*. Philadelphia, Blakiston.

Heil, M., Rosler, F., Hennighausen, E. (1994). Dynamics of activation in long-term memory: The retrieval of verbal, pictorial, spatial, and color information. *Journal of Experimental Psychology: Learning, Memory, and Cognition* 20:185–200.

Hermann, J. K., Perry, J., van der Kolk, V. A. (1989). Childhood trauma in borderline personality disorder. *American Journal of Psychiatry* 148:490–495.

Heuer, F., Reisberg, D. (1992). Emotion, arousal and memory for detail. In: Christianson, S. Å., ed. *The Handbook of Emotion and Memory: Research and Theory*. Hillsdale, N.J., Lawrence Erlbaum Associates.

Hickling, E. J., Sison, G. F. P., Jr., Vanderploeg, R. D. (1986). Treatment of posttraumatic stress disorder with relaxation and biofeedback training. *Biofeedback Self-Reg.* 11:125–134.

Hilgard, E. R. (1977). *Divided Consciousness: Multiple Controls in Human Thought and Action*. New York, Wiley.

Hoffman, H. S., Selekman, W., Fleishler, M. (1966). Stimulus aspects of aversive controls: Long term effects of suppression procedures. *Journal of Experimental Analysis of Behavior* 1:659–662.

Hogben, G. L., Cornfield, R. B. (1981). Treatment of war neurosis with phenelzine. *Archives of General Psychiatry* 38:440–445.

Horowitz, M. J. (1976). *Stress Response Syndromes*. New York, Aronson.

———. (1975). Intrusive and repetitive thoughts after experimental stress. *Archives of General Psychiatry* 32:1457–1463.

Janet, P. (1889). *L'automatisme psychologique: Essai de psychologie experimentale sur les formes inférievres de l'activité humaine*. Paris, Alcan.

Kalivas, P. W., Duffy, P. (1989). Similar effects of daily cocaine and stress on mesocorticolimbic dopamine neurotransmission in the rat. *Biological Psychiatry* 25:913–928.

Kalivas, P. W., Duffy, P., Abhold, R., Dilts, R. P. (1990). Sensitization of mesolimbic dopamine neurons by neuropeptides and stress. In: Kalivas, P. W., Barnes, C. D., eds. *Sensitization in the Nervous System*. Caldwell, N.J., Telford Press, pp. 119–124.

Kalivas, P. W., Striplin, C. D., Steketee, J. D., Klitenick, M. A., Duffy, P. (1992). Cellular mechanisms of behavioral sensitization to drugs of abuse. *Annals of the New York Academy of Sciences* 654:128–135.

Kardiner, A. (1941). *The Traumatic Neuroses of War*, Psychosomatic Monograph II-III. Washington, D.C., National Research Council.

Keane, T. M., Fairbank, J. A., Caddell, J. M., Zimering, R. T. (1989). Implosive therapy reduces symptoms of PTSD in Vietnam combat veterans. *Behavioral Therapeutics* 20:245–260.

Kihlstrom, J. F. (1983). Instructed forgetting: Hypnotic and nonhypnotic. *Journal of Experimental Psychology: General* 112:73–79.

Kim, J. J., Fanselow, M. S. (1992). Modality-specific retrograde amnesia of fear. *Science* 256:675–677.

Kline, N. A., Rausch, J. L. (1985). Olfactory precipitants of flashbacks in posttraumatic stress disorder: case reports. *Journal of Clinical Psychiatry* 46:383–384.

Kluft, R. F. (1987). An update on multiple personality disorder. *Hospital and Community Psychiatry* 38:363–373.

Krystal, H. (1968). *Massive Psychic Trauma*. New York, International Universities.

———. (1978). Trauma and affects. *Psychoanalytic Study of the Child* 33:81–116.

———. (1988). *Integration and Self-Healing: Affect, Trauma, Alexithymia*. Hillsdale, N.Y., Analytic Press.

Krystal, J. H., Bennett, A., Bremner, J. D., Southwick, S. M., Charney, D. S. (in press). Toward a cognitive neuroscience of dissociation and altered memory functions in Post-Traumatic Stress Disorder. In: Friedman, M. J., Charney,

D. S., Deutch, A. Y., eds. *Neurobiological and Clinical Consequences of Stress: From Normal Adaptation to PTSD*. New York, Raven Press.

Krystal, J. H., Kosten, T. R., Perry, B. D., Southwick, S., Mason, J. W., Giller, E. L., Jr. (1989). Neurobiological aspects of PTSD: Review of clinical and preclinical studies. *Behavioral Therapeutics* 20:177–198.

Krystal, J. H., Woods, S. W., Hill, C. L., Charney, D. S. (1988). Characteristics of self-defined panic attacks. *1988 New Research Program and Abstracts*. Washington, D.C., American Psychiatric Assoc. NR 263.

Krystal, J. H., Karper, L. P., Seibyl, J. P., Freeman, G. K., Delaney, R., Bremner, J. D., Heninger, G. R., Bowers, M. H., Jr, Charney, D. S. (1994). Subanesthetic effects of the NMDA antagonist, ketamine, in humans: Psychotomimetic, perceptual, cognitive, and neuroendocrine effects. *Archives of General Psychiatry* 51:199–214.

Lang, P. J. (1977). Imagery in therapy: An information processing analysis of fear. *Behavioral Therapy* 8:862–886.

Laurence, J. R., Perry, C. (1983). Hypnotically created memory among highly hypnotizable subjects. *Science* 222:423–524.

LeDoux, J. E. (1987). Emotion. In: Plum, V. F., ed. *Handbook of Physiology—The Nervous System*. Washington, D.C., American Physiological Society, pp. 419–459.

LeDoux, J. E., Cicchetti, P., Xagoraris, A., Romanski, L. M. (1990). The lateral amygdaloid nucleus: Sensory interface of the amygdala in fear conditioning. *Journal of Neuroscience* 10:1062–1069.

LeDoux, J. E., Romanski, L., Xagoraris, A. (1989). Indelibility of subcortical emotional memories. *Journal of Cognitive Neuroscience* 1:238–243.

Litz, B. T. (1992). Emotional numbing in combat-related post-traumatic stress disorder. *Clinical Psychology Review* 12:417–432.

Litz, B. T., Keane, T. M. (1989). Information processing in anxiety disorders: Application to the understanding of post-traumatic stress disorder. *Clinical Psychology Review* 9:243–257.

Lowenstein, R. J., Hornstein, N., Farber, B. (1988). Open trial of clonzaepam in the treatment of post traumatic stress symptoms in multiple personality disorder. *Dissociation* 1:3–12.

Macmillan, T. M. (1991). Post-traumatic stress disorder and severe head injury. *British Journal of Psychiatry* 159:431–433.

Malloy, P. F., Fairbank, J. A., Keane, T. M. (1983). Validation of a multimethod assessment of post-traumatic stress disorders in Vietnam veterans. *Journal of Consulting and Clinical Psychology* 51:488–494.

Mayer-Gross, W. (1935). On depersonalization. *British Journal of Medical Psychology* 15:103–126.

McAllister, W. R., McAllister, D. E. (1988). Reconditioning of extinguished fear after a one-year delay. *Bulletin of the Psychosomatic Society* 26:463–466.

McDougle, C. J., Southwick, S. M. (1990). Emergence of an alternate personality in combat-related posttraumatic stress disorder. *Hospital and Community Psychiatry* 41:554–556.

McFall, M. F., Murburg, M. M., Ko, G. M., Veith, R. C. (1990). Autonomic responses to stress in Vietnam veterans with post traumatic stress disorder. *Biological Psychology* 27:1165–1175.

McGee, R. (1984). Flashbacks and memory phenomena: A comment on "flashback phenomena-clinical and diagnostic dilemmas." *Journal of Traumatic Stress* 6:33–41.

McNally, R. J., Kaspi, S. P., Riemann, B. C., Zeitlin, S. R. (1990). Selective processing of threat cues in posttraumatic stress disorder. *Journal of Abnormal Psychology* 99:398–402.

McNally, R. J., Luedke, D. L., Besyner, J. K., Peterson, R. A., Bohm, K., Lips, O. J. (1987). Sensitivity to stress relevant stimuli in post traumatic stress disorder. *Journal of Anxiety Disorders* 1:105–116.

Mellman, T. A., Davis, G. C. (1985). Combat-related flashbacks in post-traumatic stress disorder: Phenomenology and similarity to panic attacks. *Journal of Clinical Psychiatry* 46:379–382.

Nisenbaum, L. K., Zigmand, M. J., Sved, A. F., Abercrombie, E. D. (1991). Prior exposure to chronic stress results in enhanced synthesis and release of hippocampal norepinephrine in response to a novel stressor. *Journal of Neuroscience* 11:1478–1484.

Orr, S. P. (1990). Psychophysiologic studies of post traumatic stress disorder. In: Giller, E. L., ed. *Biological Assessment and Treatment of Post Traumatic Stress Disorder*. Washington, D.C., American Psychiatric Press, Inc.

Paige, S. T., Reid, G. M., Allen, M. G., Newton, J. E. O. (1990). Psychophysiological correlated posttraumatic stress disorder in Vietnam veterans. *Biological Psychiatry* 27:419–430.

Paivio, A. (1971). *Imagery and verbal processes*. New York, Holt, Rinehart, and Winston.

Pallmeyer, T. P., Blanchard, E. B., Kolb, L. C. (1986). The psychophysiology of combat-induced post-traumatic stress disorder in Vietnam veterans. *Behavior Research and Therapy* 24:645–652.

Pavlov, J. P. (1927). *Conditioned Reflexes*. Oxford, Oxford University Press.

Phillips, R. G., LeDoux, J. E. (1992). Differential contribution of amygdala and hippocampus to cued and contextual fear conditioning. *Behavioral Neuroscience* 106:274–285.

Pitman, R. K., Altman, B., Greenwald, E., Longpre, R. E., Macklin, M. L., Poire, R. E., Steketee, G. S. (1991). Psychiatric complications during flooding therapy for posttraumatic stress disorder. *Journal of Clinical Psychiatry* 52:17–20.

Pitman, R. K., Orr, S. P., Forgue, D. F., deJong, J. B., Claiborn, J. M. (1987). Psychophysiologic assessment of post-traumatic stress disorder in Vietnam combat veterans. *Archives of General Psychiatry* 44:970–975.

Post, R. M. (1992). Transduction of psychosocial stress into the neurobiology of recurrent affective disorders. *American Journal of Psychiatry* 149:999–1010.

Putnam, F. W., Guroff, J. J., Silberman, E. K., Barban, L., Post, R. M. (1986). The clinical phenomenology of multiple personality disorder: Review of 100 recent cases. *Journal of Clinical Psychiatry* 47:285–293.

Pynoos, R. S., Frederick, C. J., Nader, K., Arroyo, W., Steinberg, A., Eth, S., Nunez, F., Fairbanks, L. (1987). Life threat and posttraumatic stress disorder in school-age children. *Archives of General Psychiatry* 44:1057–1063.

Rainey, J. M., Jr, Alteem, A., Ortiz, A., Yeeragani, V., Pohl, R., Beerchou, R. (1987). A laboratory procedure for the induction of flashbacks. *American Journal of Psychiatry* 144:1317–1319.

Rasmussen, K., Marilak, D. A., Jacobs, B. L. (1986). Single unit activity of the locus coeruleus in the freely moving cat. I: During naturalistic behaviors and in response to simple and complex stimuli. *Brain Research* 371:324–334.

Rescola, R. A., Heth, C. D. (1975). Reinstatement of fear to extinguished conditioned stimulus. *Journal of Experimental Psychology: Animal Behavior Processes* 104:88–96.

Saletu, B., Grunberger, J., Linzmayer, L. (1986). Acute and subacute CNS effects of milacemide in elderly people: Double-blind placebo-controlled quantitative EEG and psychometric investigations. *Archives of Gerontology and Geriatrics* 5:165–181.

Sapolsky, R. M. (1992). *Stress, the Aging Brain, and the Mechanisms of Neuron Death*. Cambridge, Mass., MIT Press.

Schwartz, B. L., Hashtroudi, S., Heerting, R. L., Hnaderson, H., Keutsch, S. I. (1991). Glycine prodrug facilitates memory retrieval in humans. *Neurology* 41:1341–1343.

Smith, M. A., Banerjee, S., Gold, P. W., Glowa, J. (1992). Induction of c-fos in mRNA in rat brain by conditioned and unconditioned stressors. *Brain Research* 578:135–141.

Solomen, Z., Garb, K., Bleich, A., Grupper, D. (1987). Reactivation of combat related post traumatic stress disorder. *American Journal of Psychiatry* 144:51–55.

Southwick, S. M., Krystal, J. H., Morgan, C. A., Johnson, D., Nagy, L. M., Nicolaou, A., Heninger, G. R., Charney, D. S. (1993). Abnormal noradrenergic function in post traumatic stress disorder. *Archives of General Psychiatry* 50:266–274.

Southwick, S. M., Krystal, J. H., Morgan, A., Nagy, L. M., Dan, E., Johnson, D., Bremner, D., Charney, D. S. (1991). Yohimbine and m-chlorophenylpiperazine in PTSD. *New Research Program and Abstracts: American Psychiatric Association, 144th Annual Meeting,* NR348.

Spiegel, D., Cardena, E. (1991). Disintegrated experience: The dissociative disorders revisited. *Journal of Abnormal Psychology* 100:366–378.

Spiegel, D., Hunt, T., Dondershine, H. E. (1988). Dissociation and hypnotizability in posttraumatic stress disorder. *American Journal of Psychiatry* 145:301–305.

Stuss, D. T. (1992). Biological and psychological development of executive function. *Brain and Cognition* 20:8–23.

Stutker, P. B., Winstead, D. K., Galina, Z. H., Allain, A. N. (1991). Cognitive deficits and psychopathology among former prisoners of war and combat veterans of the Korean conflict. *American Journal of Psychiatry* 148:67–72.

Tanaka, M., Ida, Y., Tsuda, A., Nagasaki, N. (1986). Involvement of brain noradrenaline and opioid peptides in emotional changes induced by stress in rats. In: Oomura, Y., ed. *Emotions: Neural and Chemical Control*. Tokyo, Scientific Societies Press, pp. 417–427.

Teich, A. H., McCabe, P. M., Gentile, C. C., Schneiderman, L. S., Winters, R. W., Liskowsky, D. R., Schneiderman, N. (1989). Auditory cortex lesions prevent extinction of Pavlovian differential heart rate conditioning to tonal stimuli in rabbits. *Brain Research* 480:210–218.

Terr, L. C. (1983). Time sense following psychic trauma: A clinical study of ten adults and twenty children. *American Journal of Orthopsychiatry* 53:244–261.

Thygesen, P., Heermann, K., Willanger, R. (1970). Concentration camp survivors in Denmark: Persecution, disease, compensation. *Danish Medical Bulletin* 17:65–108.

Tsaltas, E., Gray, J. A., Fillenz, M. (1987). Alleviation of response suppression to conditioned aversive stimuli by lesions of the dorsal noradrenergic bundle. *Behavioural Brain Research* 13:115–127.

Tulving, E., Thomson, D. M. (1973). Encoding specificity and retrieval processes in episodic memory. *Psychological Review* 80:352–373.

van der Kolk, B. A., Ducey, C. P. (1989). The psychological processing of traumatic experience. Rorschach patterns in PTSD. *Journal of Traumatic Stress* 2:259–274.

VanDyke, C., Zilberg, N. J., MacKinnon, J. A. (1985). Post traumatic stress disorder: A thirty year delay in a World War II veteran. *American Journal of Psychiatry* 142:1070–1073.

Wagenaar, W. A., Groeneweg, J. (1990). The memory of concentration camp survivors. *Applied Cognitive Psychology* 4:77–87.

Weingartner, H., Miller, H., Murphy, D. L. (1977). Mood-state dependent retrieval of verbal associations. *Journal of Abnormal Psychology* 86:276–284.

Weiss, S. R. B., Post, R. M., Pert, A., Woodward, R., Murman, D. (1989). Context-dependent cocaine sensitization: Differential effect of haloperidol on development versus expression. *Pharmacology, Biochemistry and Behavior* 34:655–661.

Yuille, J. C., Cutshall, J. L. (1989). Analysis of the statements of victims, witnesses and suspects. In: Yuille, J. C., ed. *Credibility Assessment*. Norwell, Mass., Kluwer Academic.

Zeitlin, S. B., McNally, R. J. (1991). Implicit and explicit memory bias for threat in post-traumatic stress disorder. *Behavior Research and Therapy* 29:451–457.

Mood-congruent Memory Biases in Anxiety and Depression

Susan Mineka
Kathleen Nugent

Researchers from a variety of areas have generally accepted the idea that cognition and emotion are closely intertwined, although the exact nature of their relationship is currently being debated. From a psychoevolutionary perspective, Plutchik (1984) has argued that "cognitions have largely evolved in the service of emotions" (p. 209). That is, the function of cognitive processes is to allow an individual to predict the future of emotion-related events, specifically the future location and availability of food, a mate, and predators. According to Plutchik, the interaction of cognition with emotion allows emotional behavior to be an adaptive response to biologically significant events. A related argument has been put forth by Gray (1990), who suggests the presence of a "genuine interweaving of emotional and cognitive processes in the workings of the brain" (p. 271). Gray argues that over time human beings were selected for their ability to learn information about reinforcing events (e.g., food, mate, predator). He further argues that if one accepts the common assumption that emotional states are those that are elicited by reinforcing events, then consequently, the function of cognition (i.e., the appraisal of reinforcing events) is linked to the experience of emotion. Gray also cites research that attributes important emotion- and cognition-related functions to the same neuroanatomical structures and systems in the brain (e.g., the hippocampal formation and the amygdala).

The understanding that the cognitive and emotional systems in human beings are closely related has had an important influence on research on the emotional disorders (i.e., the anxiety and depressive disorders). A number of theories postulate that biased cognitive processes are central to the emotional disorders. One important line of work on selective associations in fear conditioning has contributed substantially to our understanding of why fears and phobias do not tend to occur to a random, arbitrary group of objects or situations associated with trauma. To explain these observations, Seligman and Öhman have argued that human and nonhuman primates appear to have evolutionarily based predispositions to acquire fears and phobias of certain objects or situations that may once have been dangerous or posed a threat to our early ancestors (Öhman, Dimberg, and Öst, 1985; Öhman, 1986; Seligman, 1971). Human experiments on this topic typically find superior conditioning in subjects conditioned with fear-relevant conditioned stimuli (such as snakes or spiders, or angry faces) paired with mild electric shocks, relative to what is seen in subjects conditioned with fear-irrelevant stimuli (such as flowers or mushrooms, or happy faces) paired with shocks (Öhman et al., 1985; Öhman, 1986). One can conceive of such selective associations as involving a kind of memory distortion, probably occurring at encoding, in that subjects seem to selectively remember certain types of CS-US pairings (e.g., fear-relevant stimuli and aversive outcomes) and not others (e.g., fear-irrelevant stimuli and aversive outcomes). It is widely thought that this type of memory distortion contributes substantially to the nonrandom distribution of fears and phobias seen clinically.

One controversial issue in these human experiments on selective associations in fear conditioning has been whether these effects derive from phylogenetic as opposed to ontogenetic factors (Delprato, 1980), with the latter possibility stemming from the fact that human subjects in these experiments all have prior associations to the CSs used in the experiments. However, recent research using laboratory-reared rhesus monkeys as subjects has strongly implicated phylogenetic factors in these selective associations (Cook and Mineka, 1989, 1990, 1991). In these experiments, observer monkeys watched videotapes of wild-reared model monkeys behaving fearfully either with fear-relevant toy snakes (or a toy crocodile) or with fear-irrelevant artificial flowers (or a toy rabbit). In all three experiments, observer monkeys who watched model monkeys showing fear to fear-relevant objects acquired a fear of those objects, whereas observer monkeys who watched model monkeys showing fear to fear-irrelevant objects did not acquire a fear of those objects. Given that the observer monkeys had not had any prior exposure to the objects used as CSs (fear-relevant or fear-irrelevant), it seems highly likely that phylogenetic factors accounted for the observed differences in conditionability of these objects (Cook and Mineka, 1989, 1990, 1991). Thus, it seems reasonable to describe these associative biases as involving a kind of evolutionary memory (Mineka, 1992).

More central to the topic of this chapter is work deriving from information processing research on the emotion-cognition interaction. In the past 15 years there has been an explosion of interest in demonstrating attentional and memory biases for mood-congruent material. Theories by Bower (1981) and Beck (1967, 1976; Beck and Emery, 1985) have received the greatest attention. Bower's semantic associative network model outlines a network of interconnected, yet separate, nodes which represent concepts, emotions, and experiences. The spread of activation from one node to adjacent nodes occurs automatically. For example, mood-congruent memory effects are hypothesized to occur when an emotion node is activated and this activation spreads to related nodes.

Beck's alternative theory postulates that both anxiety and depression are characterized by systematic distortions in information processing. In particular, Beck employs the construct of schema to understand the distortions seen in anxiety and depression. Schemata are organized representations of prior knowledge which guide the current processing of information (e.g., Rumelhart and Ortony, 1977). Overactivation of certain maladaptive schemata is thought to be characteristic of both disorders. This overactivation is believed to lead to a greater degree of perceptual sensitivity and memory bias for information congruent with one's predominant schema(ta). The two emotional disorders are thought to differ regarding the content of the maladaptive schemata. Beck and his colleagues hypothesize that negative self-schemata are central to depression, and that danger schemata are characteristic of anxiety. Thus, individuals with negative self-schemata will attend to and remember more negative information, which will lead to and maintain negative affect and depression. Similarly, individuals with highly active danger schemata will attend to and remember more threatening stimuli, which will foster and maintain anxiety.

Although Beck's and Bower's models differ in a number of important ways, the two models each predict that anxious and depressed individuals should demonstrate attentional *and* memory biases for information that is consistent with their emotional state. Specifically, depressed persons should demonstrate attentional and memory biases for depressive stimuli and information, typically concerning loss and failure, and anxious individuals should demonstrate similar biases for stimuli concerning threat and danger (see MacLeod and Mathews, 1991; Mineka and Sutton, 1992). Further, these biases are thought to play a role in the maintenance of these disorders because the biases serve to increase the saliency of loss and danger stimuli for the individual.

The main goal of this chapter is to present the research literature on memory biases in the emotional disorders and to discuss the implications of these biases for the etiology, maintenance, and severity of these disorders. It is important to note that the memory biases we will discuss are related to the selective or non-veridical processing of emotionally relevant information (Mineka and Tomarken, 1989). In this sense they represent one of the myriad types of memory distortions discussed in this volume. The negative effects of anxiety and depression on general memory functioning will not be discussed (see MacLeod and Mathews, 1991, for a review). Before proceeding, however, we will briefly review the research literature on attentional biases in anxiety and depression. Given that Beck's and Bower's models each make predictions about both attention and memory, and given the fact that one must attend before one can remember, we feel it is appropriate and informative to summarize the attentional bias literature before proceeding with a more detailed discussion of memory biases in emotional disorders.

Attentional Biases: A Brief Summary

Anxiety. Strong research evidence exists demonstrating that individuals with anxiety disorders show an attentional bias that results in attention being directed toward potential sources of threat when there is a mixture of threatening and nonthreatening information. These results have been found with a variety of paradigms (e.g., dichotic listening, dot-probe detection, modified emotional Stroop). Moreover, not only is the attentional bias in anxious subjects present across a variety of tasks, but it also appears to be operating early during information processing and outside of awareness (see MacLeod and Mathews, 1991, for a review).

In a prototypical experiment, MacLeod, Mathews, and Tata (1986) had subjects read aloud the upper of two briefly presented (500 msec) words on a computer screen; some of the words were neutral in content and some were threat-relevant. On some trials one of the two words was followed by a dot probe, and subjects were to press a response key as soon as they saw the probe. In general, the latency to respond to the probe was faster when it appeared over the word to which the subjects were already attending. Clinically anxious subjects demonstrated the fastest response times when the probe replaced threat words (regardless of position on the screen), indicating that their attention had actually shifted toward threat words when they appeared on the screen. In contrast, nonanxious controls tended to direct their attention away from the threat cues.

Although a general consensus exists that anxiety is associated with an attentional bias for threat-related information, the exact nature of this bias and the variables that influence it are currently being debated. For example, MacLeod and Mathews (1988) reported that high state anxiety (induced by upcoming final medical school exams) had different effects on attentional functioning in low and high trait anxious individuals (who differ in chronic levels of anxiety). High trait anxious individuals demonstrated an increased attentional bias for threat words under high state anxiety, but low trait anxious persons in this condition diverted their attention away from threat words. However, other researchers have found a somewhat different pattern of results under more acutely stressful situations (e.g., Mogg, Mathews, Bird, and McGregor-Morris, 1990). In addition, the specificity of the attentional bias is still being examined. It is unclear, for example, whether the bias is for all emotional stimuli, all negative stimuli, only threatening stimuli, or only stimuli that are relevant to an individual's anxious concerns. Although the research results are mixed, it seems that the attentional bias is most likely for negative or threat-related stimuli.

Depression.   In contrast to the relatively robust results indicating the presence of an attentional bias in anxiety, there is little strong evidence in support of a similar bias in depression. Although a number of studies using the modified emotional Stroop paradigm have reported increased interference with negative mood-congruent stimuli, the validity of the Stroop task as a measure of attention has been questioned (e.g., Kahneman and Chajczyk, 1983; Mathews, 1993). In addition, the comorbidity of anxiety in the depressed subjects in these studies has not been assessed. Consequently, it is unclear whether the attentional bias found in some studies of depressed individuals is due to depression or to concomitant anxiety. No evidence of an attentional bias in depressed subjects was found using subliminal stimuli with the Stroop (Mogg, Bradley, Williams, and Mathews, 1993), or using the dot-probe reaction task (MacLeod et al., 1986). Yet, these paradigms produce clear evidence of a bias in anxious subjects.

Overall, the current research results do not appear to completely support the predictions from Bower's and Beck's theories that attentional biases should be present in both anxiety and depression. As predicted, anxiety, in particular generalized anxiety disorder (GAD), is characterized by a preconscious, automatic attentional bias for threat-related stimuli when there is a mixture of threatening and non-threatening information. However, little evidence of an attentional bias in depressed individuals exists (see MacLeod and Mathews, 1991, for a review).

Memory Biases

As we begin the presentation of the research literature on memory biases in anxiety and depression, several issues should be noted. The first issue is the type of memory that is assessed. Over the last ten years, the distinction between explicit and implicit memory has been highlighted. Traditional measures of memory can be classified as explicit (e.g., free recall, recognition). On explicit memory tasks, subjects are instructed to consciously retrieve previously studied material. In contrast, implicit memory tasks assess memory indirectly by, for example, asking subjects to complete word stems with the first word that comes to mind. Dramatic examples of dissociations on these two kinds of memory tests come from studies of amnesic patients, who show severe deficits on explicit memory tests but relatively normal performance on tests of implicit memory (see Roediger, 1990; Schacter, 1987, for reviews). In presenting the research literature on memory biases, we will examine results from studies employing explicit and implicit memory tasks.

A second issue that is central to understanding the role of memory biases in the emotional disorders is the specificity of the memory bias (e.g., all emotional stimuli versus all negative stimuli versus only threat stimuli). As discussed above for attentional biases, specificity of the stimulus materials that elicit a bias should be assessed. Finally, a third related issue is whether differences in retrieval of positive versus negative memories found using autobiographical memory paradigms are due to the person's affective state or to possible real differences in past experiences.

Depression. In general, the study of mood-congruent memory in depression involves comparing individuals who experience high levels of depression with matched nondepressed controls. A self-referential encoding task is usually employed consisting of target words and a list which vary in their affective content (see Blaney, 1986; MacLeod and Mathews, 1991, for reviews; see Matt, Vazquez, and Campbell, 1992, for a meta-analysis). Numerous studies have found that clinically depressed subjects show a strong bias to recall negative, especially self-referential, information. The bias is present both with negative autobiographical and experimentally presented stimulus materials. This bias is in contrast with that usually exhibited by nondepressed subjects, who tend to favor a recall of positive material (see MacLeod and Mathews, 1991; see Matt et al., 1992, for a meta-analysis). Subclinically depressed subjects tend to show an intermediate "even-handed" memory, remembering approximately equal amounts of positive and negative material (Matt et al., 1992).

The memory bias associated with clinical depression appears to be specific to depression-relevant words. For example, Watkins, Mathews, Williamson, and Uller (1992) included physical threat words as well as depression-relevant words, and only found the bias for the depression-relevant words. Bellew and Hill (1990) report a related finding in that depressed subjects demonstrated a recall bias for self-esteem threatening words, but not for negative words in general.

Further, most studies of autobiographical memory seem to suggest that it is the affective state, rather than any differences in experiences, that drives the bias. In an experiment assessing autobiographical memory, subjects are usually presented with either neutral, positive, or negative word cues and are asked to retrieve a specific autobiographical memory. Typical findings are that depressed subjects, but not normal controls, take longer to respond to positive than to negative cues, and retrieve less specific (i.e., more general) positive memories (e.g., Lloyd and Lishman, 1975; Teasdale and Fogarty, 1979; Richards and Whittaker, 1990; Williams and Scott, 1988). To determine whether these differences reflect real differences in past experiences, several studies have tested subjects on several occasions, seeking to establish whether the same retrieval pattern is observed in different affective states as would be expected if the "different experiences" hypothesis were true. For example, Clark and Teasdale (1982) studied diurnal depressives at different points in time and found that, as the subject's depression level increased during the day, the probability of retrieving a negative autobiographical memory in response to a neutral cue word increased, and the probability of retrieving a positive memory decreased. Similarly, the finding that mood-congruent biases seem to disappear when depression remits does not support the "different experiences" hypothesis (e.g., see Bradley and Mathews, 1988). Related findings were also reported by Bullington (1990) using mood-induction techniques (see also Parrott, 1991; Singer and Salovey, 1989).

Most of the studies referred to above have employed explicit memory measures. At present there are only three published studies with depressed patients as subjects that have used implicit memory measures. All of these studies found no significant evidence of a mood-congruent memory bias for negative information using implicit memory tests (although they all replicated the standard explicit mood-congruency effects) (Hertel and Hardin, 1990; Denny and Hunt, 1992; Watkins et al., 1992; see Roediger and McDermott, 1992, for a review and commentary). However, there are now important reasons to believe that none of these studies has provided an adequate test of whether implicit mood-congruent biases may exist with depression.

In their commentary on the three studies which have examined this issue in depressed subjects, Roediger and McDermott (1992) noted that just as there are important dissociations between performance on implicit and explicit tasks, so too are there important dissociations between different types of implicit memory tasks. These authors base their argument on transfer-appropriate processing theory—a theory which can account for dissociations both between explicit and implicit memory tests, and among implicit memory tests (see Roediger, 1990). Roediger and McDermott proposed that dissociations found on explicit and implicit memory tests are a result of the different cognitive processes required to complete the different tests. Roediger hypothesizes that the greater the overlap between the processes utilized during encoding and at retrieval, the better the memory performance on a particular test. Encoding tasks in which subjects simply read a word or count the letters in a word are classified as data-driven or perceptual; encoding tasks are classified as conceptual if subjects elaborate on the meaning of the words. Those memory tests on which subjects rely on the perceptual similarity of the encoded words in obtaining the correct answer are classified as data-driven or perceptual; memory tests that require subjects to draw on the meaning of the encoded material are classified as conceptual. Most studies on mood-congruent memory biases have used a conceptual encoding task and a perceptual implicit memory task. One would not expect a high level of priming with a conceptually driven encoding task and a perceptually driven implicit task given the extensive research findings on implicit memory performance in normal populations. Therefore, Roediger and McDermott hypothesize that the reason that little evidence of mood-congruent implicit memory biases exists at present may be due to the mismatch between the nature of the encoding task and the memory tests that have been used in *all* studies to date on mood-congruent implicit memory. Moreover, there is no particular reason to expect that perceptually driven tasks would be sensitive to mood-congruency effects, given that it is the semantic *meaning* of mood-congruent words that is so salient to emotionally disordered individuals.

In summary, there is currently good evidence for explicit memory biases for negative mood-congruent information in depression. In the case of autobiographical memory the bias seems to most likely reflect differences in affective state rather than differences in experience. Unfortunately, however, the present negative evidence regarding implicit memory biases is inconclusive.

Anxiety. In contrast to the strong evidence for mood-congruent memory biases in depression, the majority of research studying anxious individuals has not found a memory bias for threatening information (see MacLeod and Mathews, 1991; Mathews, 1993, for reviews). Further, when significant findings have been obtained, they have often failed to be replicated. For example, Mogg, Mathews, and Weinman (1987) reported a tendency for generally anxious patients (GADs) to recall *less* threatening information than controls, and this appeared to be due to a reduced sensitivity for such information rather than to different response biases across groups. Similarly, Watts, McKenna, Sharrock, and Trezise (1986) and Watts and Dagleish (1991) found that spider phobics demonstrated *poorer* explicit (recall and recognition) memory for spiders than did controls. Thus, some studies have found *poor* memory for threatening stimuli.

By contrast, other studies have simply found no significant differences in memory for threatening versus neutral information. For example, Mathews, Mogg, May, and Eysenck (1989) found no evidence for an explicit recall bias in a sample of GADs, and Nugent and Mineka (1994) in two studies found no consistent evidence of a recall bias for threatening information in high trait anxious subjects (whose levels of trait anxiety were comparable to that in the Mathews et al. [1989] study). (See also Richards and French, 1991, for another failure to find explicit memory bias in high trait anxious subjects.) Moreover, in a study that looked only at recognition memory, Mogg and colleagues (1992) also found no evidence for mood-congruency effects in GADs relative to normal controls, and Foa, McNally, and Mur-dock (1989) found no evidence for superior memory of anxiety-relevant words in speech anxious subjects undergoing a state anxiety induction procedure.

Further complicating the picture are several studies that *did* find evidence for a memory bias for threatening information. For example, Watts and Coyle (1992) failed to replicate their earlier findings of inferior memory for spider words in spider phobics, and in fact found that spider phobics recalled *more* phobia-related than control words (although they did not recall more phobia-related words than control subjects). Rusted and Dighton (1991) also found that spider phobics show *enhanced* recall for prose material re-lated to spiders. In addition, Mogg and Mathews (1990) found superior mood-congruent recall in GADs relative to controls, although this appeared to be attributable to response bias because the GADs also showed more threat intrusions. Thus, although generalized anxiety is clearly characterized by an attentional bias for threatening material, there is little consistent evi-dence of biases for threatening information when explicit memory tests are used. One possible interpretation of this pattern of findings, which we will discuss more fully below, is that although GADs clearly show heightened vigilance for threat, they may *avoid* further elaborative rehearsal that would be necessary to produce concomitant explicit memory biases.

As with depression, researchers have been interested in whether mood-congruent biases in *implicit* memory can be demonstrated with anxiety. Mathews and colleagues (1989) reported results suggesting that anxious pa-tients may show a relative bias in implicit (but not in explicit) memory for threatening information. It is not clear how reliable this effect is, however, given that Mathews (personal communication) has recently reported a fail-ure to replicate that effect in his laboratory, and that our own recent studies (Nugent and Mineka, 1994) have failed to find evidence for an implicit mem-ory bias for threatening information in very high trait anxious subjects. However, as with depression, Roediger and McDermott's (1992) commen-tary suggests that these negative results may stem from the fact that all stud-ies to date have involved a mismatch between the nature of the encoding task and the tests that have been used to assess mood-congruent implicit memory. Thus, the actual status of mood-congruent implicit memory biases in anxiety remains undetermined, and additional research needs to be car-ried out that utilizes conceptual encoding *and* memory tests.

Thus, although there are isolated findings of superior memory for threat-ening material in GAD or phobic subjects, the majority of studies have not found such a bias even though highly similar studies have been conducted to those that do consistently find a bias in depressed subjects. There are two possible exceptions to this conclusion. One comes from the study of autobiographical memory in anxious subjects. The second exception comes from the study of subjects with panic disorder (with or without agoraphobia). Panic disorder is another category of anxiety disorder in which an individual experiences occasional unexpected attacks of acute anxiety (panic attacks) and generally develops considerable anticipatory anxiety about the occurrence of possible future attacks. Agoraphobic avoidance of situations in which such attacks might occur often develops as an additional complication of panic disorder.

Regarding autobiographical memory, there are now two studies suggesting that anxious subjects may show superior autobiographical memory for anxiety-relevant material. In one study, Richards and Whittaker (1990) asked high and low trait anxious subjects to generate a personal memory at the presentation of either an anxious or a happy cue word; state anxiety was also manipulated through showing newspaper photographs depicting various moods. Results indicated that both high trait anxiety and the state anxiety induction caused a faster response to the anxious cue words; state anxiety was most predictive of enhanced retrieval to the anxiety cue words in a regression analysis. Similarly, Burke and Mathews (1992) found that GADs judged the memories they recalled to neutral cues as more consistent with "nervous" than with pleasant emotions, although blind judges did not rate the memories recalled by GADs as having more threatening content. The GADs also responded to the request to recall anxious memories more rapidly than to the request to recall non-anxious memories, whereas controls did not differ on this measure. GADs also produced more memories when instructed to provide anxious events than when otherwise instructed; controls showed a reverse trend that was nonsignificant.

The results of these studies are at least suggestive that clearer memory bias effects may be observed with autobiographical material. However, no attempt has yet been made, as has been done in the depression literature, to determine whether this effect might occur because anxious subjects may actually experience more threat or because they encode more events as threatening. The biased encoding hypothesis seems quite plausible given the prominent attentional biases for threatening material associated with anxiety briefly reviewed above, as well as interpretive biases leading to a tendency for anxious individuals to interpret ambiguous information in a threatening manner (see MacLeod and Mathews, 1991, for a review).

In contrast to the generally negative pattern of results for mood-congruent memory biases with generalized anxiety, preliminary evidence suggests a more consistent pattern of positive findings for mood-congruent memory biases in panic disorder. For example, in one study of nonclinical panickers (defined by experiencing at least one panic during the past year), Norton, Cairns, Wozney, and Malan (1988) found that the nonclinical panickers recalled more anxiety-relevant words than did nonpanickers, and more anxiety words than neutral words. However, the methods used in this study were highly unusual (including participating in a group mood induction task), and so should be interpreted with caution. In addition, Nunn, Stevenson, and Whalen (1984) compared agoraphobics with normal controls, with both groups exposed to word lists that supposedly contained both threatening and nonthreatening items. They found that the agoraphobics, unlike the controls, showed superior recall of the threatening words. This study has been criticized by MacLeod and Mathews (1991), however, because many of the "threatening" words would not have been at all threatening to normal controls (e.g., cinema, travel, street) and so the results may reflect that memory is sometimes better for emotional than for neutral information (Bower, 1981). However, in a better controlled study, McNally, Foa, and Donnell (1989) used a self-referenced encoding paradigm and tested for memory of anxiety-relevant and neutral words in subjects with panic disorder and normal controls. Their results indicated that whereas panickers recalled more anxiety-relevant words than neutral words, controls showed the opposite pattern. Finally, Becker, Rinck, and Margraf (1994) tested both implicit and explicit memory biases in panic disordered subjects and controls. On the explicit task, panickers recalled more threat words than other types of words, and more threat words than normals. Unfortunately, their implicit memory results were uninterpretable because of the failure to include an unprimed word list in their implicit task. Thus, although there are as yet relatively few studies, the results seem somewhat more consistent in finding evidence for memory bias in panic disorder than in GAD.

Why might panic disorder and GAD differ in this regard given that anticipatory anxiety is a prominent symptom of panic? One possibility suggested by McNally (personal communication) is that because panic disordered patients are often more severely incapacitated, they may be less capable of cognitively avoiding the kind of elaborative processing that fosters good memory traces which lead to memory biases. Another possibility is that the relevance of the adjectives used in memory studies of panic disorder to the panic patients may be especially high relative to the anxiety words used in the study of GAD. As McNally has suggested, the diversity of worries in GAD is so broad that it may be that many nominally threatening words do not tap the concerns of all GADs, and so they do not engage in elaborative processing necessary to produce explicit memory biases. This interpretation would not necessarily be inconsistent with evidence of the preconscious attentional biases seen in GAD given that at the very early stages of processing where attentional biases occur, research suggests that there is only a sensitivity to valence (e.g., Mogg et al., 1993).

The research results summarized above strongly indicate that the emotional disorders are associated with biased cognitive processing. However, the specific cognitive bias differs for depression and anxiety. Although a selective attentional bias is a robust finding for anxiety, scant evidence exists for a similar attentional bias in depression. In contrast, strong support for an explicit memory bias for depression-relevant information has been found in depression, but no consistent evidence for an explicit memory bias for threatening information has been found in anxiety. The results for mood-congruent implicit memory biases for both anxiety and depression should be considered inconclusive at present given that no published studies have yet used conceptual implicit memory tasks (see Roediger and McDermott, 1992).

Cognitive Biases: Etiology, Maintenance, and Outcome

Although research indicates that cognitive biases are associated with the emotional disorders, albeit different processes with different disorders, the role of these biases in etiology and maintenance of the disorders is less clearly delineated. Several studies have suggested that the biases documented above tend to diminish during remission of the emotional disorder. Mood congruent memory biases, Stroop interference effects, and differences on dichotic listening task differences for negative material were not present following recovery from a depressive episode (see MacLeod and Mathews for review, 1991; Gotlib and Cane, 1987; McCabe and Gotlib, 1993). It should be noted, however, that normal subjects experiencing an induced depressed mood demonstrate some of these biases. Thus, it would be important to explore the strength of a memory bias following a negative mood-induction in individuals with remitted depression in order to provide information about cognitive biases serving as a potential vulnerability to relapse.

There is also evidence that these cognitive biases play a role in the onset of anxiety and depression and may serve the function of reinforcing or enhancing the emotional state (Mineka and Tomarken, 1989; Mineka and Sutton, 1992; Mineka, 1992). One published study has found that information processing biases predict the onset of depression. Using a prospective design, Bellew and Hill (1991) assessed 156 pregnant women with the Beck Depression Inventory (a widely used self-report measure of depressive symptoms) and a measure of recall bias, in which subjects were given an incidental recall task with positive, negative, and self-esteem threatening (SET) words. Subjects who recalled more SET than positive words were considered to be susceptible to depression, and those who recalled more positive than SET words were considered non-susceptible to depression. The two groups did not differ antenatally with respect to BDI scores. When subjects were assessed three months postnatally, susceptible subjects who had experienced stressful life events showed an increase in levels of depressive symptoms; all other groups showed a decrease. Thus, the recall bias for SET events was a significant and useful predictor of depression in subjects who experienced stressful life events. In addition, Bellew and Hill (1990) showed that nonde-pressed subjects who were also categorized as "susceptible" based on the recall bias just described were also more susceptible to a depressive mood induction procedure.

In addition to the Bellew and Hill (1991) study which demonstrated the predictive power of cognitive biases for onset of an emotional disorder, there are also several studies which highlight the predictive value of cognitive biases for the course of a disorder. Dent and Teasdale (1988) conducted a study in which depressed women rated the degree to which each of 26 trait words (some positive, some negative) were descriptive of their personality, a task similar to that used by Derry and Kuiper (1981). The subjects then completed an incidental recall task for these words. Dent and Teasdale reported a high correlation (.8) between the number of negative trait words that were endorsed as self-descriptive and the number of such words recalled on the incidental recall task, and that both of these measures predicted how severely depressed the subjects would be five months later. Even though there were a large number of predictor variables, the number of negative trait words endorsed was the only variable, other than initial level of depression, to significantly predict levels of depression five months later. However, because the self-descriptive rating task and recall measure were so highly correlated, the authors chose not to examine the predictive validity of the incidental recall measure by itself. Future studies using a mood-congruent memory bias index would allow for more direct examination of those variables which predict future depression levels. Such results, in conjunction with results showing judgmental and interpretive biases in depression, have led Teasdale (1988) to propose a vicious cycle of depression. He hypothesizes that if someone is already depressed, then the depression will be perpetuated by a memory bias for remembering the bad events that have happened to him and a tendency to interpret ambiguous events in a negative way.

In another more recent study, Brittlebank, Scott, Williams, and Perrier (1993) followed a sample of 22 patients with Major Depressive Disorder (MDD) for seven months and administered the Hamilton Depression scale (1960; a clinician-administered scale assessing severity of depression), the Dysfunctional Attitudes Scale (the DAS, which is hypothesized to measure underlying depressogenic assumptions and schemas), and a test of auto-biographical memory at initial assessment and at three- and seven-month follow-up. Although the DAS did not predict outcome, overgeneral recall on the autobiographical memory test at the initial assessment (especially for positive memories) was highly correlated with failure to recover from depression. Indeed, overgeneral responses to positively toned words accounted for 33% of the variance in the final Hamilton depression scores; initial Hamilton scores and the DAS were *not* significant predictors.

Theories of Cognition and the Emotional Disorders: Revisions in Light of Current Research

From the review of the research literature it appears that cognitive biases play a prominent role in the emotional disorders. Further, these biases may not only be concomitants of anxiety and depression, but may play a causal role in the onset and course of anxiety and depressive episodes. However, the pattern of these biases is not exactly what was predicted by the theories of Beck and Bower. Although these two models are quite different, both predict that attentional and memory biases should be present in both anxiety and depression as a result of a hypothesized common cognitive mechanism that accounts for mood congruency effects. As the preceding review has demonstrated, neither of these theories can fully account for the current pattern of research findings. Fortunately, in recent years Mathews, Mac-Leod, Watts, and Williams have begun to develop models that can better account for the differential cognitive biases in anxiety and depression (e.g., MacLeod and Mathews, 1991; Mathews, 1993; Williams, Watts, MacLeod, and Mathews, 1988).

The Williams et al. model uses the distinction drawn by Graf and Mandler (1984) between the *activation* or *integration* of mental representations, which is a relatively automatic process, and the *elaboration* of mental representations, which is a more strategic process. Exposure to a stimulus automatically activates an associated schema, leading to a strengthening of the internal organization of the schema which results in the integration of that schema as proposed by Graf and Mandler (1984). The activated schema and its components are more readily accessible, facilitating perception of schema-congruent information and implicit memory performance. It does not, however, necessarily facilitate explicit memory (e.g., recall or recognition) because explicit memory requires more elaborative processing. Elaboration involves developing and strengthening connections between the schema and other contextual cues at encoding, and with other associated representations in memory. Graf and Mandler propose that integration is reflected by performance on implicit memory tests, and that elaboration is reflected by explicit memory test performance.

Building upon the integration/elaboration distinction of Graf and Mandler, Williams et al. (1988) also incorporate Oatley and Johnson-Laird's proposal (1987) that there may be unique modes of cognitive operation associated with each primary emotion. Based on their reading of the pattern of findings on mood-congruent attentional and memory biases discussed above, Williams et al. (see also MacLeod and Mathews, 1991; Mathews, 1993) have proposed that anxiety selectively activates mood-congruent (e.g., threatening) representations, but reduces the tendency to elaborate mood-congruent representations. This would account for the consistent pattern of preconscious (i.e., automatic) attentional biases for threatening material seen in anxious subjects, and the relatively sparse findings for explicit memory biases for threatening material seen in anxious subjects. Indeed, as reviewed above, there is some suggestion that significant biases *against* remembering mood-congruent material are characteristic of anxiety. This theory would also predict the occasional findings of implicit mood-congruent biases in anxiety (e.g., Mathews et al., 1989), but has difficulty explaining the inconsistency of such results unless this inconsistency stems from the failure to use conceptual implicit memory tests in any studies published to date.

In contrast, depression, according to Williams et al. (1988), is characterized by a tendency to elaborate mood-congruent material to a disproportionate degree, but this elaboration does not stem from any special early activation of mood-congruent material. This overelaboration of depression-relevant material would account for the consistent evidence seen in the depression literature for mood-congruent explicit memory biases (but not implicit memory biases), and the relatively sparse and inconsistent evidence for attentional biases for negative information.

The idea that anxiety is characterized by an early, selective attentional bias for threat and avoidance of more elaborate processing of this threat, and that depression is associated with greater elaboration of and memory for depression-relevant information, is consistent with psychoevolutionary theories of cognition and emotion. As discussed earlier, it is believed that cognition has developed as a means of shaping and regulating the adaptive function of emotions. Given that the environmental pressures which shaped the development of depression and anxiety were most likely quite different, it seems likely that distinct modes of information processing would facilitate the function of different emotions (e.g., Mathews, 1993; Oatley and Johnson-Laird, 1987). For example, anxiety, like fear, is associated with the continuous monitoring of the environment for signals of potential threat (e.g., Beck and Emery, 1985; Tellegen, 1985; Gray, 1987), and would require a cognitive system that could quickly scan for and perceive cues for danger. In contrast, depression is associated with reflection on those factors which resulted in failure and/or loss (e.g., Beck, 1967, 1976; Bowlby, 1980; Rehm and Naus, 1990; Tellegen, 1985), and thus would require a cognitive system adept at remembering vital information concerning loss and failure to facilitate reflection (see Mineka, 1992, for further discussion of these issues).

Summary and Suggestions for Future Research

Overall, strong support exists for the belief that biased information processing is characteristic of the emotional disorders. Further, contrary to the two most widely accepted theories about the effects of cognition in the emotional disorders, it appears that anxiety and depression can be differentiated by the nature of the cognitive bias which characterizes each disorder. Selective attentional, but probably not memory, biases for threat or danger strongly characterize the anxiety disorders. In contrast, explicit memory, but probably not attentional, biases for depression-related information are central to depression. Recently, Mathews, MacLeod, Watts, and Williams have begun to formulate models which would account for these contrasting results. For example, the model presented by Williams et al. (1988) can be seen as highly promising in that it provides a better account than do Beck's or Bower's models for the pattern of findings reviewed above for mood-congruent memory and attentional biases associated with anxiety and depression. However, much work remains to be done to test this model and to further understand the role of cognition in the etiology and maintenance of the emotional disorders.

In conclusion, we would like to outline briefly several areas of research on cognitive biases and the emotional disorders that deserve further attention. Presently, most studies examining cognitive biases in anxiety and depression have not included both anxious and depressed individuals within the same study. It is always dangerous to draw strong conclusions based on comparisons of studies conducted with different paradigms and materials. Similarly, no studies have assessed the presence of both attention and memory functioning within the same subject, be s/he anxious or depressed. Thus, it is presently unclear, for example, whether the same anxious individual who demonstrates an attentional bias also does not demonstrate a memory bias. Consequently, future studies must assess both anxious and depressed subjects with the same materials, and examine both memory and attentional processing within the same subject.

The inclusion of both depressed and anxious subjects within the same study as separate subject groups will force researchers to confront the very real issue of the high comorbidity between anxiety and depression. It is somewhat puzzling that anxious and depressed subjects appear to exhibit such distinct patterns of cognition given the high levels of comorbidity of anxiety and depressive symptoms at both the symptom and the syndrome level (e.g., Clark and Watson, 1991a and b). Future research explicitly examining the comorbidity issue will allow one to determine whether comorbid individuals (that is, those who qualify for both an anxiety and a depressive diagnosis) will demonstrate both memory and attentional biases, or whether one bias will dominate. Alternatively, such individuals may exhibit a completely different pattern of information processing.

The role of state versus trait effects in the emotional disorders also needs to be examined more closely. It is currently unclear whether cognitive biases disappear completely upon remission or are merely dormant and become reactivated when a dysphoric or anxious mood is induced. This type of information would not only provide a better understanding of vulnerability to relapse, but could provide insight regarding initial onset of the disorders.

Finally, an individual's cognitive processing abilities (biased and unbiased) probably develop over a period of time, and, in the case of clinical subjects, may change dramatically as an individual moves from a period of crisis to a period of remission. To fully understand the causal role of cognitive biases in the emotional disorders, longitudinal studies should be undertaken that would examine the nature and content of cognitive processing for individuals who have experienced or are at risk for experiencing an emotional disorder.

References

Beck, A. T. 1967. *Depression: Clinical, experimental, and theoretical aspects*. New York: Harper and Row.

Beck, A. T. 1976. *Cognitive therapy and the emotional disorders*. New York: International Universities Press.

Beck, A. and Emery, G. 1985. *Anxiety disorders and phobias: A cognitive perspective*. New York: Basic Books.

Becker, E., Rinck, M., and Margraf, J. 1994. "Memory bias in panic disorder." *Journal of Abnormal Psychology*, 103, 396–399.

Bellew, M. and Hill, B. 1991. "Schematic processing and the prediction of depression following childbirth." *Personality and Individual Differences*, 12, 943–949.

Bellew, M. and Hill, B. 1990. "Negative recall bias as a predictor of susceptibility to induced depressive mood." *Personality and Individual Differences*, 11, 471–480.

Blaney, P. H. 1986. "Affect and memory: A review." *Psychological Bulletin*, 99, 229–246.

Bower, G. H. 1981. "Mood and memory." *American Psychologist*, 36, 129–148.

Bowlby, J. 1980. *Attachment and loss, vol. 3: Loss: Sadness and depression*. Harmondsworth, England: Penguin.

Bradley, B. and Mathews, A. 1988. "Memory bias in recovered clinical depressives." *Cognition and Emotion*, 2, 235–246.

Brittlebank, A. D., Scott, J., Williams, J. M., and Perrier, I. N. 1993. "Autobiographical memory in depression: State or trait marker?" *British Journal of Psychiatry*, 162, 118–121.

Bullington, J. C. 1990. "Mood congruent memory: A replication of symmetrical effects for both positive and negative moods." *Journal of Social Behavior and Personality*, 5, 123–134.

Burke, M. and Mathews, M. 1992. "Autobiographical memory and clinical anxiety." *Cognition and Emotion*, 6, 23–35.

Clark, L. A. and Watson, D. 1991a. "Theoretical and empirical issues in differentiating depression from anxiety." In J. Becker and A. Kleinman (Eds.), *Psychosocial aspects of depression*. Hillsdale, N.J.: Erlbaum.

Clark, L. A. and Watson, D. 1991b. "Tripartite model of anxiety and depression: Psychometric evidence and taxonomic implications." *Journal of Abnormal Psychology,* 100, 316–336.

Clark, D. M. and Teasdale, J. D. 1982. "Diurnal variation in clinical depression and accessibility of memories of positive and negative experiences." *Journal Abnormal Psychology,* 91, 87–95.

Cook, M., and Mineka, S. 1989. "Observational conditioning of fear to fear-relevant versus fear-irrelevant stimuli in rhesus monkeys." *Journal of Abnormal Psychology,* 98, 448–459.

Cook, M., and Mineka, S. 1990. "Selective associations in the observational conditioning of fear in monkeys." *Journal of Experimental Psychology: Animal Behavior Processes,* 16, 372–389.

Cook, M., and Mineka, S. 1991. "Selective associations in the origins of phobic fears and their implications for behavior therapy." In P. Martin (Ed.), *Handbook of behavior therapy and psychological science: An integrative approach.* New York: Pergamon.

Delprato, D. 1980. "Hereditary determinants of fears and phobias." *Behavior Therapy,* 11, 79–103.

Denny, E. and Hunt, R. 1992. "Affective valence and memory in depression: Dissociation of recall and fragment completion." *Journal of Abnormal Psychology,* 101, 575–582.

Dent, J. and Teasdale, J. 1988. "Negative cognition and the persistence of depression." *Journal of Abnormal Psychology,* 97, 29–34.

Derry, P. and Kuiper, N. 1981. "Schematic processing and self-reference in clinical depression." *Journal of Abnormal Psychology,* 90, 286–297.

Eysenck, M. 1989. "Anxiety and cognition: Theory and research." In T. Archer and L. G. Nilsson (Eds.), *Aversion, avoidance and anxiety.* Hillsdale, N.J.: Erlbaum.

Foa, E., McNally, R., and Murdock, T. 1989. "Anxious mood and memory." *Behaviour Research and Therapy,* 27, 141–147.

Gotlib, I. H. and Cane, D. B. 1987. "Construct accessibility and clinical depression: A longitudinal approach." *Journal of Abnormal Psychology,* 96, 199–204.

Graf, P. and Mandler, G. 1984. "Activation makes words more accessible, but not necessarily more retrievable." *Journal of Verbal Learning and Verbal Behaviour,* 23, 553–568.

Gray, J. A. 1987. *The psychology of fear and stress.* New York: Cambridge University Press.

Gray, J. A. 1990. "Brain systems that mediate both emotion and cognition." *Cognition and Emotion,* 4, 269–288.

Hamilton, M. 1960. "A rating scale for depression." *Journal of Neurology, Neurosurgery and Psychiatry,* 12, 56–62.

Hertel, P. and Hardin, T. 1990. "Remembering with and without awareness in a depressed mood: Evidence for deficits in initiative." *Journal of Experimental Psychology: General,* 119, 45–59.

Kahneman, D. and Chajczyk, D. 1983. "Tests of the automaticity of reading: dilution of Stroops effects by color-irrelevant stimuli." *Journal of Experimental Psychology: Human Experimental Psychology,* 9, 497–509.

Lloyd, G. and Lishman, W. 1975. "Effects of depression on the speed of recall of pleasant and unpleasant experiences." *Psychological Medicine, 5,* 173–180.

MacLeod, C., Mathews, A., and Tata, P. 1986. "Attentional biases in emotional disorders." *Journal of Abnormal Psychology, 95,* 15–20.

MacLeod, C. and Mathews, A. M. 1991. "Cognitive-experimental approaches to the emotional disorders." In P. Martin (Ed.), *Handbook of behavior therapy and psychological science.* New York: Pergamon Press, pp. 116–150.

MacLeod, C. and Mathews, A. 1988. "Anxiety and the allocation of attention to threat." *Quarterly Journal of Experimental Psychology: Human Experimental Psychology, 38,* 659–670.

Mathews, A., Mogg, K., May, J., and Eysenk, M. 1989. "Implicit and explicit memory bias in anxiety." *Journal of Abnormal Psychology, 98,* 236–240.

Mathews, A. 1993. "Anxiety and the processing of emotional information." In L. Chapman, J. Chapman, and D. Fowles (Eds.), *Models and methods of psychopathology: Progress in experimental personality and psychopathology research.* New York: Springer.

Mathews, A., May, J., Mogg, K., and Eysenk, M. 1990. "Attentional bias in anxiety: Selective search or defective filtering." *Journal of Abnormal Psychology, 99,* 166–173.

Matt, G., Vazquez, C., and Campbell, W. K. 1992. "Mood-congruent recall of affectively toned stimuli: A meta-analytical review." *Clinical Psychology Review,* 12, 227–255.

McCabe, S. B. and Gotlib, I. H. 1993. "Attentional processing in clinically depressed subjects: A longitudinal investigation." *Cognitive Therapy and Research,* 17, 359–377.

McNally, R. J., Foa, E. B., and Donnell, C. D. 1989. "Memory bias for anxiety information in patients with panic disorder." *Cognition and Emotion, 3,* 27–44.

Mineka, S. 1992. "Evolutionary memories, emotional processing and the emotional disorders." In D. Medin (Ed.), *The psychology of learning and motivation, vol. 28.* New York: Academic Press, pp. 161–206.

Mineka, S. and Tomarken, A. 1989. "The role of cognitive biases in the origins and maintenance of fear and anxiety disorders." In T. Archer and L. Nilsson (Eds.), *Aversion, avoidance, and anxiety: Perspectives on aversively motivated behavior.* Hillsdale, N.J.: Erlbaum, pp. 195–221.

Mineka, S. and Sutton, S. 1992. "Cognitive biases and the emotional disorders." *Special Section on Emotion in Psychological Science, 3,* 65–69.

Mogg, K., and Mathews, A. 1990. "Is there a self-referent mood-congruent bias in anxiety?" *Behaviour Research and Therapy, 28,* 91–92.

Mogg, K., Mathews, A., and Weinman, J. 1987. "Memory bias in clinical anxiety." *Journal of Abnormal Psychology, 96,* 94–98.

Mogg, K., Mathews, A., Bird, C., and McGregor-Morris, R. 1990. "Effects of stress and anxiety on the processing of threat stimuli." *Journal of Personality and Social Psychology, 59,* 1230–1237.

Mogg, K., Bradley, B. P., Williams, R., and Mathews, A. 1993. "Subliminal processing of emotional information." *Journal of Abnormal Psychology, 102,* 304–311.

Mogg, K., Gardiner, J. M., Stavroy, A., and Golombok, S. 1992. "Recollective experience and the recognition memory for threat in clinical anxiety states." *Bulletin of the Psychonomic Society,* 30, 109–112.

Norton, R. G., Cairns, S. L., Wozney, K. A., and Malan, J. 1988. "Panic attacks and psychopathology in nonclinical panicker." *Journal of Anxiety Disorders,* 2, 319–331.

Nugent, K. and Mineka, S. 1994. "The effects of high and low trait anxiety on implicit and explicit memory tasks." *Cognition and Emotion,* 8, 147–163.

Nunn, J., Stevenson, R., and Whalen, G. 1984. "Selective memory effects in agoraphobic patients." *British Journal of Clinical Psychology,* 23, 195–201.

Oatley, K. and Johnson-Laird, P. 1987. "Towards a cognitive theory of emotions." *Cognition and Emotion,* 1, 29–50.

Öhman, A. 1986. "Face the beast and fear the face: Animal and social fears as prototypes for evolutionary analyses of emotion." *Psychophysiology,* 23, 123–145.

Öhman, A., Dimberg, U., and Öst, L.-G. 1985. "Animal and social phobias: Biological constraints on learned fear responses." In S. Reiss and R. Bootzin (Eds.), *Theoretical issues in behavior therapy.* New York: Academic Press.

Parrott, W. G. 1991. "Mood induction and instructions to sustain moods: A test of the subject compliance hypothesis of mood congruent memory." *Cognition and Emotion,* 5, 41–52.

Plutchik, R. 1984. "Emotions: A general psychoevolutionary theory." In K. Scherer and P. Ekman (Eds.), *Approaches to emotion.* Hillsdale, N.J.: Erlbaum.

Rehm, L. and Naus, M. 1990. "A memory model of emotion." In R. Ingram (Ed.), *Contemporary psychological approaches to depression.* New York: Plenum Press.

Richards, A. and French, C. 1991. "Effects of encoding and anxiety on implicit and explicit memory performance." *Personality and Individual Differences,* 12, 131–139.

Richards, A. and Whittaker, T. 1990. "Effects of anxiety and mood manipulation in autobiographical memory." *British Journal of Clinical Psychology,* 29, 145–154.

Roediger, H. and McDermott, K. 1992. "Depression and implicit memory: A commentary." *Journal of Abnormal Psychology,* 101, 587–591.

Roediger, H. 1990. "Implicit memory: Retention without remembering." *American Psychologist,* 45, 1043–1056.

Rumelhart, D. E. and Ortony, A. 1977. "The representation of knowledge in memory." In R. C. Anderson, R. Shapiro, and W. Montague (Eds.), *Schooling and the acquisition of knowledge.* Hillsdale, N.J.: Erlbaum.

Rusted, J. M. and Dighton, K. 1991. "Selective processing of threat-related material by spider phobics in a prose recall task." *Cognition and Emotion,* 5, 123–132.

Schacter, D. L. 1987. "Implicit memory: History and current status." *Journal of Experimental Psychology: Learning, Memory, and Cognition,* 13, 501–518.

Seligman, M. 1971. "Phobias and preparedness." *Behavior Therapy,* 2, 307–320.

Singer, J. and Salovey, P. 1988. "Mood and memory: Evaluating the network theory of affect." *Clinical Psychology Review,* 8, 211–251.

Teasdale, J. D. 1988. "Cognitive vulnerability to persistent depression." *Cognition and Emotion*, 2, 247–274.

Teasdale, J. D. and Fogarty, S. 1979. "Differential effects of induced mood on retrieval of pleasant and unpleasant events from episodic memory." *Journal of Abnormal Psychology*, 88, 248–257.

Tellegen, A. 1985. "Structures of mood and personality and their relevance to assessing anxiety, with an emphasis on self-report." In A. H. Tuma and J. D. Maser (Eds.), *Anxiety and the anxiety disorders*. Hillsdale, N.J.: Erlbaum, pp. 681–706.

Watkins, P., Mathews, A., Williamson, D. A., and Uller, R. D. 1992. "Mood-congruent memory in depression: Emotional priming or elaboration?" *Journal of Abnormal Psychology*, 101, 581–586.

Watts, F. N. and Coyle, K. 1992. "Recall bias for stimulus and response anxiety words in spider phobics." *Anxiety Research*, 4, 315–323.

Watts, F., McKenna, F. P., Sharrock, R., and Trezise, L. 1986. "Processing of phobic stimuli." *British Journal of Clinical Psychology*, 25, 253–261.

Watts, F., and Dagleish, T. 1991. "Memory for phobia-related words in spider phobics." *Cognition and Emotion*, 5, 313–329.

Williams, M., Watts, F., MacLeod, C., and Mathews, A. 1988. *Cognitive psychology and the emotional disorders*. Chichester, England: Wiley.

Williams, M. and Dritschel, B. 1988. "Emotional disturbance and the specificity of autobiographical memory." *Cognition and Emotion*, 2, 221–234.

Williams, M., and Scott, J. 1988. "Autobiographical memory in depression." *Psychological Medicine*, 12, 63–70.

Neuropsychological Perspectives

Biological Foundations of Accuracy and Inaccuracy in Memory

Larry R. Squire

> I had during many years followed a golden rule, namely, that whenever a published fact, a new observation or thought, came across me which was opposed to my general results, to make a memorandum of it without fail and at once; for I had found by experience that such facts and thoughts were far more apt to escape from the memory than favorable ones.
>
> *Charles Darwin, 1876*

Some empirical questions are difficult to answer because they are not readily approached with simple and straightforward experiments. Others are difficult because impressions from personal experience, sociopolitical issues, or religious beliefs complicate the science. The contemporary study of memory provides some interesting illustrations of this problem—apparently simple questions that have nevertheless become the subject of debate. Are memories usually accurate? Are memories readily vulnerable to distortion? Are memories ever really lost, or are they only subject to degrees of inaccessibility, which can potentially be reversed? Can memories be apparently lost for a lengthy period and then resurface as accurate recollections of the past?

It seems reasonable to suppose that a useful starting point for examining these matters is to ask how the brain actually accomplishes learning and memory. Memory is a fundamental adaptive capacity of organisms. Animals inherit in the structure of their nervous systems many behavioral adaptations that were developed during millions of years of evolution. They also inherit the potential to adapt or change as the result of events occurring during an individual lifetime. Because of this adaptation, the experiences that an animal has can modify its nervous system, and it will later behave differently as a result. This ability to change gives animals the capacity for learning and memory. Understanding the biology of learning and memory should provide a useful, and perhaps essential, foundation for addressing the questions about memory and memory distortion that form the subject matter of this volume.

This chapter focuses on three aspects of the biology of memory that are relevant to discussions of accuracy and inaccuracy in recall. The first topic is the fundamental idea that memory is not a single faculty but consists of different systems that depend on different brain structures and connections. The key distinction is between the capacity for conscious recall of facts and events (declarative memory) and a heterogeneous collection of nonconscious learning abilities that are expressed through performance (nondeclarative memory). In the context of the topic of memory distortion, the distinction between kinds of memory raises questions about what it means to have a nonconscious memory, how conscious and nonconscious memories might (or might not) interact, and whether or not a nonconscious memory could provide the basis, i.e., a cue, for consciously recollecting an event that would otherwise be inaccessible.

The second topic is the almost century-old concept of memory consolidation. Consolidation refers to the idea that memory is not fixed at the time of learning but continues to change and be reorganized as time passes. In recent years the consolidation concept has become more concrete and specific. Consolidation has been related to declarative memory, to the medial temporal lobe memory system, and to the discovery that the function of this brain system is only temporary. It is needed for a limited period of time after learning, i.e., during the consolidation process. In the context of the topic of memory distortion, the facts of memory consolidation are relevant to questions about the malleability of memory as time passes after original learning.

The third topic concerns the observation that one can sometimes recall a fact, a name, or an idea without being able to remember where or when the information was acquired. It has recently been appreciated that this phenomenon, termed "source amnesia," is related to frontal lobe pathology and that it can occur independently of the strength of the memory itself—that is, source amnesia is not a simple consequence of weak memory. In the context of the topic of memory distortion, the phenomenon of source memory is relevant to questions about the process by which recollections of past events are distinguished from visual images, dreams, and other mental content.

To approach these three issues—multiple memory systems, consolidation, and source memory—it is useful to review first some key principles about memory and the brain, including the special importance of the medial temporal lobe for declarative memory.

Visual Perception and Visual Memory.   Figure 7.1 shows a diagram of visual information processing in the primate neocortex. The visual system is organized such that visual processing begins caudally and then moves rostrally through many stations, both in series and in parallel. A ventral stream of processing continues forward to the inferotemporal cortex (area TE), a higher-order cortical visual area that is concerned with achieving representa-

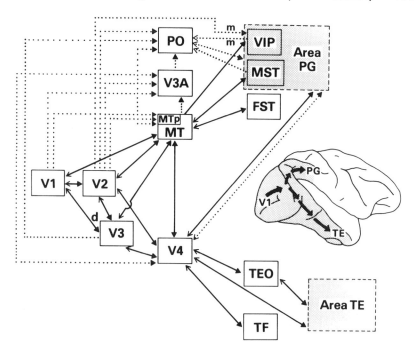

Figure 7.1 Schematic diagram of the cortical visual areas in the macaque monkey and their interconnections. There are two major routes from striate cortex (V1): One follows a ventral route into the temporal lobe via area V4, and the other follows a dorsal route into the parallel lobe via MT. Solid lines indicate projections involving all portions of the visual field representation in an area, whereas dotted lines indicate projections limited to the representation of the peripheral visual field. The projections between V4 and PG are heavier from the peripheral visual field. Heavy arrowheads indicate "forward" projections, and light arrowheads indicate "backward" projections. Two reciprocal arrowheads indicate intermediate projections. "d" indicates projections limited to the dorsal portion of V3. "m" indicates projections limited to the medial portions of PO and VIP. (From Desimone and Ungerleider, 1989.)

tions about the visual quality of objects. A dorsal stream continues forward to the parietal cortex (area PG) and is concerned with achieving representations about the location of objects in space and the computations needed to reach these locations (Cavanagh, 1993; Goodale, 1983; Merigan and Maunsell, 1993; Ungerleider and Mishkin, 1982; Van Essen, Anderson, and Felleman, 1992; Young, 1992). Current understanding is that long-term, permanent memory is stored in the same distributed assembly of structures that are needed to process and analyze what is to be remembered (Mishkin, 1982; Squire, 1987). Memory is a normal consequence of perception, and memories are stored as outcomes of perceptual analysis.

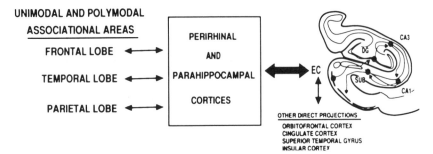

Figure 7.2 Schematic representation of the medial temporal lobe memory system in the monkey. The width of the arrows corresponds to the relative proportion of cortical inputs from the areas indicated. Abbreviations: EC, entorhinal cortex; DG, dentate gyrus; SUB, subicular complex; CA3 and CA1, fields of the hippocampus proper. (From Squire et al., 1990.)

The information processed in the visual cortex reaches a number of cortical and subcortical targets—including for example the amygdala, the striatum, the pons, the orbital frontal cortex, and (what is important for the present purposes) the entorhinal cortex and related structures of the medial temporal lobe. One important hint about the brain organization of memory functions comes from the finding that, whereas damage to or removal of visual processing areas (e.g., V4 or MT) results in specific visuoperceptual deficits, damage to or removal of structures within the medial temporal lobe produces a memory impairment. The medial temporal lobe is a major target of neocortical processing, and it works in concert with the neocortex to permit the lasting effects of perceptual experience that we call memory.

The Medial Temporal Lobe Memory System.   The importance of the medial temporal lobe for human memory functions has been appreciated since the 1950s (Scoville and Milner, 1957). However, identifying the specific structures and connections within this region that are important for memory became possible only after the development in the early 1980s of an animal model of human amnesia in the monkey (Mishkin, 1982; Squire and Zola-Morgan, 1983; Mahut and Moss, 1984). Cumulative experimental work with monkeys based on this animal model, together with occasional new data from memory-impaired patients, has indicated that the important structures are the hippocampus (including the hippocampus proper, dentate gyrus, and subicular complex) and adjacent, anatomically related cortex (entorhinal, perirhinal, and parahippocampal cortices) (Squire and Zola-Morgan, 1991; Zola-Morgan and Squire, 1993; see Figure 7.2).

Human Amnesia.   While studies of experimental animals have been essential to identify anatomical substrates of memory, many important insights about the functional organization of memory have come from the study of

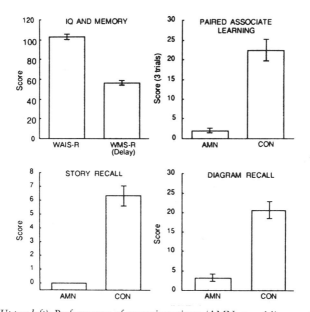

Figure 7.3 (Upper left): Performance of amnesic patients (AMN, n = 14) on a standard intelligence test (Full Scale WAIS-R Wechsler Adult Intelligence Scale–Revised) and on a standard memory test (WMS-R, Wechsler Memory Scale–Revised Delay Index). In the normal population, both tests yield average scores of 100 with a standard deviation of 15. Also shown is performance of the same amnesic patients and 8 control subjects (CON) on three tests of new learning ability. *(Upper right):* Paired-associated learning measures the ability to learn unrelated word pairs by reporting the second word in a pair when cued with the first word (10 pairs, 3 trials, maximum score = 30). *(Lower left):* Story recall measures delayed (12 min) retention of a short prose passage consisting of 21 meaning segments (maximum score = 21). *(Lower right):* Diagram recall measures the ability to reconstruct a complex line drawing (Rey-Osterreith figure) from memory after a 12-min delay (maximum score = 36). Brackets show S.E.M. See Squire and Shimamura (1986) for additional description of these tests. (From Squire et al., 1990.)

memory impairment in neurological patients. This condition, termed amnesia, can occur following surgery, head injury, stroke, ischemia, anoxia, or disease (Mayes, 1988; Shimamura, 1989; Squire Knowlton, and Musen, 1993). The modern era of these studies began in the 1950s with the demonstration that profound memory impairment sometimes occurs in isolation from other cognitive impairment (Scoville and Milner, 1957). In such cases the memory deficit extends to both verbal and nonverbal material, and across all sensory modalities. Language and general intellectual ability are intact (Figure 7.3). This dissociation between memory and intellectual ability demonstrates that the brain has to some extent separated its perceptual and intellectual functions from its capacity to lay down in memory the records that ordinarily result from engaging in perceptual and intellectual work.

Altogether, one can identify three features of human amnesia, which indicate that the deficit is best understood as belonging to the domain of memory and not some other aspect of cognition (Alvarez, Zola-Morgan, and Squire, 1994). First, amnesia is a multi-modal deficit that affects memory regardless of the sensory modality that initially processes the information. Second, immediate memory (or short-term memory) is intact. The difficulty in amnesia is in placing new information into long-term memory, a deficit best demonstrated by testing material after a delay of a few minutes or more. Third, retrograde amnesia (i.e., the loss of premorbid memories) is typically temporally-graded, affecting recent memory but leaving more remote memories intact. These same three features identify the memory impairments exhibited by rats and monkeys (Squire, 1992).

Functional Amnesia.   It is worth distinguishing the neurological form of amnesia, just described, from functional (or psychogenic) amnesia. Functional amnesia has been popularized in literature and film but is much rarer than the kinds of amnesia that result from neurological injury or disease. Functional amnesias typically do not impair new learning capacity. In such cases, patients are usually able to store a continuing record of ongoing events, from the moment they are encountered by the clinician. The principal symptom of functional amnesia is retrograde amnesia, which can even include an inability to recall one's own name. Some patients with functional amnesia have partial retrograde memory loss that includes autobiographical memories but spares memory for public events and facts about the world. Other patients have retrograde memory loss that covers a particular time period (for a representative case, see Schacter, Wang, Tulving, and Freedman, 1982). In any case, functional amnesias belong to the realm of psychiatry and dissociative disorders (Kenny, 1986; Nemiah, 1989), not to the realm of neurology and the memory systems of the brain.

Multiple Memory Systems

One of the profound insights about memory to emerge in the past decade is that memory is not a single entity but is composed of several different abilities (Squire, 1982; Weiskrantz, 1987; Mishkin, et al., 1984; Tulving, 1985; Schacter, 1987; Schacter and Tulving, 1994). This idea is true not just in a philosophical or a semantic sense but in the specific biological sense that different kinds of memory have different brain organizations and depend on different brain systems. Prior to this development, memory was understood to vary in strength and accessibility, but it could be conceptualized as a single biological and psychological phenomenon. Psychology has

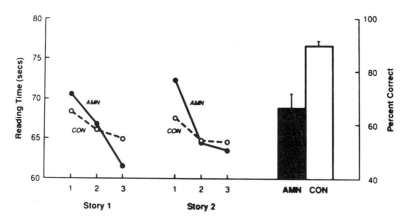

Figure 7.4 Time required to read aloud two different stories, each presented three times in succession (AMN, amnesic patients, n = 8; CON, control subjects, n = 9). Each story contained about 20 lines of text. The bars show the performance of each group on a test of story content given immediately after the final reading of the second story (chance = 33%). Brackets show S.E.M. (From Musen et al., 1990.)

emerged from its reliance on intuition and introspection, which characterized much of psychological argument in the nineteenth and early twentieth centuries. During the past few decades, with the emergence of neuroscience, psychology has begun to be informed by progress in the understanding of brain systems.

Some of the most compelling evidence for the newer view came from the finding that amnesic patients, who are severely impaired on conventional memory tests that assess recall or recognition, are nevertheless fully intact on many other kinds of learning and memory. A few examples serve to illustrate the kinds of memory tasks that amnesic patients can accomplish. In one study (Musen, Shimamura, and Squire, 1990), subjects were asked to read aloud a passage of prose (about 20 lines). When normal subjects read the same passage three times in succession, they read it a little faster each time. Amnesic patients improved their reading speed at the same rate as normal subjects (Figure 7.4). It is also important to note that, when normal subjects and amnesic patients attempted a second prose passage, they returned initially to a slower reading speed and then improved on the second passage. This finding shows that the facilitation in reading speed is not a result of some nonspecific effect, such as becoming gradually more comfortable reading aloud. Rather, the facilitation is text-specific, i.e., specific to the words and perhaps to the ideas and associations in the text.

In contrast to their normal and intact learning, as measured by reading speed, amnesic patients were markedly impaired in comparison to normal subjects on a multiple-choice test that asked subjects about the content of the stories they had just read. This test was given immediately after the patients completed the third reading of the second passage. The results suggest that the kind of memory that subjects used to read the story faster each time is fundamentally different from the kind of memory subjects used to remember the content of the story.

A second example of preserved memory performance comes from the domain of priming. Priming refers to a facilitation in the ability to detect or identify stimuli based on their recent presentation (Shimamura, 1986; Tulving and Schacter, 1990; Schacter et al., 1993). Amnesic patients exhibit fully intact priming effects, whether the test materials are written words, spoken words, familiar objects, nonwords, novel objects, or line patterns. In a typical experiment, subjects see lists of words, drawings of objects, or nonverbal material. Subsequently, subjects are tested with both old and new items and asked to name items, produce items from fragments, or to make rapid decisions about items. Priming is demonstrated by the finding that performance is better on old items than new items.

In one study, amnesic patients and control subjects studied words and nonwords and were then given a perceptual identification test with briefly presented new and old items. Amnesic patients exhibited entirely normal priming for both words and nonwords (Haist, Musen, and Squire, 1991). In contrast, the amnesic patients were impaired at recognizing as familiar the items that had appeared on the priming test. That is, they were impaired at discriminating the words that had appeared on the test from other words.

The final example of preserved memory in amnesia grew out of efforts to extend to human subjects the kind of habit learning that has been studied in experimental animals, for example, win-stay, lose-shift tasks of operant conditioning in which information is acquired gradually across many trials. The challenge had been that human subjects attempt to memorize whatever material they are given to learn, i.e., they attempt to use the kind of memory that is impaired in amnesia. To determine whether human subjects can accomplish habit learning independently of this kind of memory, a task was adopted that had been used previously to study probabilistic classification learning (Gluck and Bower, 1988). Because the associations between stimuli and responses are probabilistic, information from a single trial is unreliable and efforts at trial-by-trial memorization cannot be very successful.

The task was presented to subjects as a problem of weather prediction (Knowlton, Squire, and Gluck, 1994; see Figure 7.5). Subjects had to learn which of two outcomes (rain or shine) was predicted by combinations of 1, 2, or 3 out of 4 different cues. Each cue was independently associated to each outcome with a fixed probability. The four cues were associated with sunshine approximately 75%, 57%, 43%, or 25% of the time. With the two cues shown in the sample trial of Figure 7.5, sunshine is the outcome 82% of the time. On each trial, subjects were told to guess whether the

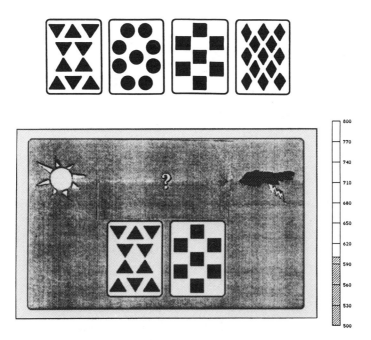

Figure 7.5 (Top): Four cues used to test probabilistic classification learning. *(Bottom):* The appearance of the computer screen on a typical trial of the same task. Subjects had to decide whether the display of cards predicted rain or shine. Feedback (correct or incorrect) was given after each response, and the vertical scale to the right increased one unit for each correct response and decreased by one unit for each incorrect response.

pattern of cards predicted rain or shine. Immediately after making each choice, subjects were told whether they were right or wrong.

Figure 7.6 shows the results for three different experiments involving three different variations of the same basic task (weather prediction using the four stimuli shown in Figure 7.5, weather prediction using different stimuli, or diagnosis of fictitious diseases using four symptoms). The probabilistic relationship between the 4 cues and the 2 outcomes was always the same, as described above. Amnesic patients exhibited the same gradual improvement as normal subjects during the first 50 trials of training. Performance improved from about 50% correct to about 65% correct. The verbal reports of the subjects suggested that they understood very little about what they had learned. Many felt they were simply guessing. In contrast to the good performance of the amnesic patients on the habit learning task, the amnesic patients performed very poorly on multiple-choice tests that asked about the training episode itself (Figure 7.7).

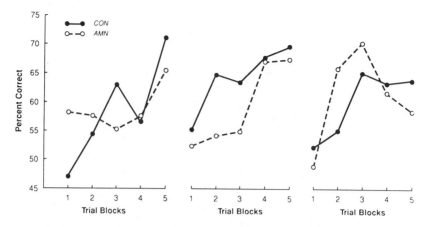

Figure 7.6 Percentage of correct performance for the control subjects (CON) and the amnesic patients (AMN) during 50 learning trials (5 blocks of 10 trials) on each of three different tasks of probabilistic classification learning. The first task was the one illustrated in Figure 7.5, and the other two were structurally similar. Chance performance = 50%. (From Knowlton and Squire, 1994.)

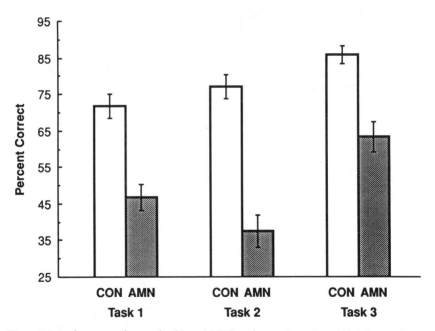

Figure 7.7 Performance of control subjects (CON) and amnesic patients (AMN) on a 4-choice, multiple-choice test given immediately after each of three tasks of probabilistic classification learning. The tests asked about the training session, e.g., the layout of the screen, the nature of the stimuli, and the number of trials that had been given. Brackets show S.E.M. (From Knowlton and Squire, 1994.)

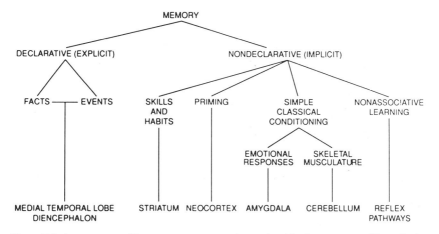

Figure 7.8 A taxonomy of long-term memory and associated brain structures. (From Squire and Knowlton, 1994.)

A Taxonomy of Memory.   Figure 7.8 distinguishes two major forms of long-term memory—declarative and nondeclarative. Several lines of evidence suggest that amnesia has revealed a biologically natural division in how the nervous system acquires, stores, and retrieves information. Declarative memory is dependent on the brain system damaged in amnesia. However, the distinction is not defined simply by listing what amnesic patients can and cannot do. Declarative memory has different operating characteristics than nondeclarative memory (Sherry and Schacter, 1987; Squire, 1994). Declarative memory is fast, specialized for one-trial learning and for forming associations between arbitrarily different stimuli (as in paired-associate learning). Declarative memory refers to the capacity for having conscious recollections of recently occurring facts and events.

In contrast to declarative memory, nondeclarative memory is not a brain-systems construct. Rather, nondeclarative memory refers to a heterogeneous collection of abilities, all of which are independent of the structures damaged in amnesia. Nondeclarative memory refers to ways in which performance can change but without requiring access to any conscious memory content. In this sense, nondeclarative memory is nonconscious. Information is acquired as changes within perceptual or response systems, or as changes encapsulated as habits, skills, or conditioned responses, and these changes are expressed through performance without any sense of memory being involved, without any sense of "pastness."

Many forms of nondeclarative memory can be related to particular brain systems (see Figure 7.8). Accordingly, one would not expect to find a condition in which all nondeclarative memory is impaired, while declarative memory is spared. At the same time, it is possible for particular forms of nonde-clarative memory to be impaired without affecting declarative memory (Packard, Hirsh, and White, 1989; Saint-Cyr, Taylor, and Lang, 1988; Hein-del, Salmon, and Butters, 1991; Zola-Morgan, Squire, and Mishkin, 1982).

Figure 7.8 introduces a number of terms, most importantly declarative and nondeclarative, or explicit and implicit. Bernard Katz once quoted his colleague, William Feldberg, as saying: "There is a type of scientist who, if given the choice, would rather use his colleague's toothbrush than his terminology" (Katz, 1969, p. 41). In this context, it is perhaps worth empha-sizing that terminology is not the important issue. Rather, the issue is that what is here termed declarative memory is a brain-systems construct, a kind of memory dependent on the integrity of the medial temporal lobe-diencephalic brain system that is damaged in amnesia. In other words, the distinction between one kind of memory and other kinds is prominently reflected in the organization of brain systems.

It has sometimes been proposed that distinctions between forms of mem-ory are better understood as reflecting different processes that can be en-gaged to access a common memory trace (Blaxton, 1989; Jacoby, 1988; Masson, 1989; Roediger, 1990; Shanks and St. John, 1994). However, the available biological information shows not only that different brain systems support different kinds of memory but that the physical locus of the long-term memory trace can be separate and distinct from one kind of memory to another (Squire et al., 1993; Schacter, 1992; Squire, Hamann, and Knowl-ton, 1994). Accordingly, when the discussion of memory systems is broad-ened to include not only behavioral data from normal subjects but also anatomy, physiology, behavioral neuroscience, and neuropsychology, the systems view of memory seems to be the correct one.

Interaction between Memory Systems?   The idea that memory is supported by both conscious and nonconscious systems raises questions about what opportunities might exist for interaction between these systems. In consider-ing how past experience can affect ongoing cognition and behavior, it is significant what view one takes about the nature of memory. By the tradi-tional view, memory is a single faculty of the mind, and memory varies mainly in strength and accessibility. By this formulation, information that is unconscious is below some threshold of accessibility and could potentially be made available to awareness. In contrast, according to the view that there are multiple forms of memory, the unconscious does not become conscious. Thus, information might be stored as a habit—as a disposition to behave in a particular way—but without affording any conscious memory content. Experience cumulates in altered perceptions, dispositions, preferences, and conditioned responses, but expression of these behaviors does not carry with it any awareness that behavior is in fact being influenced by past experience.

One might acquire new habits or change the stimuli that elicit a behavior. However, one does not become aware of the content of the habit nor experience it as a memory.

Although nondeclarative memory does not itself become declarative, one can ask whether nondeclarative memory might facilitate declarative memory by providing a cue for its retrieval. Can nondeclarative memory provoke a conscious recollection? For example, in the case of priming, can the fluency that one gains from item presentation subsequently provide a basis for judging the word familiar? Can word priming cause words to be consciously remembered? Along these lines, some investigators have suggested that subjects might sometimes use perceptual fluency as a heuristic to judge an item as familiar, even when that item has not been presented previously (Jacoby and Whitehouse, 1989; Johnston, Hawley, and Elliott, 1991; Mandler, 1980; Whittlesea, 1993).

A recent study addressed these issues by asking whether in ordinary recognition memory tasks the recognition responses are supported in part by perceptual fluency, i.e., priming. If priming can support recognition performance to any significant extent, then the relationship between recognition and recall performance should be different in amnesic patients than in normal subjects. In both subject groups, recognition should be superior to recall because it is typically easier to recognize recently presented items than to recall them. However, in amnesic patients recognition memory should be disproportionately better than would be expected from the level of recall.

In the study (Haist, Shimamura, and Squire, 1992), subjects were tested on 12 different occasions over a period of two years. On each test occasion they were presented with 20 words and then were tested for retention of the words at a variable interval from 15 seconds to 8 weeks. Six of the retention tests were tests of free recall, and six were tests of forced-choice, two-choice recognition memory. The left side of Figure 7.9 shows that amnesic patients were impaired at both recall and recognition. The right side of this figure shows that their performance on the recognition test was strictly proportional to their performance on free recall. If recognition were supported at all by priming, which is intact in amnesia, then recognition performance should have been disproportionately spared.

The results show that recognition memory does not ordinarily draw any special support from nondeclarative, nonconscious memory. Stated differently, the potential contribution of nonconscious memory processes to recognition performance is no greater than the contribution of nonconscious processes to free recall. Thus, the evidence suggests that priming does not cause words to be consciously recollected. Similar conclusions were reached in a recent study using a different method (Knowlton and Squire, 1994).

On reflection, it is perhaps advantageous that nonconscious memory, for example, perceptual fluency, does not lead ordinarily to a feeling of familiar-

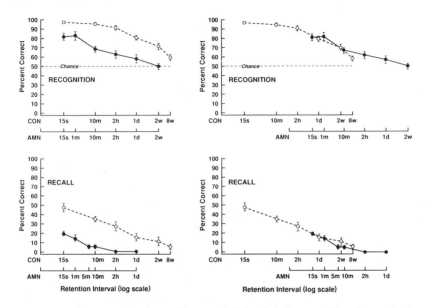

Figure 7.9 Performance of patients with amnesia (*closed circles,* n = 12) and control subjects (*open circles,* n = 19), on tests of recognition (12-alternative, forced choice; *upper panels*) or free recall *(lower panels).* Memory for a different 20-word list was tested at each of the indicated delays after learning. Control subjects were tested at relatively long intervals after learning so that their performance could be evaluated at a time when it was as poor as that of the amnesic patients. *Left panels:* Impaired performance of the amnesic patients as measured by both free recall and recognition. *Right panels:* The curves in the two left panels have been redrawn such that the performance of amnesic patients on the recognition test approximately equaled that of control subjects. When the recognition scores matched, the performance curves for free recall also matched (i.e., the amnesic patients tested 15s, 1 min, and 10 min after learning matched the control subjects tested 1 day and 2 weeks after learning). The results show that recognition does not draw support from nondeclarative memory any more than recall does. Brackets show standard errors of the mean. No error bar indicates < 2%. (From Haist, Shimamura, and Squire, 1992.)

ity. Rapid detection of a perceptual object does not reliably signal that the object has been encountered recently, i.e., that it is familiar. An object might be detected rapidly because it moved or because one has a long-standing preference for such an object. At the same time, it should be recognized that nonconscious memory processes do have the potential to evoke conscious mental states, for example, because perceptual fluency draws one's attention to an object, or because one makes an unexpected response to a stimulus, or a surprising emotional response to some object. Indeed, one could say that the neocortex is available to interpret any conscious mental content that is produced. It is then a separate question whether such content refers to a memory or not, and, if a memory, whether the memory is accurate or inaccurate. The remaining topics to be discussed, memory consolidation and source memory, identify some of the factors that make declarative memory prone to inaccuracy.

Memory Consolidation

It has long been appreciated that memory is not fixed at the time of learning but takes time to develop its permanent form. This process takes longer than the time needed for protein synthesis to occur and for neuronal growth processes to be initiated. In other words, the fixation process does not simply mark the time needed for a short-term biological process to give way to a more enduring one. Rather, changes continue within long-term memory itself.

An appreciation of this dynamic process, usually referred to as memory consolidation, began in the nineteenth century with the observation that in cases of retrograde amnesia, remote memory tends to be less vulnerable to disruption than recent memory.

> This law, which I shall designate as the *law of regression or reversion* seems to me to be a natural conclusion from the observed facts . . . This loss of memory is, as the mathematicians say, inversely as the time that has elapsed between any given incident and the fall [injury] . . . the new perishes before the old, the complex before the simple. (Ribot, 1881, pp. 122, 126, 127)

When the consolidation hypothesis was first proposed, it was based on the phenomenon of retroactive interference in normal subjects, i.e., the fact that recently learned material remains vulnerable for a time to interference by the presentation of similar material (Müller and Pilzecker, 1900). Nevertheless, it was recognized almost immediately that strong support for the consolidation idea could be found in the facts of retrograde amnesia (McDougall, 1901), and the idea that memory takes a long time to be fixed was stated clearly at about the same time.

> In normal memory a process of organization is continually going on—a physical process of organization and a psychological process of repetition and association. In order that ideas may become a part of permanent memory, time must elapse for these processes of organization to be completed. (Burnham, 1903, p. 396)

Studies of remote memory in neurological patients necessarily rely on retrospective methods and imperfect tests. Accordingly, it is not surprising that the early development of consolidation theory, and the experimental study of retrograde amnesia, depended heavily on work with experimental animals (Glickman, 1961; McGaugh and Herz, 1972). At the same time, human studies helped to demonstrate that memory consolidation is a con-

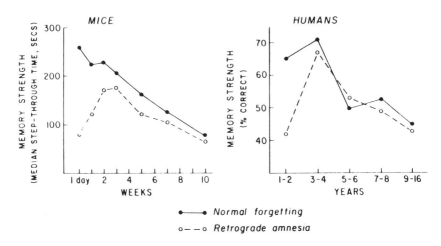

Figure 7.10 Temporally limited retrograde amnesia in mice given electroconvulsive shock (ECS) and in depressed psychiatric inpatients prescribed electroconvulsive therapy (ECT). *(Left):* Mice were given a single training trial and then ECS or sham treatment (four treatments at hourly intervals) at one of seven times after training (1 to 70 days). Retention was always tested 2 weeks after ECS. *(Right):* Patients were given a test about single-season television programs (from 1 to 16 years old) before the first and after the fifth in a prescribed course of bilateral ECT. In both cases, the abscissa shows the age of the memory at the time of treatment. Retrograde amnesia covered a substantial portion of the lifetime of the memory. *Closed circles* = normal forgetting; *open circles* = retrograde amnesia. Abbreviation: Mdn, median. (From Squire, 1986.)

cept about long-term memory, not about the transition from short-term to long-term memory. For example, for psychiatric patients prescribed electroconvulsive therapy for depressive illness, a gradient of retrograde amnesia was obtained in which the remote past was remembered normally (and better than the recent past), and the gradient extended across a time period of a few years (Squire, Slater, and Chace, 1975; see Figure 7.10, right side). Similarly, prospective tests of mice given electroconvulsive shock on one day, between one day and ten weeks after one-trial learning, demonstrated a gradient of retrograde amnesia covering about three weeks (Squire and Spanis, 1984; see Figure 7.10, left side). However, results with convulsive stimulation cannot be directly related to neuroanatomy or to the brain systems involved in learning and memory.

Prospective studies of animals with surgical lesions have led to a more specific version of the consolidation hypothesis, a version that relates consolidation to the time-limited role of the hippocampal formation in declarative memory. In one study, monkeys learned 100 different pairs of objects prior to removal of the hippocampal formation bilaterally (Zola-Morgan and

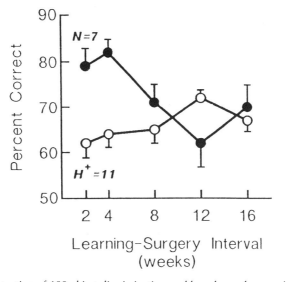

Figure 7.11 Retention of 100 object discrimination problems learned approximately 2, 4, 8, 12, and 16 weeks before hippocampal surgery (20 pairs per time period). Retention was assessed 2 weeks after surgery in monkeys with hippocampal formation (H$^+$) lesions or after an equivalent interval in unoperated animals (N). Brackets show standard error of the mean. (From Zola-Morgan and Squire, 1990.)

Squire, 1990). One member of each object pair was consistently rewarded, and 20 pairs were learned at each of five preoperative time periods (16, 12, 8, 4, and 2 weeks before surgery). After surgery, memory was tested by presenting all 100 object pairs in a mixed order for a single trial. Only a single trial was given so that the measure of remote memory was not confounded with the difficulty animals would be expected to have in relearning the object pairs (Zola-Morgan, Squire, and Amaral, 1989). Normal monkeys remembered objects learned recently better than objects learned 12–16 weeks earlier (Figure 7.11). Operated monkeys exhibited the opposite pattern, remembering objects learned long before surgery better than objects learned recently. In addition, memory for remotely learned objects was normal. Similar temporal gradients have now been demonstrated for other species and tasks, using different methods for producing a hippocampal formation lesion (Figure 7.12; Kim and Fanselow, 1992; Winocur, 1990; Cho et al., 1993).

On the basis of these recent findings, we have developed a simple computational model of memory consolidation to show concretely how the process might operate (Figure 7.13; Alvarez and Squire, 1994). Two similar ideas have also been proposed recently (Milner, 1989; McClelland, McNaughton,

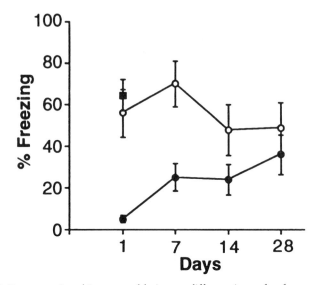

Figure 7.12 Rats were given hippocampal lesions at different times after fear conditioning. In control animals *(open circles)*, context-specific freezing was observed at each retention interval 1 to 28 days after learning. The lesions *(closed circles)* entirely disrupted context-specific freezing when it was made one day after learning, but the lesion had no effect when it was delayed by 28 days. The square symbol shows that a cortical control lesion did not affect conditioned fear. Brackets show standard error of the mean. (From Kim and Fanselow, 1992.)

and O'Reilly, 1994). The medial temporal lobe memory system serves as a temporary store, and long-term memory is stored in the neocortex. The key features of the model can be summarized in five statements:

(1) The crucial event for the formation, maintenance, and retrieval of long-term, declarative memory is an interaction between multiple, geographically separated areas of the neocortex and the structures of the medial temporal lobe. (2) The neocortex communicates with the medial temporal lobe via reciprocal connections with entorhinal, perirhinal, and parahippocampal cortices. The latter two areas in turn are reciprocally connected to entorhinal cortex, which communicates with the hippocampus. (3) Within the neocortex, the key event in consolidation is the gradual binding together of the multiple, geographically disparate cortical regions which together store the representation of a whole event. This gradual linking is the biological substrate of consolidation. (4) The medial temporal lobe learns quickly but has limited capacity. The neocortex learns slowly (i.e., disparate regions become bound together slowly) and has a large capacity. In both cases, learning proceeds according to the same simple (Hebbian) rules for changing synaptic strength. (5) Consolidation occurs when neural activity within the

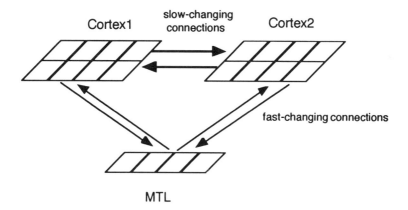

Figure 7.13 Schematic diagram of a simple computational model of memory consolidation involving an interaction between the medial temporal lobe (MTL) and putative repositories of long-term, permanent memory in the neocortex. Areas Cortex1 and Cortex2 represent association neocortex. Each unit in each of the areas (4 in MTL and 8 in Cortex1 and Cortex2) is reciprocally connected to each unit in the other areas. There are no connections within areas, only a form of winner-take-all inhibition. A key feature of the model is that connections to and from the MTL area (thin lines) change much faster than connections between the two cortical areas (thick lines). (From Alvarez and Squire, 1994.)

medial temporal lobe co-activates separate regions of the neocortex. These areas of the neocortex are initially linked only weakly but become more strongly connected as a function of repeatedly being activated simultaneously by the medial temporal lobe.

Although the neural events underlying consolidation are not known, gradual changes in synaptic connectivity are likely involved, perhaps as a result of structural modifications in neuronal morphology. There is a precedent for neuronal growth and rearrangement in the adult mammal in response to specific manipulations. For example, during the months following binocular retinal lesions in the adult cat, there is functional reorganization and sprouting of axonal terminals in the visual cortex (Darian-Smith and Gilbert, 1994). Immediately after the lesions, unit activity along a 7.5 mm length of visual cortex could not be driven by visual stimuli, i.e., there was a scotoma covering about 15 degrees of the visual field. After about nine months, functional reorganization had occurred such that about 5 mm of the cortical scotoma recovered visually-driven activity. Quantitative studies showed that horizontally projecting intracortical neurons, within the reorganized portion of cortex, increased their fiber density 57–88%. These structural changes were apparently gradual, implying a slow-developing and eventually substantial increase in the number of synaptic connections onto target neurons.

Another example comes from studies in adult rats. Following 5.6 to 8.6 hours of total training time distributed across 30 days, rats trained to traverse a difficult, elevated, narrow path had about 25% more synapses per Purkinje cell in the paramedian lobule of the cerebellum than animals who engaged in more physical exercise but did not learn motor skills (Black, Isaacs, Anderson, Alcantara, and Greenough, 1990).

These examples show that neurons can remodel themselves in response to specific perturbations, even when the perturbations are behavioral events. By analogy to these phenomena, it seems possible that memory consolidation is also based on gradual growth and change in the neocortex, and that the growth response is driven by rapidly developing, and relatively short-lived, plastic changes that are established within the medial temporal lobe at the time of learning.

Source Memory

In everyday situations of remembering, one often recalls a fact or an idea but forgets the source of the information (i.e., where or when the fact was encountered). This phenomenon has been termed "source amnesia" (Evans and Thorn, 1966; Schacter, Harbluk, and McLachlan, 1984). For normal subjects, source amnesia is common when freshly learned information is tested after a retention interval of many weeks (Shimamura and Squire, 1991). However, studies of amnesic patients and patients with frontal lobe lesions have demonstrated that source amnesia cannot be explained simply by supposing that source information is a fragile and readily forgotten element of a remembered event. Source memory is a dissociable component of a recollection that can occur independently of the strength of the recollection itself.

In one series of studies (Shimamura and Squire, 1987; Janowsky, Shimamura, and Squire, 1989), subjects were given the answers to 20 general-information questions: for example, What is the name of the town through which Lady Godiva supposedly made her famous ride? [Coventry]; What is the name of the goldfish in the Pinocchio story? [Cleo]. Two presentations of the material were given, followed by a test session either 2 hours later in the case of amnesic patients, or 7 days later for four other groups (patients with frontal lobe lesions, alcoholic control subjects, elderly control subjects, and middle-aged control subjects). During the test, no reference was made to the earlier study phase; subjects were simply asked questions. First, recall was tested for the 20 facts that had been studied, together with 10 other equally obscure facts and 10 "easy" facts. (The easy facts were included so that when subjects were subsequently asked to identify the source of the remembered information, not all of it would have originated in the experimental situation.) Whenever a subject recalled a fact correctly, the subject was asked to report when he/she had first heard this information (source

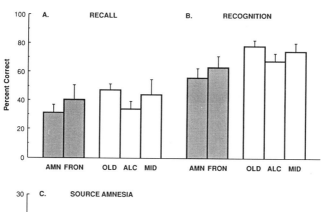

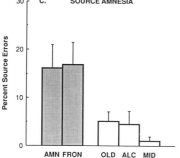

Figure 7.14 A. Recall of 20 recently learned facts. B. Forced-choice, 8-alternative recognition of the same factual information. C. Percent source amnesia, i.e., subjects recalled a fact but failed to recollect when or where the information was acquired. AMN = 11 amnesic patients; FRON = 7 patients with frontal lobe lesions; OLD = 9 elderly control subjects; ALC = 10 alcoholic control subjects; MID = 7 middle-aged subjects. The amnesic patients were tested after a 2-hr retention interval. The other groups were tested after a 7-day retention interval. Brackets show standard error of the mean. (From Shimamura and Squire, 1987; Janowsky, Shimamura, and Squire, 1989.)

memory). A source error was recorded when a subject claimed that one of the 20 studied facts had been learned from an outside source, or when a subject claimed incorrectly that one of the 20 nonstudied facts had been learned from the experimenter. Finally, recognition memory for the 20 studied facts was tested with an 8-alternative, multiple-choice test.

The main finding was that all of the subject groups remembered the facts about equally well whether memory was measured by recall or by recognition (Figure 7.14A and B). Yet, the groups differed markedly in their source memory ability. Whereas source memory errors were uncommon among the control groups (1–5%), in the patient groups source errors were made for about 15 percent of the facts that were correctly recalled. Not only did the pattern of performance across groups dissociate source memory from fact memory, this dissociation was also observed within groups. Specifically, patients who made many source errors recalled and recognized about the same number of facts as patients who made few source errors. Thus, source memory is not a simple consequence of poor memory.

One difference between the source memory performance of amnesic patients and patients with frontal lobe lesions was that, whereas both amnesic patients and frontal patients frequently misattributed study facts to sources outside the experimental session, only the frontal patients misattributed nonstudied facts to the experimental session. The amnesic patients probably did not commit the latter kind of source error because memory was very poor for the test session in which the facts were learned.

The conclusion is that source memory impairment depends in part on frontal lobe pathology (Janowsky, Shimamura, and Squire, 1989; Schacter, Harbluk, and McLachlan, 1984). This idea is also supported by the finding that elderly subjects tend to make more source memory errors than younger subjects (Schacter, Osowiecki, Kaszniak, Kihlstrom, and Valdiserri, 1994; Janowsky et al., 1989; Experiment 2), and the severity of source memory impairment in the elderly correlates with neuropsychological signs of frontal lobe dysfunction (Craik, Morris, Morris, and Loewen, 1990). The data also suggest that source amnesia, whether exhibited by amnesic patients, patients with frontal lobe lesions, or the healthy elderly, reflects a specific deficit in the association of remembered information with its context, i.e., the deficit is a source disconnection rather than source amnesia per se. Indeed, amnesic patients who commit source memory errors demonstrate in separate tests that they remember the earlier learning event at about the same (impaired) level as amnesic patients who do not commit source errors (Shimamura and Squire, 1991).

Comment

The final section of this chapter considers the relevance of multiple memory systems, memory consolidation, and source memory to the topic of accuracy and inaccuracy in memory. The fact that there are multiple memory systems, some of them nonconscious, means that humans express dispositions, habits, and preferences that are inaccessible to conscious recollection but that nevertheless arise from experience and influence our behavior. In other words, some of our actions and feelings, even though based on experience, are expressed implicitly without access to any conscious memory content. Declarative memory may be available in parallel to these implicit expressions of memory, and declarative memory might therefore be able to provide an account of how and when a disposition or a habit or a preference was established. However, if declarative memory is weak, it may be difficult to do more than guess about it.

The facts of memory consolidation can be related to the gradual morphological growth and change that are thought to provide ultimately the permanent substrate for long-term memory (Greenough and Bailey, 1988). By this view, there is continuing competition for synaptic strength, and both gains and losses of synaptic connections. Connections that are used are strengthened, and others are weakened through disuse (Purves, 1988; Recanzone and Merzenich, 1991; Merzenich and Sameshima, 1993). Thus, the beneficial effects of rehearsal on memory strength, and the weakening effects of the passage of time, i.e., forgetting, are best understood in terms of synaptic change. For example, in the case of forgetting, although direct information is not available about its biological basis in the mammalian brain, in invertebrates there is a literal reversal of some of the synaptic changes produced by learning (Bailey and Chen, 1989).

The facts of source amnesia demonstrate that autobiographical memory for the time and place when a particular event occurred is easily disconnected from the factual knowledge acquired during the event. This distinction (between fact knowledge and event memory) is well known in the psychological literature (Tulving, 1983). Recent neuropsychological work suggests that this distinction reflects the fact that both event memory and fact memory depend on medial temporal lobe and diencephalic structures, and that event memory depends additionally on the frontal lobes (Shimamura and Squire, 1987; Tulving, 1989; Knowlton and Squire, submitted).

The frontal lobes are slow to mature during development (Huttenlocher, 1990; Smith, Kates, and Vriezen, 1992) and are especially vulnerable to aging (Haug, Barmwater, Eggers, Fischer, Kuhl, and Sass, 1983). Correspondingly, source memory errors are common in young children (Gopnik and Graf, 1988; Lindsay, Johnson, Kwon, 1991) and in the elderly (Craik et al., 1990; Schacter et al., 1994). It seems reasonable to expect that source memory impairment would make it difficult to distinguish between a past perception and something that was simply imagined. This difficulty arises because the same regions of the brain in the occipital, temporal, and parietal lobes that appear to be important for visual imagery are also important for the processing of perceptual objects and for visual information storage (Farah, 1988; Kosslyn, 1994). That is, the reconstruction of a memory and the creation of a visual mental image appear to involve some of the same brain mechanisms. The frontal lobes provide the possibility of placing oneself autobiographically within a particular past episode. This link to spatial and temporal context provides one way to distinguish recollections of experienced events from images, dreams, and thoughts that do not refer to any experienced event.

If one emphasizes the dynamic aspects of long-term memory—forgetting and consolidation, gradual gains and losses in synaptic connectivity, and a continuous resculpting of neural networks after learning—then one begins to provide a biological account of what psychologists have long understood about memory. Declarative memory is imperfect, subject to error and reconstruction, distortion, and dissociations between confidence and accuracy (Ceci, Chapter 3 of this volume; Loftus, Chapter 1 of this volume; Winograd and Neisser, 1992). Our species seems best adapted for accumulating knowledge—for inference, approximation, concept formation, and classification—not for the literal retention of the individual exemplars that lead to and support general knowledge. Freud (1901) wrote: "Normal forgetting takes place by way of condensation. In this way it becomes the basis for the formation of concepts." In view of the ease with which humans form concepts and generalize about specific experiences, perhaps the remarkable thing about declarative memory is that it can so often be accurate.

References

Alvarez, P. and Squire, L. R. (1994). Memory consolidation and the medial temporal lobe: A simple network model. *Proceedings of the National Academy of Sciences,* in press.

Alvarez, P., Zola-Morgan, S., and Squire, L. R. (1994). The animal model of human amnesia: Long-term memory impaired and short-term memory intact. *Proceedings of the National Academy of Sciences,* in press.

Bailey, C. H. and Chen, M. (1989). Time course of structural changes at identified sensory neuron synapses during long-term sensitization in *Aplysia. Journal of Neuroscience, 9,* 1774–1781.

Black, J. E., Isaacs, K. R., Anderson, B. J., Alcantara, A. A., and Greenough, W. T. (1990). Learning causes synaptogenesis, whereas motor activity causes angiogenesis, in cerebellar cortex of adult rats. *Proceedings of the National Academy of Sciences, 87,* 5568–5572.

Blaxton, T. A. (1989). Investigating dissociations among memory measures: Support for a transfer appropriate processing framework. *Journal of Experimental Psychology: Learning, Memory and Cognition, 15,* 657–668.

Burnham, W. H. (1903). Retroactive amnesia: Illustrative cases and a tentative explanation. *American Journal of Psychology, 14,* 382–396.

Cavanagh, P. (1993). The perception of form and motion. *Current Opinion in Neurobiology, 3,* 177–182.

Ceci, S. (1995). False beliefs: Some developmental and clinical considerations. In: D. L. Schacter, J. T. Coyle, G. D. Fischbach, M.-M. Mesulam, and L. E. Sullivan (Eds.), *Memory Distortion.* Cambridge, Mass.: Harvard University Press.

Cho, Y. H., Beracochea, D., and Jaffard, R. (1993). Extended temporal gradient for the retrograde and anterograde amnesia produced by ibotenate entorhinal cortex lesions in mice. *Journal of Neuroscience, 13,* 1759–1766.

Craik, F. I. M., Morris, L. W., Morris, R. G., and Loewen, E. R. (1990). Relations between source amnesia and frontal lobe functioning in older adults. *Psychology and Aging, 5,* 148–151.

Darien-Smith, C. and Gilbert, C. D. (1994). Axonal sprouting accompanies functional reorganization in adult cat striate cortex. *Nature, 368,* 737–740.

Desimone, R. and Ungerleider, L. G. (1989). Neural mechanisms of visual process in monkeys. In: F. Boller and J. Grafman (Eds.), *Handbook of Neuropsychology,* vol. 2 (pp. 267–299). Amsterdam: Elsevier.

Evans, F. J. and Thorn, W. A. F. (1966). Two types of posthypnotic amnesia: Recall amnesia and source amnesia. *International Journal of Clinical and Experimental Hypnosis, 14,* 162–179.

Farah, M. J. (1988). Is visual imagery really visual: Overlooked evidence from neuropsychology. *Psychological Review, 95,* 307–317.

Freud, S. (1901). The psychopathology of everyday life. In: J. Strachey (Ed.), *Standard Edition of the Complete Psychological Works of Sigmund Freud,* Vol. 6 (p. 134). London: Hogarth Press.

Glickman, S. W. (1961). Perseverative neural processes and consolidation of the memory trace. *Psychological Bulletin, 58,* 218–233.

Gluck, M. A. and Bower, G. M. (1988). Evaluating an adaptive network model of human learning. *Journal of Memory and Language, 27,* 166–195.

Goodale, M. A. (1993). Visual pathways supporting perception and action in the primate cerebral cortex. *Current Opinion in Neurobiology, 3,* 578–585.

Gopnik, A. and Graf, P. (1988). Knowing how you know: Young children's ability to identify and remember the sources of their beliefs. *Child Development, 59,* 1366–1371.

Greenough, W. T. and Bailey, C. H. (1988). The anatomy of a memory: Convergence of results across a diversity of tests. *Trends in Neurosciences, 11,* 142–146.

Haist, F., Musen, G., and Squire, L. R. (1991). Intact priming of words and nonwords in amnesia. *Psychobiology, 19,* 275–285.

Haist, F., Shimamura, A. P., and Squire, L. R. (1992). On the relationship between recall and recognition memory. *Journal of Experimental Psychology: Learning, Memory and Cognition, 18,* 492–508.

Haug, H., Barmwater, U., Eggers, R., Fischer, D., Kuhl, S., and Sass, N. L. (1983). Anatomical changes in aging brain: Morphometric analysis of the human prosencephalon. In: J. Cervos-Navarro and H. I. Sarkander (Eds.), *Brain Aging: Neuropathology and Neuropharmacology (Aging, vol. 21).* New York: Raven Press.

Heindel, W. C., Salmon, D. P., and Butters, N. (1991). The biasing of weight judgments in Alzheimer's and Huntington's disease: A priming or programming phenomenon? *Journal of Clinical and Experimental Neuropsychology, 13,* 189–203.

Huttenlocher, P. R. (1990). Morphometric study of human cerebral cortex. *Neuropsychologia, 28,* 512–527.

Jacoby, L. L. (1988). Memory observed and memory unobserved. In: U. Neisser and E. Winograd (Eds.), *Remembering Reconsidered* (pp. 145–177). New York: Cambridge University Press.

Jacoby, L. L. and Whitehouse, K. (1989). An illusion of memory: False recognition influenced by unconscious perception. *Journal of Experimental Psychology: General, 118,* 126–135.

Janowsky, J., Shimamura, A. P., and Squire, L. R. (1989). Source memory impairment in patients with frontal lobe lesions. *Neuropsychologia, 27,* 2043–2056.

Johnston, W. A., Hawley, K. J., and Elliot, M. G. (1991). Contribution of perceptual fluency to recognition judgments. *Journal of Experimental Psychology: Learning, Memory, and Cognition, 17,* 210–223.

Katz, B. (1969). The release of neural transmitter substances. In: *The Sherrington Lectures X.* Liverpool: Liverpool University Press.

Kenny, M. G. (1986). *The Passion of Ansel Bourne: Multiple personality in American culture.* Washington, D.C.: Smithsonian Institution Press.

Kim, J. J. and Fanselow, M. S. (1992). Modality-specific retrograde amnesia of fear. *Science, 256,* 675–677.

Knowlton, B. J. and Squire, L. R. (in press). Remembering and knowing: Two different expressions of declarative memory. *Journal of Experimental Psychology, Learning, Memory and Cognition.*

Knowlton, B. J., Squire, L. R. and Gluck, M. (1994). Probabilistic classification learning in amnesia. *Learning and Memory, 1,* 106–120.

Kosslyn, S. M. (1994). *Image and Brain: The Resolution of the Imagery Debate.* Cambridge: MIT Press.

Lindsay, D. S., Johnson, M. K., and Kwon, P. (1991). Developmental changes in memory source monitoring. *Journal of Experimental Child Psychology, 52,* 297–318.

Loftus, E. F., Feldman, J., and Dashiell, R. (1995). The reality of illusory memories. In: D. L. Schacter, J. T. Coyle, G. D. Fischbach, M.-M. Mesulam, and L. E. Sullivan (Eds.), *Memory Distortion.* Cambridge, Mass.: Harvard University Press.

Mahut, H. and Moss, M. (1984). Consolidation of memory: The hippocampus revisited. In: L. R. Squire and N. Butters (Eds.), *Neuropsychology of Memory* (pp. 297–315). New York: Guilford Press.

Mandler, G. (1980). Recognizing: The judgment of previous occurrence. *Psychological Review, 87,* 252–271.

Masson, M. E. J. (1986). Identification of typographically transformed words: Instance-based skill acquisition. *Journal of Experimental Psychology: Learning, Memory and Cognition, 12,* 479–488.

Mayes, A. (1988). *Human Organic Memory Disorders.* New York: Oxford University Press.

McClelland, J. L., McNaughton, B. L., and O'Reilly, R. C. (1994). *Technical Report PDP.CNS.94.* Pittsburgh: Carnegie Mellon University.

McDougall, W. R. (1901). Experimentelle beitrage zur lehre vom Gedachtniss [Experimental contributions to the theory of memory] by G. E. Muller and A. Pilzecker. *Mind, 10,* 388–394.

McGaugh, J. L. and Herz, M. J. (1972). *Memory Consolidation,* San Francisco: Albion.

Merigan, W. H. and Maunsell, J. H. R. (1993). How parallel are the primate visual pathways? *Annual Review of Neuroscience, 16,* 369–402.

Merzenich, M. M. and Sameshima, K. (1993). Cortical plasticity and memory. *Current Opinion in Neurobiology, 3,* 187–196.

Milner, P. (1989). A cell assembly theory of hippocampal amnesia. *Neuropsychologia, 27,* 23–30.

Mishkin, M. (1982). A memory system in the monkey. *Phils. R. Soc. Lond. [Biol.], 298,* 85–92.

Mishkin, M., Malamut, B., and Bachevalier, J. (1984). Memories and habits: Two neural systems. In: G. Lynch, J. L. McGaugh and N. M. Weinberger (Eds.), *Neurobiology of Learning and Memory* (pp. 65–77). New York: Guilford.

Müller, G. E. and Pilzecker, A. (1900). Experimentelle beitrage zur lehre vom Gedachtniss. *Zeitschrift fur Psychologie Erganzungsband, 1,* 1–288.

Musen, G., Shimamura, A. P., and Squire, L. R. (1990). Intact text-specific reading skill in amnesia. *Journal of Experimental Psychology: Learning, Memory and Cognition, 6,* 1068–1076.

Nemiah, J. C. (1989). Dissociative disorders (hysterical neuroses, dissociative type). In: H. T. Kaplan and B. J. Sadock (Eds.), *Comprehensive Textbook of Psychiatry/V* (pp. 1028–1044). Baltimore: Williams and Wilkins.

Packard, M. G., Hirsh, R., and White, N. M. (1989). Differential effects of fornix and caudate nucleus lesions on two radial maze tasks: Evidence for multiple memory systems. *Journal of Neuroscience, 9,* 1465–1472.

Purves, D. (1988). *Body and Brain.* Cambridge, Mass.: Harvard University Press.

Recanzone, G. H. and Merzenich, M. M. (1991). Alterations of the functional organization of primary somatosensory cortex following intracortical microstimulation or behavioral training. In: L. R. Squire, N. M. Weinberger, G. Lynch, and J. L. McGaugh (Eds.), *Memory: Organization and Locus of Change* (pp. 217–238). New York: Oxford University Press.

Ribot, T. 1881. *Les Maladies de la Mémoire [Diseases of Memory].* New York: Appleton-Century-Crofts.

Roediger, H. (1990). Implicit memory: Retention without remembering. *American Psychologist, 45,* 1043–1056.

Saint-Cyr, J. A., Taylor, A. E., and Lang, A. E. (1988). Procedural learning and neostriatal dysfunction in man. *Brain, 111,* 941–959.

Schacter, D. L. (1987). Implicit memory: History and current status. *Journal of Experimental Psychology: Learning, Memory and Cognition, 13,* 501–518.

Schacter, D. L. (1992). Understanding implicit memory: A cognitive neuroscience approach. *American Psychologist, 47,* 559–569.

Schacter, D. L., Chiu, C. Y., and Ochsner, K. N. (1993). Implicit memory: A selective review. *Annual Review of Neuroscience, 16,* 159–182.

Schacter, D. L., Harbluk, J. L., and McLachlan, D. R. (1984). Retrieval without recollection: An experimental analysis of source amnesia. *Journal of Verbal Learning and Verbal Behavior, 23,* 593–611.

Schacter, D. L., Osowiecki, D., Kaszniak, A. W., Kihlstrom, J. F., and Valdiserri, M. (1994). Source memory: Extending the boundaries of age-related deficits. *Psychology and Aging, 9,* 81–89.

Schacter, D. and Tulving, E. (Eds.). (1994). *Memory Systems: 1994.* Cambridge, Mass.: MIT Press.

Schacter, D., Wang, P. L., Tulving, E., and Freedman, P. C. (1982). Functional retrograde amnesia: A quantitative case study. *Neuropsychologia, 20,* 523–532.

Scoville, W. B. and Milner, B. (1957). Loss of recent memory after bilateral hippocampal lesions. *J. Neurol. Neurosurg. Psychiatry, 20,* 11–21.

Shanks, D. R. and St. John, M. F. (1994). Characteristics of dissociable human learning systems. *Behavioral and Brain Sciences,* in press.

Sherry, D. F. and Schacter, D. L. (1987). The evolution of multiple memory systems. *Psychological Review, 94,* 439–454.

Shimamura, A. P. (1989). Disorders of memory: The cognitive science perspective. In: F. Boller and J. Grafman (Eds.), *Handbook of Neuropsychology,* Vol. 3 (pp. 35–73). New York: Elsevier.

Shimamura, A. P. and Squire, L. R. (1987). A neuropsychological study of fact memory and source amnesia. *Journal of Experimental Psychology: Learning, Memory, and Cognition, 13,* 464–473.

Shimamura, A. P. and Squire, L. R. (1991). The relationship between fact and source memory: Findings from amnesic patients and normal subjects. *Psychobiology, 19,* 1–10.

Smith, M. L., Kates, M. H., and Vriezen, E. R. (1992). The development of frontal-lobe functions. In: F. Boller and J. Grafman (Eds.), *Handbook of Neuropsychology,* Vol. 7 (pp. 309–330). Amsterdam: Elsevier.

Squire, L. R. (1982). The neuropsychology of human memory. *Annual Review of Neuroscience, 5,* 241–273.

Squire, L. R. (1986). Mechanisms of memory. *Science, 232,* 1612–1619.

Squire, L. R. (1987). *Memory and Brain.* New York: Oxford University Press.

Squire, L. R. (1992). Memory and the hippocampus: A synthesis from findings with rats, monkeys, and humans. *Psychological Review, 99,* 195–231.

Squire, L. R. (1994). Declarative and nondeclarative memory: Multiple brain systems supporting learning and memory. In: D. Schacter and E. Tulving (Eds.), *Memory Systems: 1994.* Cambridge, Mass.: MIT Press.

Squire, L. R., Hamann, S., and Knowlton, B. (1994). Dissociable learning and memory systems of the brain. *Behavioral and Brain Sciences,* in press.

Squire, L. R. and Knowlton, B. J. (1994). Memory, hippocampus and brain systems. In: M. Gazzaniga (Ed.), *The Cognitive Neurosciences.* Cambridge, Mass.: MIT Press.

Squire, L. R., Knowlton, B., and Musen, G. (1993). The structure and organization of memory. *Annual Review of Psychology, 44,* 453–495.

Squire, L. R. and Shimamura, A. P. (1986). Characterizing amnesic patients for neurobehavioral study. *Behavioral Neuroscience, 100,* 866–877.

Squire, L. R., Slater, P. C., and Chace, P. M. (1975). Retrograde amnesia: Temporal gradient in very long-term memory following electroconvulsive therapy. *Science, 187,* 77–79.

Squire, L. R. and Spanis, C. W. (1984). Long gradient of retrograde amnesia in mice: Continuity with the findings in humans. *Behavioral Neuroscience, 98,* 345–348.

Squire, L. R. and Zola-Morgan, S. (1983). The neurology of memory: The case for correspondence between the findings for human and nonhuman primate. In: J. A. Deutsch (Ed.), *The Physiological Basis of Memory* (pp. 199–268). New York: Academic Press.

Squire, L. R. and Zola-Morgan, S. (1991). The medial temporal lobe memory system. *Science, 253,* 1380–1386.

Squire, L. R., Zola-Morgan, S., Cave, C. B., Haist, F., Musen, G., and Suzuki, W. (1990). Memory: Organization of brain systems and cognition. In: *Cold Spring Symp. Quant. Biol. 55* (pp. 1007–1023). New York: Cold Spring Harbor.

Tulving, E. (1983). *Elements of Episodic Memory*. New York: Oxford University Press.

Tulving, E. (1985). How many memory systems are there? *American Psychologist, 40*, 385–398.

Tulving, E. (1989). Remembering and knowing the past. *American Scientist, 77*, 361–367.

Tulving, E. and Schacter, D. L. (1990). Priming and human memory systems. *Science, 247*, 301–306.

Ungerleider, W. and Mishkin, M. (1982). Two cortical visual systems. In: D. J. Ingle, M. A. Goodale and R. J. W. Mansfield (Eds.), *The Analysis of Visual Behavior* (pp. 549–586). Cambridge, Mass.: MIT Press.

Van Essen, D. C., Anderson, C. H., and Felleman, D. J. (1992). Information processing in the primate visual system: An integrated systems perspective. *Science, 255*, 419–423.

Weiskrantz, L. (1987). Neuroanatomy of memory and amnesia: A case for multiple memory systems. *Human Neurobiology, 6*, 93–105.

Whittlesea, B. W. A. (1993). Illusions of familiarity. *Journal of Experimental Psychology: Learning, Memory and Cognition, 19*, 1235–1253.

Winocur, G. (1990). Anterograde and retrograde amnesia in rats with dorsal hippocampal or dorsomedial thalamic lesions. *Behavioral Brain Research, 38*, 145–154.

Winograd, E. and Neisser, U. (Eds). (1992). *Affect and Accuracy in Recall*. Cambridge: Cambridge University Press.

Young, M. P. (1992). Objective analysis of the topological organization of the primate cortical visual system. *Nature, 358*, 152–254.

Zola-Morgan, S. and Squire, L. R. (1990). The primate hippocampal formation: Evidence for a time-limited role in memory storage. *Science, 250*, 288–290.

Zola-Morgan, S. and Squire, L. R. (1993). Neuroanatomy of memory. *Annual Review of Neuroscience, 16*, 547–563.

Zola-Morgan, S., Squire, L. R., and Amaral, D. G. (1989). Lesions of the hippocampal formation but not lesions of the fornix or the mammillary nuclei produce long-lasting memory impairment in monkeys. *Journal of Neuroscience, 9*, 898–913.

Zola-Morgan, S., Squire, L. R., and Mishkin, M. (1982). The neuroanatomy of amnesia: Amygdala-hippocampus versus temporal stem. *Science, 218*, 1337–1339.

Acknowledgments

Preparation of this chapter was supported by grants from the Medical Research Service of the Department of Veterans Affairs, NIMH, the Office of Naval Research, and the McKnight Foundation.

Confabulation

8

Morris Moscovitch

Memory distortion, rather than memory loss, occurs because re-membering is often a reconstructive process. To convince oneself of this, one only has to try to remember yesterday's events and the order in which they occurred; or even, as sometimes happens, what day yesterday was. Damage to neural structures involved in the storage, retention, and automatic recovery of encoded information produces memory loss which in its most severe form is amnesia (see Squire, 1992; Squire, Chapter 7 of this volume). Memory distortion, however, is no more a feature of the memory deficit of these patients than it is of the benign, and all too common, memory failure of normal people. When, however, neural structures involved in the reconstructive process are damaged, memory distortion becomes prominent and results in confabulation, even though memory loss may not be severe. Though flagrantly distorted and easily elicited, confabulations nonetheless share many characteristics with the type of memory distortions we all produce. Studying confabulation from a cognitive neuroscience perspective, of interest in its own right, may also contribute to our understanding of how memories are normally distorted.

Confabulation is a symptom that accompanies many neuropsychological disorders and some psychiatric ones, such as schizophrenia (Enoch, Trethowan, and Baker, 1967; Joseph, 1986). What distinguishes confabulation from lying is that typically there is no intent to deceive and the patient is unaware of the falsehoods. It is an "honest lying." Confabulation is simple to detect when the information the patient provides is patently false, self-contradictory, bizarre, or at least highly improbable. These are called fantastic confabulations (Kopelman, 1987). Just as often, however, the tale fabricated by the patient is coherent, internally consistent, and relatively commonplace. It is identified as a confabulation only by consulting with the patient's friends or relatives or by cross-checking it with information provided by the patient on other occasions.

Confabulations also are not systematic in the sense that they are subordinated to a single theme. When confronted with the truth, the patient either clings to the story despite its implausibility or inconsistency, or readily abandons it in deference to the examiner. The indifference or apathy with which either course is taken, and the lack of thematic cohesiveness, stand in contrast to the attitude of some delusional psychiatric patients who fiercely defend their elaborately structured system of beliefs. In my experience, the only time indifference gives way to willfulness and tenacity is when confabulation is wedded to action. In such circumstances, the patient's attempt to carry out a plan of action consistent with the confabulation is not always easily thwarted or deflected. This last point suggests that confabulations are not restricted to verbal statements (Talland, 1961, 1965; Berlyne, 1972) but can include action and non-verbal depictions such as drawings (Joslyn, Grundvig, and Chamberlain, 1978; Kern, Van Gorp, Cummings, Brown, and Osato, 1992). The treatment by one of our patients of the nursing staff as office help and another patient's repeated attempts to leave the hospital for home in the evening indicated, as strongly as their verbal statements, that they mistook the hospital for their workplace.

Before proceeding further, I think it best to illustrate what confabulations are like with an example. On the basis of my own work, and of reports in the literature, I will then list what I think are the primary features of confabulation. The rest of this chapter will be devoted to a discussion of its causes, both structural and functional, and of the possible contribution that studies of confabulation can make to theories of normal and pathological memory, and to research on memory distortion. Finally, I will present two models that can accommodate the findings.

Excerpt from an Interview with Patient HW

HW is a 61-year-old right-handed man who had a sub-arachnoid hemorrhage clipped. Clipping near the anterior communicating artery (ACoA) was followed by widespread bilateral frontal ischemia and infarction. CAT scans confirmed widespread frontal damage with sparing of the temporal lobes medially and laterally. The interview took place in 1987. More detailed information about HW and his deficits appears in Moscovitch, 1989.

Q. Can you tell me a little bit about yourself? How old are you?
A. I'm 40, 42, pardon me, 62.
Q. Are you married or single?
A. Married.

Q. How long have you been married?
A. About 4 months.
Q. What's your wife's name?
A. Martha.
Q. How many children do you have?
A. Four. (He laughs.) Not bad for 4 months!
Q. How old are your children?
A. The eldest is 32, his name is Bob, and the youngest is 22, his name is Joe.
   (These answers are close to the actual age of the boys.)
Q. (He laughs again.) How did you get these children in 4 months?
A. They're adopted.
Q. Who adopted them?
A. Martha and I.
Q. Immediately after you got married you wanted to adopt these older
   children?
A. Before we were married we adopted one of them, two of them. The eldest
   girl Brenda and Bob, and Joe and Dina since we were married.
Q. Does it all sound a little strange to you, what you are saying?
A. (He laughs.) I think it is a little strange.
Q. Your record says that you've been married for over 30 years. Does that
   sound more reasonable to you?
A. No.
Q. Do you really believe that you have been married for 4 months?
A. Yes.
Q. You have been married for a long time to the same woman, for over 30
   years. Do you find that strange?
A. Very strange.
Q. Do you remember your wedding well?
A. No, not particularly. (In other interviews he is able to describe his wedding
   in some detail.)
Q. Were your parents at the wedding?
A. Yes.
Q. How old were they?
A. My father is 95–96. My mother is 10 years younger so she is 85–86. (In
   fact, they died quite a few years ago when they were in their 70s.)
Q. So you got married the first time when you were 61 years old? You weren't
   married when you were younger?
A. This is my second marriage. The first woman was 2 years ago.
Q. That would make you how old when you got married the first time?
A. 50.
Q. What happened to your first wife?
A. Not a thing.
Q. Did you get divorced?
A. Yes.
Q. Are you Protestant or Catholic?
A. (He laughs.) I'm Catholic.
Q. That would make it pretty difficult, wouldn't it?
A. Yes, the first one was invalid.

Characteristic Features of Confabulation

With this interview in mind, it will be simple to review the prominent features of confabulation. I have used Talland's list (1965, pp. 49–50) as a guide and modified it to bring it up to date and to conform more closely to my own beliefs concerning the nature of the syndrome.

1. Confabulations are usually verbal statements but can also occur as non-verbal depictions or actions.

2. Typically, they are accounts concerning the patient but also can include non-personal information such as knowledge of historical events, fairy tales (Delbecq-Derouesné, Beauvois, and Shallice, 1990; Luria, 1976), geography (Moscovitch, 1989), and other aspects of semantic memory (Dalla Barba, 1993a; Sandson, Albert, and Alexander, 1986).

3. The account need not be coherent and internally consistent, as patient HW's belief about his marriages and the ages of his children indicates.

4. The account is false in the context in which it is related and often false in details within its own context.

5. Most often, the account is drawn fully or principally from the patient's recollection of his actual experiences, including his thoughts in the past and current musings. If the examiner is aware of the patient's history and his current concerns and perceptions, the source of the elements that enter into the patient's confabulations can be identified. HW once mistook me for an insurance salesman because we had been discussing a friend of his who was one. Talland describes a case in which a painting of a seascape in the examiner's office caught a patient's eye and served as the stimulus that launched him into a fantastic confabulation of his life as a sailor.

6. Information is presented without awareness of its distortions or of its inappropriateness and without concern when the errors are pointed out. Our patient merely laughed when confronted with the implausibility of having four children in four months; with little hesitation, he provided a preposterous explanation for this amazing feat. Indeed, the lack of awareness and concern is not confined to single accounts but extends to the patient's entire condition. In short, the patient is anosognosic (McGlynn and Schacter, 1989).

7. Usually confabulation serves no purpose; it is motivated in no other way than by the patient's attempt to relate his or her experiences. Initial or primary confabulations are not produced "to oblige the listener or to fill in gaps in their knowledge of facts" (Talland, 1965, p. 42), though "secondary" confabulations may arise to explain (away) the internal inconsistencies of the primary confabulations that are sometimes apparent even to the patient. Thus, HW's assertion that he was married for four months was a primary confabulation that was elicited as his honest answer to a question. Trying to resolve the discrepancy between that answer and the knowledge that he had four grown children, however, probably accounted for all the remaining "secondary" confabulations in his account.

8. The readiness to confabulate may be determined by the patient's "personality structure, the traits evolved in dealing with the environment and in monitoring his image" (Talland, 1965, p. 44). As Gainotti (1975) observed, demented patients with a premorbid pattern of denial or rationalization of illness and with a need for prestige and domination in interpersonal relations were two or three times more likely to confabulate than patients who did not have these traits. It is not known whether this observation also applies to patients with traumatic brain injury who are not demented.

Thus, like normal remembering, confabulation involves the reconstruction of the context and modification and combination of elements and can be influenced by personality. Confabulation occurs because one or more of the mechanisms of normal remembering are damaged. Exactly which ones are involved is a matter for later discussion. Because poor memory and reconstruction are prerequisites for memory distortion by normal people, the confabulating patient can be studied as an exaggerated example of what occurs normally. As is often the case, psychopathology can provide insight into the normal.

The Prevalence and Distribution of Confabulation in Neurological Disorders

Confabulation is not found exclusively in patients with memory disorders but can also be present in patients with other deficits. Confabulation occurs often in patients with dementia and in patients who are in a confusional state. In the latter case confabulation disappears as orientation is reestablished, but in patients with ACoA aneurysms confabulation is likely to persist (DeLuca, 1993; DeLuca and Cicerone, 1991). Confabulation has also been reported in cases of cortical blindness, hemiplegia, aphasia, and neglect that are accompanied by denial of deficit (anosognosia). In these cases, confabulation has the same characteristic as it does in patients with memory disorders (see McGlynn and Schacter, 1989), except that its manifestations are related to the particular deficit. Thus, patients with cortical blindness will assert that they see well and describe in detail the individual they believe they are observing although no one, in fact, is present (Kinsbourne, 1989). Patients with hemiplegia will deny that one of their limbs is malfunctioning and claim to be able to carry out activities that require the use of that limb. Aphasic confabulators will provide definitions for nonsense words. Our focus, however, will be on confabulations associated with memory disorders.

Locus of Lesions That Are Associated with Confabulation

Confabulation has been linked to damage to the ventromedial frontal lobes and related structures that are fed by the ACoA (see Figure 8.1). These in-

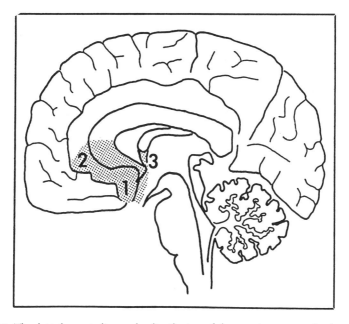

Figure 8.1 The dotted area indicates the distribution of the anterior communicating artery (ACoA) and its perforators. 1, basal forebrain; 2, anterior cingulate; 3, anterior hypothalamus. (From Parkin and Leng, 1993.)

clude the basal forebrain, septum, fornix, cingulate gyrus, cingulum, anterior hypothalamus, and the head of the caudate nucleus (Alexander and Freedman, 1984; Irle, Wowra, Kunert, Hampl, and Kunze, 1991; Vilkki, 1985). Confirmed or suspected frontal damage, especially in the right hemisphere (Joseph, 1986), is a common feature of confabulation in patients with memory disorders (Stuss, Alexander, Lieberman, and Levine, 1978; Kapur and Coughlin, 1980; Baddeley and Wilson, 1986; Moscovitch, 1989) and in patients with anosognosia related to other deficits (McGlynn and Schacter, 1989). Some authors believe, however, that confabulation is associated with lesions of the cingulate (Lhermitte and Signoret, 1976) or of the basal forebrain and hypothalamus (Luria, 1976). Their view gains support from recent reports of confabulating patients who perform normally on standard neuropsychological tests that are sensitive to frontal damage (Delbecq-Derouesné et al., 1990; Dalla Barba, 1993b). Deficits on these tests, however, are typically associated with damage to the lateral frontal cortex and not with the ventromedial cortex that is usually implicated in confabulation. Damage to the ventromedial frontal cortex may nonetheless be accompanied by deficits of executive function (Shallice and Burgess, 1992) which are not picked up by traditional tests but which may contribute to confabulation. The possibility still remains that damage restricted to the ventromedial frontal lobes, possibly on the right, may be sufficient to produce confabulation; and, even if not sufficient, ventromedial frontal damage may be a necessary condition.

Explanations and Theories of Confabulation

Compensation

Among the earliest theories of confabulation are those that can be classified as compensatory: patients confabulate as a means of compensating for a deficiency. Bonhoffer's (1901; cited in Talland, 1965) *confabulation of exigency or embarrassment* is of this type. Patients confabulate in order to cover lapses in memory or fill in gaps of knowledge (Barbizet, 1963), as much to oblige a listener as to satisfy a patient's own needs. We can see these factors operating in HW's clumsy attempt to account for his having four adult children after being married for four months. As noted earlier, these can be considered as *secondary confabulations* that are devised to reconcile beliefs, based on *primary confabulations,* that are incompatible with each other. The compensatory theory does not explain why HW said he was married for only four months in the first place.

Similarly, proposals that confabulation is attributed to suggestibility (Pick, 1905) or to psychological defense mechanisms associated with certain types of premorbid personality (Weinstein and Kahn, 1955; Gainotti, 1975) also fail to capture the cause of primary confabulations in most patients. HW, like other confabulating patients, volunteers erroneous information with little prodding and, as often as not, continues to hold onto his beliefs despite suggestions to the contrary (see interview). Admittedly, some patients with degenerative dementing disorders may confabulate in order to protect themselves from knowledge that can be devastating. Most confabulating patients with traumatic brain damage, however, are so apathetic and indifferent to their disorder that it is difficult to believe that their confabulations are a means to defend against anxiety, let alone catastrophic reactions.

Temporal Disorder and Loss of "Source" Memory

One of the more popular theories is that confabulation arises from "the disruption of [the patient's] temporal frame of reference" (Talland, 1965, p. 56; Van Der Holst, 1932, cited in Williams and Rupp, 1938). The temporal disorder prevents patients from establishing a point of reference in time around which they can place events in sequence. As a result, memories of events that are related but are widely separated in time and place become fused or are misattributed to another context. *A disturbed sense of chronology* will also lead to erroneous dating of even single events. Such a process can produce *primary confabulations* and, once produced, may give rise to *secondary confabulations* that function to reconcile discrepant beliefs.

The temporal theory is consistent with evidence that frontal lobe lesions or dysfunction lead to deficits in judgments of temporal order (Kopelman, 1989; Milner, Petrides, and Smith, 1985; Shimamura, Janowsky, and Squire, 1991; Vriezen and Moscovitch, 1990) and, perhaps, to impaired attribution of temporal or spatial context to any event (Schacter, 1987; Shimamura and Squire, 1987). "Confabulation is source amnesia (Schacter, Harbluk, and McLachlan, 1984) magnified and extended to include a lifetime of experience" (Moscovitch, 1989, p. 138).

Although a deficit in chronology and attribution of context is a prominent feature of confabulation, I do not think it is the cause of confabulation but is itself a symptom of a deeper underlying disorder. An impaired chronological mechanism cannot account for spontaneous, fantastic confabulations which are not just incorrectly reassembled memories but true inventions. Similarly, the compensatory, secondary confabulations can be so farfetched that they cannot be explained as normal reactions to conflicting beliefs caused by an impaired chronological process. Besides, implicit in this interpretation is that confabulation is restricted to the patient's personal experiences or what he or she takes to be those experiences. I will provide evidence that confabulation also involves semantic memory which includes general, rather than personal, knowledge.

Retrieval Theories

There is general agreement that confabulation is primarily a deficit in retrieval more than encoding, consolidation, or storage (Lhermitte and Signoret, 1976), "of the ability to 'ecphoria' than of engram formation" (Williams and Rupp, 1938, p. 403). The strongest evidence in favor of the retrieval hypothesis is that confabulation affects remote memories as well as those that were acquired postmorbidly. Retrieval, however, is not a simple, unitary process. The question remains as to which aspect of retrieval is impaired in patients who confabulate. Because damage is not localized to a single structure and because the symptoms, apart from confabulation, are variable, it is by no means simple to isolate the retrieval deficit that underlies confabulation.

The suggestion that confabulation is related to an *impaired ability to withhold responses* and *to monitor* those that are given (Mercer, Wapner, Gardner, and Benson, 1977; Shapiro, Alexander, Gardner, and Mercer, 1981; Stuss et al., 1978; Stuss and Benson, 1986; Talland, 1965) places the deficit at a late stage of retrieval, after the memory had been retrieved but before a response was emitted. Consistent with this proposal is that memory for content is better preserved than memory for temporal order and context.

There are indications, however, that early retrieval processes involved in memory search are also impaired. Patients do not always confabulate in response to every question which they do not answer correctly. In fact, the most common error is one of omission—they simply do not supply any answer or, if one is supplied, it is sparse in detail. In itself this is not peculiar except that such failures also occur in circumstances in which the answer would be readily available to them if only they could devise a proper strategy to retrieve it.

Strategic versus Associative/Cue Dependent Retrieval

To understand the nature of the retrieval deficit in confabulation it is necessary to distinguish between two types of retrieval processes: associative/cue dependent and strategic (see also Conway's [1992] distinction between direct and generative retrieval). The former is a relatively automatic process that is engaged when a specific, proximal cue interacts with information stored in memory, a process termed "ecphory" (Seman, 1922, cited in Schacter, Tulving, and Eich, 1978). The recovered product of that interaction is either the memory that is being sought or provides the material for subsequent, strategic retrieval processes. Strategic retrieval processes are self-initiated, goal-directed, effortful, and intelligent. When the retrieval cue is inadequate, strategic processes are involved in initiating and organizing a search that uses whatever knowledge is available, whether semantic or episodic, to reinstate the appropriate context and locate the cue that allows local, associative processes to operate. Once the memory trace is recovered, other strategic processes then monitor the output. Among other things, this would involve determining whether the recovered trace satisfies the goals of the memory search and whether it is consistent with other information in semantic and episodic memory. If not, new search processes are initiated and the entire sequence is repeated until a solution is found or the search is abandoned.

Strategic retrieval processes are essentially problem-solving routines applied to memory. They help frame the problem and recruit general and personal knowledge to constrain it further until local routines can arrive at a possible solution. The solution is then evaluated to see if it is correct.

The order in which associative and strategic retrieval processes are applied is not fixed. Sometimes a highly distinctive cue may lead to recovery of the target, and only then do strategic processes use that information to reconstruct the context in which the event occurred. At other times, the processes are reversed.

Confabulation as a Deficit in Strategic Retrieval

I wish to argue that impairment of processes involved in strategic retrieval causes the major positive and negative signs of confabulation. These can be exacerbated by two factors: (1) deficiencies in associative retrieval and (2) damage to the system from which information is recovered. In the case of memory, the system includes the medial temporal/diencephalic structures involved in engram formation and storage. A damaged system is more likely to produce faulty output when it is queried. Because strategic retrieval is itself impaired, the faulty output cannot be monitored and evaluated properly. In general terms, errors of omission occur when specific cues are inadequate and do not trigger responses, and there is a subsequent failure to initiate and implement strategic search. On the other hand, confabulation occurs when the outcome of disturbed strategic search and associative retrieval is faulty and a response is emitted without proper monitoring and evaluation.

This hypothesis is consistent with the idea that the frontal lobes are implicated in confabulation. Studies of patients with frontal damage or dysfunction suggest that the frontal lobes contribute to strategic memory functions at encoding and retrieval—the use to which memory is put rather than its mere storage and reactivation (for review see Moscovitch, 1989; Moscovitch and Winocur, 1992a, 1992b). In particular the frontal lobes have been implicated in the temporal organization of memory (Milner, Petrides, and Smith, 1985; Schacter, 1987), which may be particularly sensitive to disturbances in strategic retrieval processes (Moscovitch, 1989). This may explain why temporal disorders are such a prominent feature of confabulation.

One difficulty with this hypothesis is that much of our knowledge of the cognitive deficits that are associated with frontal lesions is based on studies of patients with damage to the dorsolateral or ventrolateral regions, whereas it is the ventromedial region that is implicated in confabulation. The extent to which damage to each of these regions contributes to the symptom complex that is characteristic of confabulation has yet to be determined. Until it is, we will work on the assumption that at least as far as memory is concerned, disorders of strategic processes are also associated with damage to the ventromedial region and related subcortical structures.

The strategic retrieval hypothesis is meant to be applied equally across all domains: episodic memory as well as semantic, recently acquired memories as well as remote ones, regardless of content. At first glance, this hypothesis would appear to have difficulty in accounting for reports that confabulation involves episodic more than semantic memory (Dalla Barba, 1993b) and that, in both cases, it is particularly temporal aspects of memory that are especially affected. There are a number of reasons why confabulation is so unevenly distributed across various domains even though the strategic retrieval hypothesis may be correct. One reason is that the semantic memory tests or questionnaires that were administered by Dalla Barba made fewer demands on strategic retrieval processes than episodic memory tests. Were the two types of tests equivalent, then performance on both tests would be similar. The other reason, which was mentioned earlier, is that damage to systems involved in associative retrieval and storage of domain-specific information will exacerbate confabulation. It may be argued that some memory disorder may be a prerequisite for confabulation. These issues will be examined in the following sections. In the remaining part of the chapter I will discuss in more detail some aspects of confabulation as well as associated memory problems.

The Domain of Confabulation
Episodic versus Semantic Memory

Dalla Barba (1993a, 1993b; Dalla Barba, Cipolotti, and Denes, 1990) reports two cases in which confabulation is confined to episodic or autobiographical memory and a third case in which it also includes semantic memory. It is significant that only episodic memory was deficient in the two former cases whereas semantic memory was also impaired in the latter.

Impaired semantic memory and aphasia were associated with semantic and lexical-semantic confabulations, respectively, in Baddeley and Wilson's (1988) and Sandson et al.'s (1986) patients. These findings are consistent with the prediction that such damage would exacerbate confabulation in the affected domain. The reason is that a damaged system is more likely to produce faulty output. Because the strategic retrieval system itself is damaged, that output cannot be monitored and evaluated properly. Patients may confabulate more about episodic than semantic memory because it is episodic memory that is more often impaired, perhaps because of the proximity of structures involved in episodic memory to those involved in strategic retrieval.

Yet another reason for the greater prevalence of confabulation about episodic memory is that retrieval of episodic memories in the laboratory and in real life is likely to make greater demands on strategic processes than retrieval of semantic memories. Examination of the 15 questions used by Dalla Barba (1993b, pp. 19–20) to probe episodic memory shows that at least 12 of them had a temporal component which requires strategic retrieval, whereas this was true of only three of the semantic memory questions. In addition, all the episodic memory questions involved a narrative that probably required strategic search processes to ferret out details, whereas more than half the semantic memory questions could be answered by a single word or sentence.

In an attempt to equate the strategic retrieval demands of semantic and episodic memory, we used a word-cue test first developed by Galton (1879) to study autobiographical memory and revived by Crovitz (1973; Crovitz and Schiffman, 1974). We devised a semantic, historical version to complement the traditional episodic memory version of the Crovitz Test (see Table 8.1). In the episodic version, the subject was presented with a set of 12 cue words, one at a time, and was asked to use it to retrieve a memory of a

Table 8.1 List of words used to cue personal (autobiographical) and historical (generic) memories in the Crovitz Test

Personal	Historical
Happy	Revolt (Rebellion)
Find	Explorer
Letter	Invention or Discovery
Throw	Saint
Lonely	Battle
Game	Assassination
Successful	Sea
Make	King or Queen
Break	Indians or Settlers
Dog	Miracle
Angry	Train
River	Fire or Natural Disaster

particular event he or she had experienced and to describe it in detail. In the semantic version, one of another set of 12 words served as cues for the subject to describe a historical event that occurred before he or she was born. We chose the Crovitz test because we thought that retrieving detailed information in response to such minimal, non-specific cues would necessarily involve strategic retrieval processes. The test was scored according to the procedure described by Zola-Morgan, Cohen, and Squire (1983, 1984). Three points were awarded for a detailed description that provided temporal information. Two points were awarded for a proper description of an event but one that lacked detail or temporal specification, and 1 point was awarded for providing general (non-specific) information in response to the cue. When no response was given to the cue or if the response was lacking in detail, subjects were prompted to provide additional information.

We tested four patients with confabulation, five amnesic patients whose memory was at least as poor as that of the confabulating patients, and twelve normal adults between the ages of 65 and 70. The results appear in Tables 8.2 and 8.3. One of the confabulating patients could not produce any response on either version, presumably because strategic search was too impaired. Significantly, she also confabulated least in daily life. As noted earlier, recovering some information is a prerequisite to confabulation. The other three confabulators scored more poorly on both the semantic and the episodic versions of the test than either amnesic patients or normal control subjects who did not differ from each other. In comparison to amnesic and control subjects, confabulators had more difficulty in producing a description of a personal episode or a historical event or personality and needed prompting, but when they did respond, confabulation was present on half

Table 8.2 Examples of the cue-word responses and the scores they received

Cue-Word	Points	Response
Personal		
ANGRY	1	I've been angry an awful lot in my life, but OK a specific incident. I've always been an angry type . . . (angry—at a person?) Don't know specifics (angry at wife?) no (what makes you angry?) I'm Irish. (is it waiting that makes you angry? or when you can't do something?) no—people. When I see somebody doing something I think they're doing it on purpose.
LONELY	2	I have been very lonely for the past 4 years since I had my cardiac arrest. I spend most of my time by myself, I used to be very active, belonged to clubs, played tennis, traveled a great deal, and I was very active. Since my cardiac arrest, I haven't done any of those things. My wife went to work shortly after my cardiac arrest so she was at work all day and the children were at school, so I was always alone. (can you think of a specific time during this period that you were especially lonely?) No . . . I was always lonely. I lost most of my friends, my best friend wasn't much of a talker and I was the one who used to keep the conversation going. But when you have two people who don't talk much it's not much fun, so I lost most of my friends that way.
LETTER	3	I wrote a letter to a lady in response to a letter she had written to me. It was unusual, it was a girlfriend I had had in Med School. She lives in Brooklyn, New York, and I was in school in New York, and I dated her. She's in New Jersey now, I think, and in the letter she told me about her family and how she is married and has I think 2 kids. I got that letter in January of this year.
Historical		
SEA/OCEAN	1	All I can think about is the Black Sea, having to do with the time of Christ, and I don't know what it's about it just came into my head.
QUEEN/KING	2	Henry VIII had 5, 6, 7, or 8 wives. Quite a few events or fights. 1500, 1600? He had his wives executed and then he would marry another one. I think he had a navy and 2 of the boats sank but others he still had. Didn't go on crusades or anything like the earlier kings . . . I don't think they had railways then.

Table 8.2   (*continued*)

Cue-Word	Points	Response
		(wives' names?) I don't know. (Why executed?) maybe he wanted things done a certain way and they didn't do it, or maybe they had friends he didn't like. He carried a sword. They had horses then. (How were wives executed?) maybe they tied them down or something, chopped off their heads with hatchets . . . before the guillotine in France.
INDIANS/ SETTLERS	3	George Custard decided he had to change to be elected president, if he could be a "hero" so he decided to destroy the "Sioux" nation as there was gold there. He cut off at a pass at the little big horn, and massacred them, Chief Crazy Horse killed Custard who they called "Golden Hair" . . . There were no survivors.

the trials. For example, in response to the word "Queen," one patient produced "Victoria." When prompted to provide additional information all he said was, "One day she didn't want to go to school so now we have a holiday named after her." Victoria Day is a holiday in Canada but it celebrates her birth. In response to "Assasination," another patient told a story about David and Goliath who had a contest involving Jesus, to see whether one could shoot as straight with a rifle as with a slingshot. Goliath was killed by accident during the match.

Data are also presented from one patient with a right dorsolateral frontal lesion who did not confabulate, though she did provide fewer, less detailed answers than controls and amnesics. This suggests that the dorsolateral fron-

Table 8.3   Average scores obtained in the personal and historical version of the Crovitz Test

Group	N	Personal Without Prompt	With Prompt	Confabulations	N	Historical Without Prompt	With Prompt	Confabulations
Controls	9	19.9	24.4	0.0	7	24.0	26.1	0.7
Mid Frontal + Amn	4	12.2	22.0	9.0	2	6.0	10.0	11.5
Lateral Frontal	1	15.0	21.0	1.0	1	12.0	12.0	0.0
Amnesic	6	24.7	31.4	1.2	3	21.6	31.2	3.6

Note: Twelve cue words were used in each version and scored separately for details given with and without prompts. Maximum score is 36 (see text for details).

tal cortex may be necessary for initiating strategic search whereas the ventro-medial frontal cortex may play a greater role in monitoring.

Comparable deficits in episodic and semantic memory tasks were observed if subjects had to date, or place in proper temporal order, events that they had experienced and historical events that were part of their semantic knowledge. For example, after having said that America was discovered in 1492 (aside from Jesus' birth, the only event that one of our patients could date correctly), he then claimed that the American Declaration of Independence was signed in 1400. On repeated tests, he thought that World War II began between 1940 and 1976 and ended as early as 1954 and as recently as 1979. What was interesting was that he dated the events that he had experienced within the time of his birth; those he had not experienced, he assigned to the distant past. Thus, when semantic and episodic memory tests are comparable, similar deficits associated with strategic retrieval processes are observed in both.

Temporal, Spatial, and Procedural Knowledge

Temporal ordering and dating may be especially prone to confabulation. Memories are not typically recovered via associative retrieval processes in a correct chronological sequence or with temporal dating tags. Instead, strategic retrieval processes operating on available episodic and semantic knowledge are used to estimate the date and temporal order of all but highly over-learned events by relating them to known landmarks. Freidman (1993) reached a similar conclusion in reviewing an extensive literature on temporal ordering and dating in normal people.

Confabulation about place is less readily elicited than that about time because associative retrieval is likely to be more effective in dealing with space than with time. Associative retrieval may be sufficient to answer the question "Where is Paris?" but not "When were you in Paris last?" which often requires a strategic search. Nonetheless, questions about place can be devised that require strategic search, and these should elicit confabulations as readily as do questions about time. Such questions usually involve locations about which the subject has imperfect knowledge. Informal tests on one of our patients confirmed this prediction. He identified the location of familiar landmarks in Toronto, claimed ignorance about unfamiliar locations, but confabulated about less familiar but recognizable places (Moscovitch, 1989).

Our hypothesis suggests that confabulation should be least likely for knowledge about procedures or skills. Strategic search is not needed to determine whether or not one has a particular skill. Despite prodding and strong suggestions to the contrary, HW insisted correctly that he could not fix a typewriter or a camera, but that he could change a tire and described how he would do it.

This does not mean that patients would not confabulate about their skills under any circumstances. If the patient had some knowledge about a task, and perhaps had even attempted to execute it, or wished that he could, then he might confabulate. Little children, whose frontal lobes are not fully developed (Diamond, 1991; Kates and Moscovitch, 1994; Smith, Vriezen, and Kates, 1992), often engage in such confabulations when they talk about their abilities or plans (see Ceci, Chapter 3 of this volume).

Correlation of Confabulation with Memory and Cognitive Function Sensitive to Frontal Damage

A number of investigators have noted that confabulation is not correlated with severity of memory loss but rather with performance on cognitive tests sensitive to frontal lobe damage (e.g., Stuss and Benson, 1986; Stuss et al., 1978; Baddeley and Wilson, 1986; Kopelman, 1987). In the case reported by Kapur and Coughlan (1980) confabulation cleared as frontal functions returned. The same may probably be true of Parkin, Leng, and Stanhope's (1988) patient who had severe memory problems with confabulation for some time after rupture of an ACoA aneurysm. Two years later when formal testing began, however, he was left with a severe memory loss but his confabulation had cleared and performance on tests of fluency and Wisconsin Card Sorting was normal.

Delbecq-Derouesné et al. (1990), however, reported that their confabulating patients performed normally on a battery of standard cognitive tests of frontal lobe function. The one exception was tests of letter fluency. Dalla Barba et al. (1990) claimed that their patient also had no frontal deficits, but the tests were far less extensive.

These two opposing patterns of results are to be expected if the ventromedial frontal cortex that is implicated in confabulation is adjacent to, but not overlapping with, areas that are involved in the cognitive tests (Johnson, O'Connor, and Cantor, 1994). Typically, damage is likely to affect both regions, but on occasion it will be restricted to the ventromedial area.

Thus, no strong predictions about general memory loss or impaired performance on non-memory tests of frontal function follow from the retrieval deficit hypothesis. What is predicted, however, is that confabulation should be associated with deficits on memory tests that have a strong strategic retrieval component. Insofar as the majority of confabulating patients perform abysmally on tests of free recall but within the normal range on tests of recognition, this prediction is upheld (see Moscovitch, 1989; Parkin and Leng, 1993).

One exception is the case reported by Delbecq-Derouesné et al. (1990), who ostensibly showed exactly the reverse pattern. Recall was normal if only hits were scored, though there were a large number of intrusions in recounting events and stories as befits a confabulating patient. Recognition was poor and characterized by a large number of false positive responses to lures. To account for these results, one would have to assume that different aspects of strategic retrieval are impaired in the patients of Delbecq-Derouesné et al. than in the others. Specifically, an initial search process may need to be distinguished from a later, post-ecphoric monitoring process. Poor performance on free recall may result from an inadequate initial search process in the majority of patients, a process which is relatively preserved in Delbecq-Derouesné et al.'s patient. Although post hoc, this explanation is consistent with the observation that it is only this patient whose frontal cognitive functions seem to be intact.

Active initial search is circumvented on recognition tests where the target can act as its own, strong associative retrieval cue and lead to good performance in most patients. To account for their patient's poor recognition, Delbecq-Derouesné et al. proposed that post-ecphoric monitoring is too impaired to distinguish between familiarity based on episodic memory (the target) and that based on semantic memory (the lures). According to this interpretation, the patient uses a familiarity heuristic on which to base recognition judgment but cannot monitor whether the item is familiar because it had been studied recently or because it is an item that is experienced often, such as a word that occurs frequently in the language. If correct, this interpretation suggests that recognition performance would have been improved had the targets and lures been infrequent so that the studied item would gain disproportionately in familiarity. Conversely, performance may have dropped significantly lower than chance if the targets had been rare but the lures frequent.

Damage to the right prefrontal cortex has been associated with confabulation and with a heightened tendency to make a large number of false alarms to novel items on tests of recognition (Delbecq-Derouesné et al., 1990; Parkin, Dunn, Lee, O'Hara, and Nussbaum, 1993; Schacter and Curran, in preparation, cited in the Introduction to this volume). The idea that the right prefrontal cortex is involved in monitoring and verifying memories (Shallice et al., 1994) is consistent with these observations and with recent evidence from PET studies of right prefrontal activation during recollection (Tulving, Kapur, Craik, Moscovitch, and Houle).

Implication for Theories of Normal and Pathological Memory
Components of Retrieval

Perhaps more than any other syndrome, confabulation provides support for theories of memory that distinguish between two types of retrieval processes or two components to retrieval. One is an automatic component in which a proximal specific cue elicits the target, what we have termed associative/ cue dependent retrieval. The other is an effortful search component in which semantic information and episodic information are recruited in response to non-specific distal cues to home in on the target or, more likely, on the proximal cue and to monitor and evaluate the outcome of this search. We have termed this second type strategic retrieval. Thus, strategic retrieval it- self consists of two components: an initial effortful, guided *memory search* and a *post-ecphoric monitoring process* that evaluates the outcome of that search.

Broadly similar proposals have been advanced in the literature on normal (e.g., Mandler, 1980; Joulia and Atkinson, 1974; Tulving, 1983; Morton, Hammersley, and Bekerian, 1985) and pathological memory (Baddeley and Wilson, 1986; Delbecq-Derouesné et al., 1990; Goldberg and Bilder, 1986; Rozin, 1976; Schacter, 1987; Shapiro et al., 1981; Shimamura, 1994; Stuss and Benson, 1986, among others).

Models of Feeling of Knowing and Confabulation

Recent studies and theories of feeling of knowing by Koriat (1993) and Met- calfe (1993) seem to capture the essence of the type of strategic retrieval process that is impaired in confabulating patients. "Feeling of knowing" refers to the condition in which the requested target is not retrieved but the individual feels that he knows the answer and would recognize it if it were provided. These theories postulate a basic memory storage system and a monitoring-control system that assesses novelty and the amount and type of information that is accessible during retrieval. Feeling-of-knowing judg- ments are based on the accessibility of pertinent, but not necessarily correct, information during retrieval. Thus, in a series of experiments Koriat (1993) has shown that it is the total amount of partial but accessible information about the target that determines feeling-of-knowing judgments and not whether the information that was accessed is correct or wrong. Using a com- posite-trace distributed model of memory, called CHARM, Metcalfe suc- cessfully simulated the performance of normal people on tests of feeling-of- knowing and release from PI. When the monitoring-control device of the model was "damaged," the output of the model resembled the impaired performance of patients with frontal lesions or dysfunction on these tests (feeling of knowing: Janowsky, Shimamura, and Squire, 1989; Shimamura and Squire, 1986; release from PI: Cermak, Butters, and Moreines, 1974; Moscovitch, 1982; Squire, 1982; Winocur, Kinsbourne, and Moscovitch, 1981). Although there are no reports on how confabulating patients per- formed on these tests, it is very likely that they would perform even more poorly than patients with frontal damage who did not confabulate. Indeed, Koriat's experiment in which normal people are led to provide high feeling-of-knowing judgments to erroneous but pertinent information approximates what I believe happens in patients with confabulation. Because their monitoring-control device is damaged, the output of erroneous retrieval becomes expressed overtly rather than being withheld, as it is in normal people, where it may give rise to a feeling-of-knowing state.

Memory Storage Is Random and Lacking in Temporal Information

The fact that confabulations often refer to actually experienced events that are chronologically distorted suggests that temporal order is a property that is conferred on memories by post-ecphoric strategic retrieval processes. The idea that memories are stored randomly, without regard to sequence except immediate contiguity, was proposed by Landauer (1975), who described how such a system would operate and give rise to a number of phenomena, such as interference, that are cue-dependent. This device, however, must be coupled with a strategic retrieval component that allows access to stored memories when local, proximal cues are inadequate, monitors recovered memories, and organizes them into proper sequence and context. We refer to this context as *historical* because that word most fully captures the temporal, spatial, and situational aspects that comprise a context.

Two Models of Memory, Functional and Neuropsychological, to Account for Confabulation

Of the various models that deal with two types of retrieval, Conway's (1992) model and my own (Moscovitch, 1989, 1992) incorporate most fully those features of strategic and associative retrieval that are discussed in this chapter. In Conway's *generative retrieval* model, strategic retrieval processes construct a context or memory description in the first phase. The second phase is an access phase which involves a search through knowledge structures such as general themes and schemas (Schank, 1982) to recreate the situation in which a particular event occurred. Specific, local cues are then used to retrieve information about details of the event from a random memory storage system which holds phenomenological records of consciously experienced events. It is significant that production of general schemas is impaired after frontal damage (Godbout and Doyon, 1994; Grafman, 1989) which would contribute to these patients' difficulties in engaging in strategic search. In the final evaluation phase, the recovered records are evaluated in terms of the original context, i.e., task demands, metaknowledge of what an appropriate outcome should be, consistency with other episodic and semantic knowledge, and so on.

In my own model, any event that is experienced consciously is automatically picked up by the hippocampus and related limbic structures in the medial temporal lobe and diencephalon. The hippocampal component helps form a memory trace of that event which is stored in cortical structures that gave rise to the conscious experience. The neural substrate that made the experience conscious is as much part of the trace as the neural substrate coding other features of the event. Thus, "consciousness" is built into the trace. Memory traces are laid down randomly and, except for simultaneity or immediate temporal contiguity, they are not organized by theme or temporal order with regard to any other event. In short, the memories lack historical context. They may, however, have *associative context,* which refers to the multimodel spatial background within which the target is embedded and which comprises an event. Recovery of memory traces involves associative cue-dependent retrieval processes (ecphory) that may activate the cortical engrams directly if the memories are fully consolidated or via the hippocampus if they are new. The frontal lobes act as "working-with-memory" structures that initiate and organize strategic retrieval search when the associative cue is inadequate. The frontal lobes are also involved in monitoring, evaluating, and verifying recovered memory traces in accordance with the goals of the memory task, and in organizing memory traces into the correct *historical context,* i.e., by the theme and temporal order. The search component is likely mediated by different regions of the prefrontal cortex than the post-ecphoric monitoring and verification component. A possible candidate for the former is the lateral frontal cortex and for the latter, the ventromedial frontal cortex, with the right side playing a more prominent role in both instances.

Implications for Research on Memory Distortion in Normal People

By now it should be apparent that confabulation is similar in many ways to the type of memory distortion observed in children and in adults in the laboratory and in real life (see, in this volume, Ceci, Chapter 3; Loftus, Chapter 1; Schacter, Introduction). Evidence from both lines of research supports the view that remembering is a reconstructive process and suggests that the more heavily recollection depends on reconstruction, the greater the possibility for distortion. This view places the primary locus of memory distortion at retrieval. Rather than discuss these and other similarities, I thought it would be more informative to focus on those findings and hypotheses that research on confabulation has produced that are distinctive or at odds with those from studies of normal people.

Research on normal people (see Schacter, Introduction) has suggested that distortion is more likely to occur if a memory is weak and its source is not known. This stands to reason because the worse the memory, the greater is the need for reconstruction in order to fill the gaps in one's memory (see Joseph, 1986). This explanation, a variant of the compensation hypothesis, may account for the type of memory distortions seen in everyday life, but it has difficulty explaining confabulations in clinical populations. Some memory loss may be a prerequisite for confabulation, as it is for any sort of memory distortion, but the upper limit for the extent and severity of memory loss as a contributing factor to confabulation is reached pretty quickly; it may not even exceed the level found in normal people. Certainly, there is no correlation between the severity of memory loss and that of confabulation. On the other hand, the evidence from confabulation identifies the ability to monitor, evaluate, and verify recovered "memories" as the critical factor that leads to gross distortions. All these are strategic memory functions that are impaired in patients with frontal-lobe damage. Likewise, loss of source, rather than being the cause of memory distortion, is itself a symptom of impaired strategic retrieval caused by frontal damage (see Schacter, 1987), though "source amnesia" may provide the occasion for yet further distortions.

Studies of confabulation also support the idea that memory traces of consciously experienced events, what Conway (1992) calls phenomenological records, are stored randomly without a temporal or thematic tag. The only relations among traces are simple contiguity and association by similarity. Temporal order and thematic organization, what I have called the historical context of memory, is conferred on recovered traces only at retrieval. If this view is correct (and I believe it is; see also Freidman, 1993), then it is easy to see why memory is so prone to distortion even if the traces themselves are intact. In a system that does not honor temporal order, the possibility of one event influencing the memory of another is very great, especially if they bear some similarity to each other. Similarly, if the assignment of events to their proper context and sequence depends on strategic retrieval, then post-event suggestions, which themselves become memory traces, can be mistaken, at yet another point in time, for true memories. In confabulating patients these distortions are frequent and exaggerated.

The question to be asked, given that the memory system is organized in this way, is why memory is as good as it is. Why don't we all confabulate? There are two answers to this question. One is that we do confabulate— all the time, but the distortions are sufficiently small so as not to matter. For most occasions our memory is good enough, though we may wish it were better. When precision of content and sequence is demanded, as it is in eyewitness testimony (see Loftus, Chapter 1 of this volume), our memory is notoriously poor and distorted.

The other answer is that what prevents gross confabulations is proper monitoring, evaluation, and verification of memory traces. These strategic retrieval operations are dependent on the prefrontal cortex. It is significant that confabulation occurs in other disorders, such as schizophrenia, that are associated with frontal dysfunction (Weinberger, Berman, and Zec, 1986; Weinberger, Berman, and Daniel, 1991) and in children whose frontal lobes are poorly developed (Diamond, 1991; Kates and Moscovitch, 1994; Smith et al., 1992). Depleting cognitive resources in normal people by manipulating attention has been shown to affect strategic retrieval associated with frontal function (Moscovitch, 1992, 1994) and to lower frontal activation associated with memory (Shallice et al., 1994). These observations suggest that such manipulations may also play a role in altering the degree of memory distortion in normal people. In a more speculative vein, these studies suggest that variation in frontal function across time in a single individual, or across individuals, may be a contributing factor to memory distortion.

Summary

Confabulation is a joint function of the accessibility of associatively retrieved memories and of the viability of the strategic retrieval process (Moscovitch, 1989). Damage to the associative retrieval system (which includes memory storage) will produce memory loss and faulty output. Impaired strategic search processes may have a similar consequence. These alone are not sufficient to produce confabulation, though they can account for errors of omission that are the most common response of patients with confabulation. Because damage to the hippocampus and related structures is spared in many patients with confabulation, and because performance improves tremendously when associative cues are adequate, I believe that the principal source of errors of omission is poor strategic search. Confabulation arises because of deficient strategic retrieval processes at output that are involved in monitoring, evaluating, and verifying recovered memory traces, and placing them in proper historical context. The ventromedial frontal cortex and related structures in the basal forebrain, cingulum, and striatum are the structures that are most likely to mediate strategic retrieval processes and whose damage leads to confabulation. As I have argued in the previous section, even with these structures intact and functioning well, the nature of the memory system is such that some distortion is likely at retrieval. When ventromedial prefrontal structures are damaged or dysfunctional, the likelihood is greatly increased that gross memory distortions typical of confabulation will occur.

References

Alexander, M. P., and Freedman, M. 1984. Amnesia after anterior communicating artery aneurysm rupture. *Neurology,* 34: 752–757.
Baddeley, A., and Wilson, B. 1986. Amnesia, autobiographical memory and confab-

ulation. In D. Rubin, ed., *Autobiographical memory*. New York: Cambridge University Press.

Barbizet, J. 1963. Defect of memorizing of hippocampal-mammillary origin: A review. *Journal of Neurology, Neurosurgery, and Psychiatry,* 26: 127–135.

Berlyne, N. 1972. Confabulation. *British Journal of Psychiatry,* 120: 31–39.

Cermak, L. S., Butters, N., and Moreines, J. 1974. Some analyses of the verbal encoding deficit in alcoholic Korsakoff patients. *Brain and Language,* 1: 141–150.

Conway, M. A. 1992. A structural model of autobiographical memory. In M. A. Conway, D. C. Rubin, H. Spinnler, and W. A. Wagenaar, eds., *Theoretical perspectives on autobiographical memory*. Amsterdam: Kluwer Academic Publishers, pp. 167–194.

Crovitz, H. November, 1973. Unconstrained search in long-term memory. Paper presented at the meeting of the Psychonomic Society, St. Louis, Mo.

Dalla Barba, G. 1993a. Confabulation: Knowledge and recollective experience. *Cognitive Neuropsychology,* 10: 1–20.

Dalla Barba, G. 1993b. Different patterns of confabulation. *Cortex,* 29: 567–581.

Dalla Barba, G., Cipolotti, L., and Deues, G. 1990. Autobiographical memory loss and confabulation in Korsakoff's syndrome: A case report. *Cortex,* 26: 525–534.

Delbecq-Derouesné, J., Beauvois, M. F., and Shallice, T. 1990. Preserved recall versus impaired recognition: A case study. *Brain,* 113: 1045–1074.

Deluca, J. 1993. Predicting neurobehavioral patterns following anterior communicating artery aneurysm. *Cortex,* 29: 639–647.

Deluca, J., and Cicerone, K. D. 1991. Confabulation following aneurysm of the anterior communicating artery. *Cortex,* 27: 417–424.

Diamond, A. 1991. Guidelines for the study of brain-behavior relationships during development. In H. S. Levin, H. M. Eisenberg, and A. L. Benton, eds., *Frontal lobe function and dysfunction*. Oxford: Oxford University Press, pp. 339–378.

Enoch, M. D., Trethowan, W. H., and Baker, J. G. 1967. *Some uncommon psychiatric syndromes*. Bristol: John Wright and Sons.

Freidman, W. J. 1993. Memory for the time of past events. *Psychological Bulletin,* 113: 44–66.

Gainotti, G. 1975. Confabulation of denial in senile dementia. *Psychiatria Clinica,* 8: 99–108.

Godbout, L., and Doyon, J. 1994. *Schematic representations of knowledge after frontal or posterior lobe lesions*. Manuscript submitted for publication.

Goldberg, E., and Bilder, R. M. 1986. Neuropsychological perspectives: Retrograde amnesia and executive deficits. In L. W. Poon, ed., *Clinical memory assessment of older adults*. Washington, D.C.: APA Press, pp. 55–68.

Grafman, J. 1989. Plans, actions, and mental sets: The role of the frontal lobes. In E. Perecman, ed., *Integrating theory and practice in clinical neuropsychology*. Hillsdale, N.J.: Erlbaum.

Incissa della Rochetta, A. 1986. Classification and recall of pictures after unilateral frontal or temporal lobectomy. *Cortex,* 22: 189–211.

Irle, E., Wowra, B., Kunert, H. J., and Kunze, S. 1992. Memory disturbances following anterior communicating artery rupture. *Annals of Neurology,* 31: 473–480.

Johnson, M. K., O'Connor, M., and Cantor, J. 1994. *Confabulation, memory deficits, and frontal dysfunction*. Manuscript submitted for publication.

Joseph, R. 1986. Confabulation and delusional denial: Frontal lobe and lateralized influences. *Journal of Clinical Psychology,* 42: 507–520.

Joslyn, D., Grundvig, J. K., and Chamberlain, C. J. 1978. Predicting confabulation from the Graham-Kendall Memory-for-Design test. *Journal of Consulting and Clinical Psychology,* 46: 181.

Kapur, N., and Coughlan, A. K. 1980. Confabulation and frontal lobe dysfunction. *Journal of Neurology, Neurosurgery, and Psychiatry,* 43: 461–463.

Kates, M. H., and Moscovitch, M. 1994. *The development of memory for temporal order: An assessment of frontal-lobe functioning in children.* Manuscript submitted for publication.

Kern, R., Van Gorp, W., Cummings, J., Brown, W., and Osato, S. 1992. Confabulation in Alzheimer's disease. *Brain and Cognition,* 19: 172–182.

Kinsbourne, M. 1989. The boundaries of episodic remembering. In H. L. Roediger and F. I. M. Craik, eds., *Varieties of memory and consciousness: Essays in honor of Endel Tulving.* Hillsdale, N.J.: Erlbaum, pp. 179–191.

Kopelman, M. D. 1987. Two types of confabulation. *Journal of Neurology, Neurosurgery, and Psychiatry,* 50: 482–487.

Kopelman, M. D. 1989. Remote and autobiographical memory, temporal context memory and frontal atrophy in Korsakoff and Alzheimer patients. *Neuropsychologia,* 27: 437–460.

Koriat, A. 1993. How do we know that we know? The accessibility model of the feeling of knowing. *Psychological Review,* 100: 609–639.

Landauer, T. K. 1975. A multicopy storage and random access model of memory. *Cognitive Psychology,* 7: 495–531.

Lhermitte, F., and Signoret, J.-L. 1976. The amnesic syndromes and the hippocampal-mammillary system. In M. R. Rosenzweig and E. L. Bennett, eds., *Neural mechanisms of learning and memory.* Cambridge, Mass.: MIT Press, pp. 44–56.

Luria, A. 1976. *The neuropsychology of memory.* New York: Wiley.

Mandler, G. 1980. Recognizing: The judgment of previous occurrence. *Psychological Review,* 87: 252–271.

McGlynn, S. M., and Schacter, D. L. 1989. Unawareness of deficit in neuropsychological syndromes. *Journal of Clinical and Experimental Neuropsychology,* 11: 143–205.

Mercer, B., Wapner, W., Gardner, H., and Benson, D. F. 1977. A study of confabulation. *Archives of Neurology,* 34: 429–433.

Metcalfe, J. 1993. Novelty monitoring, metacognition, and control in a composite holographic associative recall model: Implications for Korsakoff amnesia. *Psychological Review,* 100: 3–22.

Milner, B., Petrides, M., and Smith, M. L. 1985. Frontal lobes and the temporal organization of memory. *Human Neurobiology,* 4: 137–142.

Morton, J., Hammersley, R. H., and Bekerian, D. A. 1985. Headed records: A model for memory and its failure. *Cognition,* 20: 1–23.

Moscovitch, M. 1982a. Multiple dissociations of function in amnesia. In L. S. Cermak, ed., *Human memory and amnesia.* Hillsdale, N.J.: Erlbaum.

Moscovitch, M. 1982b. A neuropsychological approach to perception and memory in normal and pathological aging. In F. I. M. Craik and S. Trehub, eds., *Aging and cognitive processes.* New York: Plenum Press.

Moscovitch, M. 1989. Confabulation and the frontal systems: Strategic versus asso-ciated retrieval in neuropsychological theories of memory. In H. L. Roediger, III and F. I. M. Craik, eds., *Varieties of Memory and Consciousness*, Hillsdale, N.J.: Erlbaum, pp. 133–160.

Moscovitch, M. 1992. Memory and working-with-memory: A component process model based on modules and central systems. *Journal of Cognitive Neurosci-ence*, 4: 257–267.

Moscovitch, M. 1994. Cognitive resources and dual-task interference effects at re-trieval in normal people: The role of the frontal lobes and medial temporal cor-tex. *Neuropsychology*, 8: 524–534.

Moscovitch, M., Vriezen, E., and Goshen-Gottstein, Y. 1993. Implicit tests of mem-ory in patients with focal lesions and degenerative brain disorders. In H. Spinnler and F. Boller, eds., *Handbook of Neuropsychology: Volume 8*. Amster-dam: Elsevier.

Moscovitch, M., and Winocur, G. 1992a. The neuropsychology of memory and aging. In T. A. Salthouse and F. I. M. Craik, eds., *The handbook of aging and cognition*. Hillsdale, N.J.: Erlbaum.

Moscovitch, M., and Winocur, G. 1992b. Frontal lobes and memory. In L. R. Squire, ed., *Encyclopedia of learning and memory: Neuropsychology*, D. L. Schacter, section editor. New York: MacMillan Publishing Company.

Parkin, A. J., Dunn, J. C., Lee, C., O'Hara, P. F., and Nussbaum, L. 1993. Neuropsy-chological sequelae of Wernicke's Encephalopathy in a 20-year-old woman: Selec-tive impairment of a frontal memory system. *Brain and Cognition*, 21: 1–19.

Parkin, A. J., and Leng, N. R. C. 1993. Neuropsychology of the amnesic syndrome. Hove, U.K.: Erlbaum.

Parkin, A. J., Leng, N. R. C., and Stanhope, N. 1988. Memory impairment following ruptured aneurysm of the anterior comunicating artery. *Brain and Cognition*, 7: 231–243.

Parkin, A. J., Leng, N. R. C., Stanhope, N., and Smith, A. P. 1988. Memory loss following ruptured aneurysm of the anterior communicating artery. *Brain and Cognition*, 7: 231–243.

Rozin, P. 1976. The psychobiological approach to human memory. In R. M. Rosen-zweig and E. L. Bennett, eds., *Neural mechanisms of learning and memory*. Cambridge, Mass.: MIT Press, pp. 3–48.

Sandson, J., Albert, M. L., and Alexander, M. 1986. Confabulation in aphasia. *Cor-tex*, 22: 621–626.

Schaak, R. C. 1982. *Dynamic memory*. Cambridge: Cambridge University Press.

Schacter, D. L. 1987. Memory, amnesia, and frontal lobe dysfunction. *Psychology*, 15: 21–36.

Schacter, D. L., Eich, J. E., and Tulving, E. 1978. Richard Semon's theory of mem-ory. *Journal of Verbal Learning and Verbal Behavior*, 17: 721–743.

Schacter, D. L., Harbluk, J. L., and McLachlan, D. R. 1984. Retrieval without recol-lection: An experimental analysis of source amnesia. *Journal of Verbal Learning and Verbal Behavior*, 23: 593–611.

Shallice, T., and Burgess, P. W. 1992. Deficits in strategy application following fron-tal lobe damage in man. *Brain*, 114: 727–741.

Shallice, T., Fletcher, P., Frith, C. D., Grasby, P., Frackowiak, R. S. J., and Dolan, R. J. 1994. The functional anatomy of episodic memory. *Nature*, 368: 633–635.

Shapiro, B. E., Alexander, M. P., Gardner, H., and Mercer, B. 1981. Mechanisms of confabulation. *Neurology,* 31: 1070–1076.

Shimamura, A. P. 1994. Memory and frontal lobe function. In M. S. Gazzaniga, ed., *The cognitive neurosciences.* Cambridge, Mass.: MIT Press.

Shimamura, A. P., Janowsky, J. S., and Squire, L. R. 1991. What is the role of frontal lobe damage in memory disorders? In H. D. Levin, H. M. Eisenberg, and A. L. Benton, eds., *Frontal lobe functioning and dysfunction.* New York: Oxford University Press, pp. 173–195.

Smith, M. L., Kates, M. H., and Vriezen, E. R. 1992. The development of frontal-lobe functioning. In S. Segalowitz and I. Rapin, eds., *Handbook of Neuropsychology, Volume 7.* Amsterdam: Elsevier, pp. 309–330.

Squire, L. R. 1982. Comparison between forms of amnesia: Some deficits are unique to Korsakoff's syndrome. *Journal of Experimental Psychology: Learning, Memory and Cognition,* 8: 560–571.

Squire, L. R. 1992. Memory and the hippocampus: A synthesis from findings with rats, monkeys and humans. *Psychological Review,* 99: 195–231.

Stuss, D. T., Alexander, M. D., Lieherman, A., and Levine, I. I. 1978. An extraordinary form of confabulation. *Neurology,* 28: 1166–1172.

Stuss, D. T., and Benson, D. F. 1986. *The frontal lobes.* New York: Raven Press.

Talland, G. A. 1961. Confabulation in the Wernicke-Korsakoff syndrome. *Journal of Nervous and Mental Diseases,* 132: 361–381.

Talland, G. A. 1965. *Deranged memory.* New York: Academic Press.

Tulving, E. 1983. *Elements of episodic memory.* Oxford: Clarendon Press.

Tulving, E., Kapur, S., Craik, F. I. M., Moscovitch, M., and Houle, S. 1994. Hemispheric encoding/retrieval asymmetry in episodic memory: Positron emission tomography finding. *Proceedings of the National Academy of Sciences, USA,* 91: 2016–2020.

Vilkki, J. 1985. Amnesic syndrome after surgery for anterior communicating artery aneurysms. *Cortex,* 21: 431–444.

Vriezen, E., and Moscovitch, M. 1990. Temporal ordering and conditional associative learning in Parkinson's disease. *Neuropsychologia,* 28: 1283–1294.

Weinberger, D. R., Berman, K. F., and Daniel, D. G. 1991. Prefrontal cortex dysfunction in schizophrenia. In H. S. Levin, H. M. Eisenberg, and A. L. Benton, eds., *Frontal lobe function and dysfunction.* Oxford: Oxford University Press, pp. 275–287.

Weinberger, D. R., Berman, K. F., and Zec, R. F. 1986. Physiologic dysfunction of dorsolateral prefrontal cortex in schizophrenia. *Archives of General Psychiatry,* 43: 114–124.

Weinstein, E. A., and Kahn, R. L. 1955. *Denial of illness.* Springfield, Ill.: Thomas.

Williams, H. W., and Rupp, C. 1938. Observation on confabulation. *American Journal of Psychiatry,* 95: 395–405.

Wilson, B., and Baddeley, A. 1988. Semantic, episodic, and autobiographical memory in a post meningitic amnesic patient. *Brain and Cognition,* 8: 31–46.

Winocur, G., Kinsbourne, M., and Moscovitch, M. 1981. The effect of cuing on release from proactive interference in Korsakoff amnesic patients. *Journal of Experimental Psychology: Human Learning and Memory,* 7: 56–65.

Neurobiological Perspectives

Emotional Activation, Neuromodulatory Systems, and Memory

9

James L. McGaugh

Since our experiences and actions depend critically upon our re-membrances of prior experiences, it would seem essential that our memories accurately represent our experiences. But, as we know, they do not. We are good at forgetting. We often remember inaccurately: We fail to remember experiences and, under some circumstances, are confident that we remember events that we did not experience. Distortion, in the general sense of failure to reflect experiences accurately, appears to be a central feature of memory (Bartlett, 1932; Tulving, 1983; Schacter, Introduction to this volume). Weak memories seem particularly vulnerable to mis-remembering. However, as every student of memory knows, Ebbinghaus (1885) convincingly demon-strated that repetition of the to-be-remembered information increases the strength of memory and retards forgetting. We are generally quite accurate in remembering well-rehearsed and often recalled information.

Emotional Arousal and Memory

Many of our experiences are single events or brief episodes. Such experiences are generally quickly forgotten or, at best, poorly remembered. However, under some conditions events and episodes can be well-remembered even if they are not repeated. We have many lasting memories of important pleasant events such as birthdays, weddings and holiday celebrations. We also have strong memories of unpleasant events such as personal embarrassments, ac-cidents and deaths of loved ones. Some episodes in our lives appear to be almost indelibly recorded (LeDoux, 1992b). At the extreme are recurring intensely unpleasant memories that characterize the Post Traumatic Stress Syndrome (Pitman, 1989). Observations such as these have suggested that emotional arousal at the time of an experience may play a critical role in influencing memory strength (Bower, 1992). Over a century ago, William James (1890) observed that "An experience may be so exciting emotionally as almost to leave a scar on the cerebral tissues." There is now considerable evidence supporting James's conclusion. Findings of many experimental studies of human as well as animal memory suggest that the emotional arousal induced by an experience is an important determinant of the strength of memory for the event (Heuer and Reisberg, 1990; McGaugh, 1990; Bower, 1992; Revelle and Loftus, 1992). Moreover, recent findings have identified neurobiological systems that appear to play critical roles in mediating the influence of emotional arousal on memory storage. This chapter focuses on the findings and implications of experiments investigating these systems.

Modulation of Memory Storage

It is now well established that the neural traces of experiences are susceptible to modulating influences for a period of time following learning. The hypothesis (Mueller and Pilzecker, 1900) that memory traces are initially fragile and subsequently become consolidated is strongly supported by clinical as well as experimental findings indicating that retention is impaired by conditions, such as brain trauma, electrical stimulation of the brain, or drugs, that interfere with normal brain functioning shortly after learning (McGaugh and Herz, 1972). The consolidation hypothesis is also supported by extensive evidence from animal studies indicating that retention can be enhanced by posttraining electrical stimulation of the brain as well as posttraining administration of drugs affecting neuromodulatory systems normally activated by learning experiences (McGaugh and Herz, 1972; McGaugh, 1973). This evidence suggests the possibility that emotional arousal may enhance memory by activating systems involved in regulating the storage of newly acquired information. Thus, the susceptibility of memory storage processes to modulating influences occurring after learning provides the opportunity for emotional activation to regulate the strength memory traces representing important experiences (Gold and McGaugh, 1975).

Hormones and Memory Storage

There are, of course, other ways in which emotion might, and no doubt does, influence memory. Emotional arousal can affect attention at the time of learning as well as subsequent rehearsal and recall, and it can be difficult to distinguish such effects from influences on memory storage. An important implication of the hypothesis that emotional arousal has an influence on memory storage is that the hypothesis can be addressed by experiments using posttraining treatments. Because the critical alterations in such experiments are induced after the completion of training, the results of these experiments cannot, of course, be attributed to influences on attention during the learning.

The extensive evidence that memory can be enhanced by posttraining administration of drugs, such as amphetamine, that are known to affect hormonal and neurotransmitter systems (McGaugh, 1973) suggested the possibility that memory storage may normally be regulated by stress-related hormones that are released by emotionally arousing experiences (Gold and McGaugh, 1975). In the first experiment investigating this possibility (Gold and van Buskirk, 1975) rats were given inhibitory avoidance (passive avoidance) training and after training received injections of saline or low doses of the adrenal medullary hormone epinephrine (which is normally released by stressful experiences). The epinephrine injections produced dose-dependent enhancement of memory, as indicated by superior retention test performance of the epinephrine-treated rats in comparison with that of the saline controls. Furthermore, the memory enhancement was time-dependent: the epinephrine injections were most effective when administered immediately after training. Many subsequent experiments have shown that posttraining administration of epinephrine enhances memory in a variety of training tasks using appetitive as well as aversive motivation (Gold, van Buskirk, and Haycock, 1977; Borrell, de Kloet, Versteeg, and Bohus, 1983; Izquierdo and Diaz, 1983; Sternberg, Isaacs, Gold, and McGaugh, 1985; Liang, Bennett, and McGaugh, 1985; Introini-Collison and McGaugh, 1986; Flood, Garland, and Morley, 1992; Williams and McGaugh, 1993). Furthermore, epinephrine effects on memory are long-lasting: memory-enhancing effects are found on retention tests given at intervals of up to a month after training (Introini-Collison and McGaugh, 1986).

The findings of studies of the effects of epinephrine on memory are consistent with the hypothesis that memory is influenced by hormones normally released by emotionally arousing experiences. Additionally, other stress-related hormones, including vasopressin, ACTH, and corticosterone, have been reported to enhance memory when administered posttraining (Gold and van Buskirk, 1976; Ettenberg, van der Kooy, Le Moal, Koob, and Bloom, 1983; de Wied, Gaffori, van Ree, and de Jong, 1984; Micheau, Destrade, and Soumireu-Mourat, 1984; McGaugh and Gold, 1989; Koob, LeBrun, Bluthe, Dantzer, Dorsa, and LeMoal, 1991). The finding that retention is enhanced by posttraining administration of the gut peptide cholecystokinin (CCK), which is known to be released following the ingestion of food, indicates that hormonal influences on memory are not restricted to stress-related hormones (Morley and Flood, 1991). There is also extensive evidence indicating that retention is impaired by posttraining administration of opioid peptides as well as high doses of other stress-released hormones, including epinephrine (Izquierdo, Medina, Netto, and Pereira, 1991; McGaugh, Introini-Collison, and Castellano, 1993). Thus, the findings of studies of the effects of posttraining administration of hormones strongly suggest that the physiological consequences of emotional arousal affect memory by modulating consolidation processes occurring after the learning experience independently of any effects that the arousal might have on attention or other processes affecting learning. More generally, the evidence provides strong support for the hypothesis that hormones play an important role in mediating the influences of emotional arousal on memory.

Pathway of Neuromodulatory Influences

Many of the hormones found to influence memory storage do not readily enter the brain when released or administered peripherally. Ultimately, of course, the hormones must influence brain processes involved in memory. How is this accomplished? There are several possibilities. First, it may be that small quantities of hormones pass the blood-brain barrier. Second, it may be that hormones activate the release of other substances that readily enter the brain. Gold (1991) suggested, for example, that the effects of epinephrine may be mediated by initiating the release of glucose. A third possibility is that hormone influences might be initiated peripherally by activation of receptors on visceral afferents projecting to the brain. The findings of several experiments suggest that the effects of epinephrine and CCK on memory are mediated by the latter route. Flood and his colleagues (Flood, Smith, and Morley, 1987) reported that severing the vagus nerve surgically blocks the memory-enhancing effects of CCK. Vagus nerve afferents project from the periphery to the nucleus of the solitary tract (NTS) which, in turn, projects to regions of the forebrain known to be involved in memory. Functioning of the NTS appears to be critical for memory storage: inactivation of the NTS (with microinjections of lidocaine) induces retrograde amnesia (Williams and McGaugh, 1992) and blocks the effects of peripherally administered epinephrine on memory (Williams and McGaugh, 1993).

Epinephrine effects on memory appear to be initiated by activation of beta-adrenergic receptors located in the periphery, that is, outside of the brain. In several experiments (Introini-Collison, Saghafi, Novack, and McGaugh, 1992) using two aversively motivated training tasks (inhibitory avoidance and Y-maze escape tasks) we found that the memory-enhancing effects of epinephrine were selectively blocked by the beta-adrenergic antagonist sotalol, a drug which does not enter the brain when administered peripherally. Epinephrine effects on memory were not blocked by alpha-adrenergic antagonists. We also found that memory was enhanced by posttraining peripheral injections of DPE (dipivalyl epinephrine), an adrenergic agonist drug that is less polar than epinephrine and, therefore, enters the brain more readily. Furthermore, the DPE effects were not blocked by sotalol, but were blocked by propranolol, a beta-adrenergic antagonist that readily enters the brain.

These findings indicate that the memory-modulating effects of some hormones, including epinephrine and CCK, that are known to be released by training experiences are initiated by activation of peripheral afferents that project to the brain. They also indicate that memory storage processes can be influenced by compounds that directly enter the brain. The results of the studies of the effects of epinephrine and DPE clearly indicate that memory storage is influenced by activation of peripheral as well as central beta-adrenergic receptors. As discussed below, there is extensive evidence suggesting that activation of central noradrenergic systems is involved in mediating effects of many neuromodulatory influences on memory storage (McGaugh, Introini-Collison, Cahill, Castellano, Dalmaz, Parent, and Williams, 1993).

Involvement of the Amygdala

Extensive evidence from human as well as animal studies suggests that the amygdaloid complex is involved in emotionally influenced memory. The importance of the amygdala in emotion was first suggested by the pioneering findings of Kluver and Bucy (1937) and Weiskrantz (1956) showing that, in monkeys, lesions of the amygdala impaired emotional responsiveness to aversive or rewarding objects. The view that the amygdala is involved in emotion and emotionally related memory is strongly supported by subsequent research findings. In humans, emotional arousal is associated with activation of the amygdala, and electrical stimulation of the amygdala evokes emotional responses (Gloor, 1992; Halgren, 1992). Additionally, findings of recent studies of human patients with bilateral amygdala lesions suggest that such lesions induce a selective impairment in emotionally related memory (Babinsky, Calabrese, Durwen, Markowitsch, Brechtelsbauer, Heuser, and Gehlen, 1993; Markowitsch, Calabrese, Wurker, Durwen, Kessler, Babinsky, Brechtelsbauer, Heuser, and Gehlen, 1994). In animals, lesions of the amygdala impair the learning and retention of many kinds of tasks, especially (but not exclusively) tasks using emotionally arousing aversive motivation (e.g., footshock) (Kesner, Walser, and Winzenried, 1989; Cahill and McGaugh, 1990; Davis, 1992; Gaffan, 1992; LeDoux, 1992a), and posttraining electrical stimulation of the amygdala can enhance or impair retention (Kesner and Wilburn, 1974; McGaugh and Gold, 1976).

Adrenergic Influences

Several lines of evidence suggest that epinephrine and other hormones affect memory through influences involving the amygdala. The finding that the memory modulating effects of electrical stimulation of the amygdala are altered in animals whose adrenal medulla was surgically removed (and were, consequently, unable to release epinephrine) (Liang, Bennett, and McGaugh, 1985) was the first to suggest this possibility. In further support of this view, other studies have reported that lesions of the amygdala or the stria-terminalis, a major amygdala pathway, block the memory-enhancing effects of posttraining systemic injections of epinephrine (Liang and McGaugh, 1983b; Cahill and McGaugh, 1991). Furthermore, the finding that the effects of systemically administered epinephrine on memory are blocked by intra-amygdala injections of the beta-adrenergic receptor antagonist propranolol (Liang, Juler, and McGaugh, 1986) suggests that the epinephrine effects involve the release of the adrenergic neuromodulator norepinephrine (NE) within the amygdala. This suggestion is consistent with the report that epinephrine induces the release of brain NE (Gold and van Buskirk, 1978) and that stress induces the release of NE within the amygdala (Tanaka, Kohno, Nakagawa, Ida, Takeda, and Nagasaki, 1982). The hypothesis that modulation of memory storage involves noradrenergic activation within the amygdala is supported by evidence that intra-amygdala injections of beta-adrenergic antagonists impair memory and that the impairment is blocked by concurrent administration of NE (Gallagher, Kapp, Pascoe, and Rapp, 1981). The hypothesis is also supported by evidence that memory is enhanced by posttraining intra-amygdala injections of NE or the beta-adrenergic agonist clenbuterol (Liang, Juler, and McGaugh, 1986; Liang, McGaugh, and Yao, 1990; Introini-Collison, Miyazaki, and McGaugh, 1991).

Other Neuromodulatory Influences

As discussed above, memory storage is also influenced by other hormonal and neuromodulatory systems. Posttraining systemic injections of opioid peptides and opiates generally impair memory, and opiate antagonists enhance memory (McGaugh, 1989; McGaugh, Introini-Collison, and Castellano, 1993). Similarly, GABAergic agonists impair memory and GABAergic antagonists enhance memory (Castellano, Brioni, and McGaugh, 1990). Considerable evidence suggests that these influences, like those of epinephrine, involve the amygdala. As was found with epinephrine, opioid and GABAergic influences are blocked by lesions of the amygdala or stria terminalis (McGaugh, Introini-Collison, Juler, and Izquierdo, 1986; Ammassari-Teule, Pavone, Castellano, and McGaugh, 1991). Furthermore, the influences appear to be due to modulation of the release of NE within the amygdala: when administered either systemically or intra-amygdally, opiate and GABAergic influences on memory are blocked by intra-amygdala injections of beta-adrenergic antagonists (McGaugh, Introini-

Collison, and Nagahara, 1988; Introini-Collison, Nagahara, and McGaugh, 1989; McGaugh, Introini-Collison, Cahill, Castellano, Dalmaz, Parent, and Williams, 1993). Furthermore, injections of the opioid peptide beta-endorphin administered into the amygdala posttraining attenuate the memory-enhancing effects of systemic injections of the opiate antagonist naloxone, as well as those of epinephrine and CCK (Flood, Garland, and Morley, 1992). Since opiates are known to inhibit NE release (Werling, McMahon, Portoghese, Takemori, and Cox, 1989), these findings provide additional evidence that several hormonal and neuromodulatory systems have a common effect on memory by modulating noradrenergic influences in the amygdala.

It is well documented that benzodiazepines (BZDs) impair memory. In humans, BZDs impair memory when administered in doses commonly used to reduce anxiety or induce sleep (Lister and File, 1984; Lister, 1985). In rats and mice, BZDs impair memory (Cahill, Brioni, and Izquierdo, 1986; Venault, Chapouthier, Prado de Carvalho, Simiand, Morre, Dodd, and Rossier, 1986; Pereira Rosat, Huang, Godoy, and Izquierdo, 1989) and BZD inverse agonists and BZD antagonists enhance memory (Venault, Chapouthier, Simiand, Dodd, and Rossier, 1987; Pereira, Medina, and Izquierdo, 1989; Lal and Forster, 1990). The evidence indicating that BZD antagonists enhance memory suggests that the antagonism may be due to inhibition of endogenous BZDs released by stressful training (Izquierdo, Pereira, and Medina, 1990).

These findings are of particular interest in relation to the effects of GABAergic drugs on memory, since BZDs are known to enhance GABA$_A$-mediated synaptic inhibition. Extensive evidence suggests that, like GABA-ergic effects, BZD effects on memory involve the amygdala. In rats, neurotoxic lesions of either the entire amygdaloid complex or lesions restricted to the basolateral nucleus block BZD impairment of retention of inhibitory avoidance (Tomaz, Dickinson-Anson, and McGaugh, 1991, 1992). Furthermore, intra-amygdala injections of the BZD midazolam impair inhibitory avoidance retention (Dickinson-Anson and McGaugh, 1993) and, conversely, intra-amygdala injections of the BZD antagonist flumazenil enhance inhibitory avoidance retention (Da Cunha, Wolfman, Huang, Walz, Koya, Bianchin, Medina, and Izquierdo, 1991). The finding that posttraining intra-amygdala injections of the GABAergic antagonist bicuculline block the memory impairment induced by a peripherally administered BZD provides additional evidence that BZDs affect memory storage through GABAergic influences in the amygdala (Dickinson-Anson, Mesches, Coleman, and McGaugh, 1993).

Most experiments examining the effects of BZDs and GABAergic drugs on memory have used aversive stimulation, such as footshock, for motivation. The findings of recent experiments indicate that BZD and GABAergic drugs also affect memory for changes in the magnitude of food reward. When rats are first trained to run to a goal box for a large food reward and then are given a smaller amount of food, they reduce their running speeds and display emotional distress. This effect is referred to as the Crespi effect, or behavioral contrast (Crespi, 1942; Amsel, 1962, 1967). Under these conditions, the aversiveness of the training results from a decrease in the amount of an otherwise positive reward. Our findings indicating that inactivation of the amygdala with lidocaine immediately after the reduction blocks expression of the contrast effect indicates that memory of the change in reward conditions and the emotional responses to the change are susceptible to amygdala influences (Salinas, Packard, and McGaugh, 1993).

It is well known that BZDs block behavioral contrast (Rosen and Tessel, 1970; Flaherty, 1990). Findings from our laboratory (Salinas, Dickinson-Anson, and McGaugh, submitted) indicate that the effect is due to impairment of memory for the shift in reward magnitude. A BZD (midazolam) administered systemically prior to the day of the reward reduction did not block the aversive effect of the change as indicated by reduction in running speeds on that day. However, on the day following the BZD injection and reward reduction, the rats' initial running speeds were like those prior to the reward reduction. That is, they showed no evidence that they remembered that the reward had been reduced. In another experiment rats first received reward reduction and then, on the following day, the larger reward was reinstated. Midazolam administered prior to the trials in which the larger reward was once again given blocked the memory of the reinstatement. Thus, the BZD blocked memory for a positive shift in reward magnitude as well as memory for a negative (and clearly aversive) shift in reward magnitude. In similar experiments (Salinas, Dickinson-Anson, and McGaugh, submitted), the GABAergic agonist muscimol was administered immediately after the reduction or reinstatement of reward magnitude. As indicated by the rats' running speeds on the first trial of the day following the reward shifts and posttraining injections, muscimol impaired retention of both the reward reduction and the reward increase. In view of extensive evidence indicating that GABAergic influences on memory involve the amygdala, these findings provide additional evidence supporting the hypothesis that emotional influences on memory are mediated by the amygdala.

Function of the Amygdala in Memory Storage

The evidence summarized above indicates that several hormonal and neuromodulatory systems modulate memory storage by influencing activity in the amygdala. But we have not suggested that the effects are due to modulation of synaptic plasticity within the amygdala. Although there is evidence of synaptic plasticity, i.e., long-term potentiation (LTP) in the amygdala (Clugnet and LeDoux, 1990), as well as evidence suggesting that the amygdala is a locus of synaptic plasticity underlying learned fear (Davis, 1992; LeDoux, 1992b), several findings suggest that, at least for the kinds of training tasks used in the experiments summarized above, the amygdala affects retention by modulating the formation of memory traces in other brain regions. First, lesions of the amygdala induced several days after training do not block retention of inhibitory avoidance (Liang, McGaugh, Martinez, Jensen, Vasquez, and Messing, 1982) or escape training (Parent and McGaugh, submitted; Parent, Tomaz, and McGaugh, 1992). Second, the evidence that lesions of the stria terminalis block the memory-enhancing effects of posttraining intra-amygdala injections of NE (Liang, McGaugh, and Yao, 1990) suggests that the modulation involves efferent activity mediated by the stria terminalis. Third, the findings of recent experiments indicate that inactivation of the amygdala when retention is tested does not block the memory-enhancing effects of posttraining intra-amygdala drug injections (Packard, Cahill, and McGaugh, in press).

In these experiments (Packard, Cahill, and McGaugh, in press), rats were trained, in a single session, in one of two water-maze tasks, a spatial task or a visually cued task. In a first experiment, immediately after the training session the rats received injections of d-amphetamine administered into the hippocampus, caudate, or amygdala. On a retention test the following day animals given the hippocampal injections showed selective enhancement of memory for the spatial task, and animals given caudate injections showed selective enhancement of retention of the cued task. In contrast, animals given amygdala injections showed enhanced retention of both tasks. Thus, the role of the amygdala in modulating memory storage is not restricted to a specific form of memory. It is of interest that the hippocampal and caudate injections specifically affected retention of the task, spatial or cued, that is known, from the results of double-dissociation experiments, to be differentially impaired by lesions of the hippocampus or caudate, respectively. In a second experiment rats received posttraining intra-amygdala injections of saline or d-amphetamine immediately after training on one of the two tasks. Prior to the retention test on the following day, the amygdala was inactivated with lidocaine. As in the first experiment, d-amphetamine enhanced the retention of both tasks. Furthermore, and most important, the lidocaine injections administered into the amygdala prior to the retention test did not block the memory-enhancing effects of the d-amphetamine.

These findings clearly suggest that the effects, on memory storage, of drugs and hormones affecting amygdala activity are not based on long-lasting synaptic plasticity within the amygdaloid complex. Rather, they are consistent with the extensive evidence summarized above suggesting that the amygdala modulates the processes mediating memory storage in other brain regions. Available evidence provides few clues to the brain regions that serve as the permanent locus of changes modulated by the amygdala. The evidence that intra-amygdala injections of the excitatory amino acid NMDA induces the expression of c-fos in the hippocampus and caudate nucleus (Cahill and McGaugh, 1993) indicates that the amygdala is functionally connected with both of these brain regions and suggests the possibility that the amygdala may influence forms of memory differentially regulated by the hippocampus and caudate by modulating the functioning of these regions. In addition, or alternatively, the amygdala might directly modulate plasticity in the cortical brain regions mediating the long-term retention of many different forms of memory. Another potentially important clue is the evidence that the stria terminalis lesions block the effects of all neuromodulatory treatments affecting memory storage that have been investigated, including electrical stimulation of the brain (Liang and McGaugh, 1983a), as well as peripherally and intra-amygdally injected drugs and hormones. Thus, brain regions activated by amygdala efferents mediated by the stria terminalis are obviously important candidate regions for further research.

Adrenergic Involvement in Emotional Arousal and Memory

We return now to the issue of the role of emotional arousal in memory. As summarized above, the findings of studies using animals suggest that emotional arousal is accompanied by hormonal and other neuromodulatory influences on memory that converge in altering amygdala noradrenergic functioning. The finding of central importance in this regard is that when administered either peripherally or directly into the amygdala, beta-adrenergic antagonists block the memory modulating effects of many hormones and drugs. These findings suggest the possibility that activation of adrenergic systems may play a critical role in mediating the influences of emotional arousal on memory in humans. Recent experiments in our laboratory examined this issue in experiments aimed at determining whether a beta-adrenergic antagonist, propranolol, would selectively attenuate the effects of emotional arousal on memory in human subjects.

To determine the effects of emotional arousal on memory, we conducted an initial experiment using procedures generally patterned after those developed by Heuer and Reisberg (1990). In replication of their basic findings, our results indicated that emotional arousal induced by a story line accompanying a series of slides enhanced memory on retention tests given two weeks later (Cahill and McGaugh, submitted). The emotionally arousing portion of the story was selectively associated with several slides in the middle of a series of slides. The subjects were informed that the experiment concerned physiological responses to different kinds of stimuli. In the subsequent experiment (unpublished findings) replicating one of the experimental conditions used in the first experiment, subjects were shown the same series of slides accompanied by either an arousing or a non-arousing story line. One hour prior to the session, propranolol (40 mg) was administered to half of the subjects and a placebo pill was administered to the other subjects. The propranolol group was comparable to the placebo group in the degree of emotional arousal (indicated by self-ratings) induced by the arousing story line. And, on the retention tests, the propranolol and placebo groups did not differ in memory of the non-arousing information. However, the two groups did differ in memory of information concerning the emotionally arousing story: The placebo group had enhanced memory for the slides that had been associated with the emotionally arousing story. Propranolol blocked the effects of emotional arousal on memory but did not generally impair memory.

These findings fit well with those of animal experiments summarized above and provide strong support for the hypothesis suggesting that, in humans as well as animals, the influence of emotional arousal on long-term memory is based, at least in part, on activation of adrenergic systems. According to this general hypothesis, retention should be enhanced by epinephrine and drugs that activate adrenergic systems. To date, few studies have addressed this issue in studies using human subjects. In two studies reporting that epinephrine effects on memory were different from those induced by emotional arousal, only a single dose of epinephrine was used and retention was tested after a very short delay (12 minutes) (Christianson and Mjorndal, 1985; Christianson, Nilsson, Mjorndal, Perris, and Tjellden, 1986). Further research is needed to examine dose-response effects of epinephrine on long-term retention in human subjects.

Memory Selectivity and Distortion

In some sense, all of our memories are distorted: They are rarely accurate reflections of our past experiences. But all memories are not equally inaccurate. To a considerable degree, the accuracy of our memories depends upon their strength. Simply put, information that is weakly stored is quickly forgotten. Furthermore, when our memories are weak we may not only fail to remember but, perhaps more important, we may, and often do, remember inaccurately. Fortunately, much of our memory is strong and long-lasting. We usually make few, if any, errors in recalling frequently experienced and well-rehearsed information such as the names of the days of the week or the names of friends and relatives. But even such information can be forgotten—or at least can be more difficult to recall—if it is not used for long periods of time. For example, a foreign language (or even a first language) that was once fluently spoken may eventually become "rusty" if not used for many years.

Of course, even very strong memories are not immune to distortion. Each act of remembering creates new memories of old experiences (Bartlett, 1932; Schacter, Introduction to this volume). Furthermore, memory for personally experienced events can become confused with reported or imagined events. Briefly experienced events may be especially susceptible to forgetting and mis-remembering. The findings of research investigating the "flashbulb memory" hypothesis (Brown and Kulic, 1977) amply document this conclusion. The basic hypothesis is that highly surprising, important, and affectively arousing experiences produce accurate and long-lasting memories. Research investigating this hypothesis has typically studied subjects' memories of well-publicized, startling, or shocking occurrences. Although there is extensive evidence that memories for such events (and experiences associated with the events) are lasting (Brown and Kulik, 1977; Bohannon, 1988), there is also extensive evidence that they are not always accurate (Neisser and Harsch, 1992). A critical assumption of the "flashbulb memory" hypothesis is that the public event is highly surprising and important to the individual subjects included in the sample studied. More generally, the accuracy and durability of memory for public events should be expected to vary with the importance of the event to the individual subjects as well as their affective responses to the news. Recent evidence supports these implications (Conway, Anderson, Larsen, Donnelly, McDaniel, McClelland, Rawles, and Logie, 1994). When tested one year after a significant public event (the resignation of Margaret Thatcher), the memories of U.K. subjects who judged an event to be important and emotionally arousing were highly accurate. In contrast, non-U.K. subjects (for whom the event was less important) remembered less well and less accurately. A major problem with the methodology of "flashbulb memory" experiments is that the information about the novelty and importance of the event, as well as the subjects' emotional responses at the time of the event, is based solely on the subjects' retrospective reports and judgments. Such studies obviously lack precision in specifying the degree of emotional activation experienced by the subjects at the time of the event.

However, as summarized above, the general hypothesis that emotional arousal influences the memory of briefly experienced events is also strongly supported by extensive evidence provided by experiments using animal as well as human subjects in which the physiological responses activated by learning experiences were directly modulated by hormones and drugs. Moreover, such research has provided insights into the neuromodulatory systems regulating the influence of emotional arousal on memory. Hormones released by arousing experiences activate the amygdala, a brain region that is known to be involved in both emotion and memory. The amygdala, in turn, regulates the consolidation of lasting memory traces in other brain regions. The orchestration of these systems thus appears to provide a mechanism for varying the strength of memory in relation to the significance of experience. The resulting memories are distorted only in the sense that their strengths have been modulated. Moreover, recalled memories strengthened by such post-learning modulation may be less susceptible to the creative (i.e., distorting) processes of remembering.

References

Ammassari-Teule, M., Pavone, F., Castellano, C., and McGaugh, J. 1991. "Amygdala and dorsal hippocampus lesions block the effects of GABAergic drugs on memory storage." *Brain Research, 551,* 104–109.

Amsel, A. 1962. "Frustrative nonreward in partial reinforcement and discrimination learning." *Psychological Review, 69,* 306–328.

———. 1967. *Partial Reinforcement Effects on Vigor Persistence.* New York: Academic Press.

Babinsky, R., Calabrese, P., Durwen, H., Markowitsch, H., Brechtelsbauer, D., Heuser, L., and Gehlen, W. 1993. "The possible contribution of the amygdala to memory." *Behavioural Neurology, 6,* 167–170.

Bartlett, F. 1932. *Remembering: A Study in Experimental and Social Psychology.* Cambridge: Cambridge University Press.

Bohannon, J. N. 1988. "Flashbulb memories for the space shuttle disaster: A tale of two theories." *Cognition, 29,* 179–196.

Borrell, J., de Kloet, E. R., Versteeg, D. H. G., and Bohus, B. 1983. "The role of adrenomedullary catecholamines in the modulation of memory by vasopressin." In E. Endroczi, D. de Wied, L. Angelucci, and V. Scapagnini (Eds.), *Integrative Neurohumoral Mechanisms, Developments in Neuroscience,* pp. 85–90. Amsterdam: N. Holland/Elsevier.

Bower, G. 1992. "How might emotions affect language?" In S.-Ä. Christianson (Eds.), *The Handbook of Emotion and Memory,* pp. 3–32. Hillsdale, N.J.: Erlbaum.

Brown, R., and Kulik, J. 1977. "Flashbulb memories." *Cognition, 5,* 73–99.

Cahill, L., Brioni, J., and Izquierdo, I. 1986. "Retrograde memory enhancement by diazepam: Its relation to anterograde amnesia, and some clinical implications." *Psychopharmacology, 90,* 554–556.

Cahill, L., and McGaugh, J. 1993. "The functional anatomy of amygdala efferent pathways." *Society for Neuroscience Abstracts, 19,* 1226.

———. Submitted. "Enhanced long-term memory associated with emotional arousal."

———. 1990. "Amygdaloid complex lesions differentially affect retention of tasks using appetitive and aversive reinforcement." *Behavioral Neuroscience, 104,* 523–543.

———. 1991. "NMDA-induced lesions of the amygdaloid complex block the retention enhancing effect of posttraining epinephrine." *Psychobiology, 19,* 206–210.

Castellano, C., Brioni, J. D., and McGaugh, J. L. 1990. "GABAergic modulation of memory." In L. Squire and E. Lindenlaub (Eds.), *Biology of Memory*, pp. 361–378. Schattauer: Verlag.

Christianson, S.-Ä., and Mjorndal, T. 1985. "Adrenalin, emotional arousal and memory." *Scandinavian Journal of Psychology, 26,* 237–248.

Christianson, S.-Ä., Nilsson, L.-G., Mjorndal, T., Perris, C., and Tjellden, G. 1986. "Psychological versus physiological determinants of emotional arousal and its relationship to laboratory induced amnesia." *Scandinavian Journal of Psychology, 27,* 300–310.

Clugnet, M. C., and LeDoux, J. E. 1990. "Synaptic plasticity in fear conditioning circuits: Induction of LTP in the lateral nucleus of the amygdala by stimulation of the medial geniculate body." *Journal of Neuroscience, 10,* 2818–2824.

Conway, M. A., Anderson, S. J., Larsen, S. F., Donnelly, C. M., McDaniel, M. A., McClelland, A. G. R., Rawles, R. E., and Logie. 1994. "The formation of flash-bulb memories." *Memory and Cognition, 22,* 326–343.

Crespi, L. 1942. "Quantitative variation in incentive and performance in the white rat." *American Journal of Psychology, 55,* 467–515.

Da Cunha, C., Wolfman, C., Huang, C. H., Walz, R., Koya, R., Bianchin, M., Medina, J. H., and Izquierdo, I. 1991. "Effect of post-training injections of flumazenil into the amygdala, hippocampus and septum on retention of habituation and of inhibitory avoidance in rats." *Brazilian Journal of Medical and Biological Research, 24,* 301–306.

Davis, M. 1992. "The role of the amygdala in conditioned fear." In J. Aggleton (Ed.), *The Amygdala,* pp. 255–306. New York: Wiley-Liss.

de Wied, D., Gaffori, O., van Ree, J. M., and de Jong, W. 1984. "Central target for the behavioural effects of vasopressin neuropeptides." *Nature, 308,* 276–278.

Dickinson-Anson, H., and McGaugh, J. 1993. "Midazolam administered into the amygdala impairs retention of an inhibitory avoidance." *Behavioral and Neural Biology, 60,* 84–87.

Dickinson-Anson, H., Mesches, M., Coleman, K., and McGaugh, J. 1993. "Bicuculline administered into the amygdala blocks benzodiazepine-induced amnesia." *Behavioral and Neural Biology, 60,* 1–4.

Ebbinghaus, H. 1885. *Über das Gedächtnis.* Leipzig: Duncker and Humbolt.

Ettenberg, A., van der Kooy, D., Moal, M. L., Koob, G. F., and Bloom, F. E. 1983. "Can aversive properties of (peripherally-injected) vasopressin account for its putative role in memory?" *Behavioural Brain Research, 7,* 331–350.

Flaherty, C. 1990. "Effect of anxiolytics and antidepressants on extinction and negative contrast." *Pharmacology and Therapeutics, 46,* 309–320.

Flood, J., Garland, J., and Morley, J. 1992. "Evidence that cholecystokinin-enhanced retention is mediated by changes in opioid activity in the amygdala." *Brain Research, 585,* 94–104.

Flood, J. F., Smith, G. E., and Morley, J. E. 1987. "Modulation of memory processing by cholecystokinin: Dependence on the vagus nerve." *Science, 236,* 832–834.

Gaffan, D. 1992. "Amygdala and the memory of reward." In J. Aggleton (Ed.), *The Amygdala,* pp. 471–484. New York: Wiley-Liss.

Gallagher, M., Kapp, B. S., Pascoe, J. P., and Rapp, P. R. 1981. "A neuropharmacology of amygdaloid systems which contribute to learning and memory." In Y. Ben-Ari (Ed.), *The Amygdaloid Complex,* pp. 343–354. Amsterdam: Elsevier/N. Holland.

Gloor, P. 1992. "Role of the amygdala in temporal lobe epilepsy." In J. Aggleton (Ed.), *The Amygdala,* pp. 505–538. New York: Wiley-Liss.

Gold, P., and van Buskirk, R. 1978. "Posttraining brain norepinephrine concentrations: Correlation with retention performance of avoidance training with peripheral epinephrine modulation of memory processing." *Behavioral Biology, 23,* 509–520.

———. 1976. "Enhancement and impairment of memory processes with posttrial injections of adrenocorticotrophic hormone." *Behavioral Biology, 16,* 387–400.

———. 1975. "Facilitation of time-dependent memory processes with posttrial amygdala stimulation: Effect on memory varies with footshock level." *Brain Research, 86,* 509–513.

Gold, P. E. 1991. "An integrated memory regulation system: From blood to brain." In R. C. A. Frederickson, J. L. McGaugh, and D. L. Felten (Eds.), *Peripheral Signaling of the Brain: Role in Neural Immune Interactions, Learning and Memory,* pp. 391–420. Toronto: Hogrefe and Huber.

Gold, P. E., and McGaugh, J. L. 1975. "A single-trace, two process view of memory storage processes." In D. Deutsch and J. A. Deutsch (Eds.), *Short-Term Memory,* pp. 355–378. New York: Academic Press.

Gold, P. E., van Buskirk, R., and Haycock, J. 1977. "Effects of posttraining epinephrine injections on retention of avoidance training in mice." *Behavioral Biology, 20,* 197–207.

Halgren, E. 1992. "Emotional neurophysiology of the amygdala within the context of human cognition." In J. Aggleton (Ed.), *The Amygdala,* pp. 191–228. New York: Wiley-Liss.

Heuer, F., and Reisberg, D. 1990. "Vivid memories of emotional events: The accuracy of remembered minutiae." *Memory and Cognition, 18,* 496–506.

———. 1992. "Emotion, arousal, and memory for detail." In S.-Å. Christianson (Ed.), *The Handbook of Emotion and Memory,* pp. 151–180. Hillsdale, N.J.: Erlbaum.

Introini-Collison, I. B., and McGaugh, J. L. 1986. "Epinephrine modulates long-term retention of an aversively-motivated discrimination." *Behavioral and Neural Biology, 45,* 358–365.

Introini-Collison, I., Miyazaki, B., and McGaugh, J. 1991. "Involvement of the amygdala in the memory-enhancing effects of clenbuterol." *Psychopharmacology, 104,* 541–544.

Introini-Collison, I., Saghafi, D., Novack, G., and McGaugh, J. 1992. "Memory-enhancing effects of posttraining dipivefrin and epinephrine: Involvement of peripheral and central adrenergic receptors." *Brain Research, 572,* 81–86.

Introini-Collison, I. B., Nagahara, A. H., and McGaugh, J. L. 1989. "Memory-enhancement with intra-amygdala posttraining naloxone is blocked by concurrent administration of propranolol." *Brain Research, 476,* 94–101.

Izquierdo, I., and Dias, R. D. 1983. "Effect of ACTH, epinephrine, β-endorphin, naloxone, and of the combination of naloxone or β-endorphin with ACTH or epinephrine on memory consolidation." *Psychoneuroendocrinology, 8(1)*, 81–87.

Izquierdo, I., Pereira, M. E., and Medina, J. H. 1990. "Benzodiazepine receptor ligand influences on acquisition: Suggestion of an endogenous modulatory mechanism mediated by benzodiazepine receptors." *Behavioral and Neural Biology, 54*, 27–41.

Izquierdo, I., Medina, J. H., Netto, C., and Pereira, M. 1991. "Peripheral and central effects on memory of peripherally and centrally administered opioids and benzodiazepines." In R. C. A. Frederickson, J. L. McGaugh, and D. L. Felten (Eds.), *Peripheral Signaling of the Brain: Role in Neural-Immune Interactions, Learning and Memory*, pp. 303–314. Toronto: Hogrefe and Huber.

James, W. 1890. *The Principles of Psychology*. New York: Henry Holt.

Kesner, R., Walser, R., and Winzenried, G. 1989. "Central but not basolateral amygdala mediates memory for positive affective experiences." *Behavioural Brain Research, 33*, 189–195.

Kesner, R., and Wilburn, M. 1974. "A review of electrical stimulation of the brain in the context of learning and retention." *Behavioral Biology, 10*, 259–293.

Kluver, H., and Bucy, P. 1937. " 'Psychic blindness' and other symptoms following bilateral temporal lobectomy in rhesus monkeys." *American Journal of Physiology, 119*, 352–355.

Koob, G. F., Lebrun, C., Bluthe, R., Dantzer, R., Dorsa, D. M., and Moal, M. L. 1991. "Vasopressin and learning: peripheral and central mechanisms." In R. C. A. Frederickson, J. L. McGaugh, and D. L. Felten (Eds.), *Peripheral Signaling of the Brain: Role in Neural-Immune Interactions, Learning and Memory*, pp. 351–363. Toronto: Hogrefe and Huber.

Lal, H., and Forster, M. 1990. "Flumazenil improves active avoidance performance in aging NZB/BINJ and C57BL/6NNia mice." *Pharmacology, Biochemistry and Behavior, 35*, 747–750.

LeDoux, J. 1992a. "Emotion and the amygdala." In J. Aggleton (Ed.), *The Amygdala*, pp. 339–352. New York: Wiley-Liss.

———. 1992b. "Emotion as memory: Anatomical systems underlying indelible neural traces." In S.-Å. Christianson (Ed.), *The Handbook of Emotion and Memory*, pp. 269–288. Hillsdale, N.J.: Erlbaum.

Liang, K. C., Bennett, C., and McGaugh, J. L. 1985. "Peripheral epinephrine modulates the effects of posttraining amygdala stimulation on memory." *Behavioural Brain Research, 15*, 93–100.

Liang, K. C., Juler, R., and McGaugh, J. L. 1986. "Modulating effects of posttraining epinephrine on memory: Involvement of the amygdala noradrenergic system." *Brain Research, 368*, 125–133.

Liang, K. C., and McGaugh, J. L. 1983a. "Lesions of the stria terminalis attenuate the amnestic effect of amygdaloid stimulation on avoidance responses." *Brain Research, 274*, 309–318.

———. 1983b. "Lesions of the stria terminalis attenuate the enhancing effect of posttraining epinephrine on retention of an inhibitory avoidance response." *Behavioural Brain Research, 9*, 49–58.

Liang, K. C., McGaugh, J. L., Martinez, J. L., Jr., Jensen, R. A., Vasquez, B. J., and

Messing, R. B. 1982. "Posttraining amygdaloid lesions impair retention of an inhibitory avoidance response." *Behavioural Brain Research, 4*, 237–249.

Liang, K. C., McGaugh, J. L., and Yao, H. 1990. "Involvement of amygdala pathways in the influence of posttraining amygdala norepinephrine and peripheral epinephrine on memory storage." *Brain Research, 508*, 225–233.

Lister, R. 1985. "The amnesic action of benzodiazepines in man." *Biobehavioral Review, 9*, 87–94.

Lister, R., and File, S. 1984. "The nature of lorazepam-induced amnesia." *Psychopharmacology, 83*, 183–187.

Markowitsch, H. J., Calabrese, P., Wurker, M., Durwen, H. F., Kessler, J., Babinsky, R., Brechtelsbauer, D., Heuser, L., and Gehlen, W. 1994. "The amygdala's contribution to memory—a study on two patients with Urbach-wiethe disease." *NeuroReport, 5*, 1349–1352.

McGaugh, J., Introini-Collison, I., Cahill, L., Castellano, C., Dalmaz, C., Parent, M., and Williams, C. 1993. "Neuromodulatory systems and memory storage: Role of the amygdala." *Behavioural Brain Research, 58*, 81–90.

McGaugh, J., Introini-Collison, I., and Castellano, C. 1993. "Involvement of opioid peptides in learning and memory." In A. Herz, H. Akil, and E. Simon (Eds.), *Handbook of Experimental Pharmacology, Opioids, Part II*, pp. 429–447. Heidelberg: Springer-Verlag.

McGaugh, J. L. 1973. "Drug facilitation of learning and memory." *Annual Review of Pharmacology, 13*, 229–241.

———. 1989. "Involvement of hormonal and neuromodulatory systems in the regulation of memory storage." *Annual Review of Neuroscience, 12*, 255–287.

———. 1990. "Significance and remembrance: The role of neuromodulatory systems." *Psychological Science, 1*, 15–25.

McGaugh, J. L., and Gold, P. E. 1976. "Modulation of memory by electrical stimulation of the brain." In M. R. Rosenzweig and E. L. Bennett (Eds.), *Neural Mechanisms of Learning and Memory*, pp. 549–560. Cambridge, Mass.: MIT Press.

———. 1989. "Hormonal modulation of memory." In R. B. Brush and S. Levine (Eds.), *Psychoendocrinology*, pp. 305–339. New York: Academic Press.

McGaugh, J. L., and Herz, M. J. 1972. *Memory Consolidation*. San Francisco: Albion Publishing Company.

McGaugh, J. L., Introini-Collison, I. B., Juler, R. G., and Izquierdo, I. 1986. "Stria terminalis lesions attenuate the effects of posttraining naloxone and β-endorphin on retention." *Behavioral Neuroscience, 100*, 839–844.

McGaugh, J. L., Introini-Collison, I. B., and Nagahara, A. H. 1988. "Memory-enhancing effects of posttraining naloxone: Involvement of β-noradrenergic influences in the amygdaloid complex." *Brain Research, 446*, 37–49.

Micheau, J., Destrade, C., and Soumireu-Mourat, B. 1984. "Time-dependent effects of posttraining intrahippocampal injections of corticosterone in retention of appetitive learning in mice." *European Journal of Pharmacology, 106*, 39–46.

Morley, J. F., and Flood, J. F. 1991. "Gut peptides as modulators of memory." In R. C. A. Frederickson, J. L. McGaugh, and D. L. Felten (Eds.), *Peripheral Signaling of the Brain: Role in Neural Interactions, Learning and Memory*, pp. 379–390. Toronto: Hogrefe and Huber.

Mueller, G. E., and Pilzecker, A. 1900. "Experimentelle Beitrage zur Lehre vom Gedachtniss." *Zeitschrift für Psychologie, 1,* 1–288.

Neisser, U., and Harsch, N. 1992. "Phantom flashbulbs: false recollections of hearing the news about the Challenger." In E. Winograd and U. Neisser (Eds.), *Affect and Accuracy in Recall: Studies of Flashbulb Memories,* pp. 9–31. Cambridge: Cambridge University Press.

Packard, M., Cahill, L., and McGaugh, J. In press. "Amygdala modulation of
hippocampal-dependent and caudate nucleus-dependent memory processes."
Proceedings, National Academy of Sciences.

Parent, M., and McGaugh, J. Submitted. "Posttraining infusion of lidocaine into the
amygdala basolateral complex impairs retention of inhibitory avoidance
training."

Parent, M., Tomaz, C., and McGaugh, J. 1992. "Increased training in an aversively
motivated task attenuates the memory impairing effects of posttraining N-
Methyl-D-Aspartic Acid-induced amygdala lesions." *Behavioral Neuroscience,
106,* 791–799.

Pereira, M., Medina, J., and Izquierdo, I. 1989. "Effect of pre-training flumazenil
administration on the acquisition of three different tasks in rats." *Brazilian Journal of Medical and Biological Research, 22,* 1501–1505.

Pereira, M., Rosat, R., Huang, C., Godoy, M., and Izquierdo, I. 1989. "Inhibition by
diazepam of the effect of additional training and of extinction on the retention of
shuttle avoidance behavior in rats." *Behavioral Neuroscience, 103,* 202–205.

Pitman, P. 1989. "Post-traumatic stress disorder, hormones, and memory." *Biological Psychiatry, 26,* 221–223.

Revelle, W., and Loftus, D. 1992. "The implications of arousal effects for the study
of affect and memory." In S.-Å. Christianson (Ed.), *The Handbook of Emotion
and Memory,* pp. 113–150. Hillsdale, N.J.: Erlbaum.

Rosen, A., and Tessel, R. 1970. "Chlorpromazine, chlordiazepoxide, and incentive
shift performance in the rat." *Physiological Psychology, 72,* 257–262.

Salinas, J., Dickinson-Anson, H., and McGaugh, J. Submitted. "Midazolam induces
anterograde amnesia for changes in reward magnitude."

Salinas, J. A., Packard, M. G. and McGaugh, J. L. 1993. "Amygdala modulates
memory for changes in reward magnitude: Reversible post-training inactivation
with lidocaine attenuates the response to a reduction reward." *Behavioural
Brain Research, 59,* 153–159.

Sternberg, D. G., Isaacs, K., Gold, P. E., and McGaugh, J. L. 1985. "Epinephrine
facilitation of appetitive learning: Attenuation with adrenergic receptor antagonists." *Behavioral and Neural Biology, 44,* 447–453.

Tanaka, M., Kohno, Y., Nakagawa, R., Ida, Y., Takeda, S., and Nagasaki, N. 1982.
"Time-related differences in noradrenaline turnover in rat brain regions by
stress." *Pharmacology Biochemistry and Behavior, 16,* 315–319.

Tomaz, C., Dickinson-Anson, H., and McGaugh, J. 1991. "Amygdala lesions block
the amnestic effects of diazepam." *Brain Research, 568,* 85–91.

———. 1992. "Basolateral amygdala lesions block diazepam-induced anterograde
amnesia in an inhibitory avoidance task." *Proceedings, National Academy of
Sciences, 89,* 3615–3619.

Tulving, E. 1983. *Elements of episodic memory.* New York: Oxford University Press.

van der Kolk, B., Greenberg, M., Orr, S., and Pitman, R. 1989. "Endogenous opioids, stress-induced analgesia, and posttraumatic stress disorder." *Psychopharmacology Bulletin, 25,* 417–421.

Venault, P., Chapouthier, G., Carvalho, L. P. D., Simiand, J., Morre, M., Dodd, R. H., and Rossier, J. 1986. "Benzodiazepine impairs and beta-carboline enhances performance in learning and memory tasks." *Nature, 321,* 864–866.

Venault, P., Chapouthier, G., Simiand, J., Dodd, R. H., and Rossier, J. 1987. "Enhancement of performance by methyl beta-carboline-c-carboxylate, in learning and memory tasks." *Brain Research Bulletin, 19,* 365–370.

Weiskrantz, L. 1956. "Behavioral changes associated with ablation of the amygdaloid complex in monkeys." *Journal of Comparative and Physiological Psychology, 49,* 381–391.

Werling, L., McMahon, P., Portoghese, P., Takemori, A., and Cox, B. 1989. "Selective opioid antagonist effects on opioid-induced inhibition of release of norepinephrine in guinea pig cortex." *Neuropharmacology, 28,* 103–107.

Williams, C. L., and McGaugh, J. 1992. "Reversible inactivation of the nucleus of the solitary tract impairs retention performance in an inhibitory avoidance task." *Behavioral and Neural Biology, 58,* 204–210.

———. 1993. "Reversible lesions of the nucleus of the solitary tract attenuate the memory-modulating effects of posttraining epinephrine." *Behavioral Neuroscience, 107,* 1–8.

Speculations on the Fidelity of Memories Stored in Synaptic Connections

10

Rodney A. Swain

Kim E. Armstrong

Thomas A. Comery

Aaron G. Humphreys

Theresa A. Jones

Jeff A. Kleim

William T. Greenough

In this chapter we briefly outline the empirical basis for believing that one mechanism whereby memory is stored in the brain is in the pattern of its synaptic connections. We subsequently consider evidence indicating that a functional pattern of synaptic connections can be or can become occluded in the course of the normal functioning of the nervous system. Within our cellular framework, these would be the closest parallels to repressed memory, although it is probably unlikely that they would have very much to do with the human behavioral memory distortion that is the focus of this volume. Finally, we call attention to an interpretation of the broad array of changes in tissue organization that may arise in the brain as a consequence of behavioral experience and argue that terms like "brain adaptation" may be a useful supplement to the concept of memory.

Relationships between Synapse Formation and Memory

The data that support the hypothesis that alterations in the pattern of functional synaptic connections underlie at least some aspects of memory in the brain have grown increasingly convincing over the two decades or so during which this research has accumulated. The basic findings are these:

1. Synapses form in response to behavioral experiences likely to induce memories, such as rearing in complex environments. Both direct measurement of the number of synapses per neuron in visual cortex (Turner and Greenough, 1983, 1985; Bhide and Bedi, 1984) and indirect measures of dendritic field dimensions and spine density (Globus, Rosenzweig, Bennett, and Diamond, 1973; Juraska, 1984; Volkmar and Greenough, 1972) indicate dramatic synapse formation in rats reared in toy-filled cages, compared to littermates housed individually or in pairs in standard laboratory cages. A variety of evidence indicates that similar effects occur in other cerebral cortical areas (e.g., Greenough, Volkmar, and Juraska, 1973; Wallace, Kilman, Withers, and Greenough, 1992), brainstem (Fuchs, Montemayor, and Greenough, 1990) and cerebellum (Floeter and Greenough, 1979; Pysh and Weiss, 1979).

2. *Similar synaptic changes occur in adult rats.* Again, both dendritic field measures (Juraska, Greenough, Elliot, Mack, and Berkowitz, 1980; Green, Greenough, and Schlumpf, 1983) and synaptic measures (Hwang and Greenough, 1986; Kilman, Sirevaag, and Greenough, 1991) confirm that rats housed as adults in similar conditions exhibit similar changes. In very old rats, these changes may be small and sometimes insufficient to reverse a pattern of deterioration with age (e.g., Greenough, McDonald, Parnisari, and Camel, 1986).

3. *Adult rats trained on maze and motor tasks show similar phenomena.* Extensive training in the Hebb-Williams (1949) maze (Greenough, Juraska, and Volkmar, 1979) or on a reaching task (Greenough, Larson, and Withers, 1985) altered dendritic branching of neurons in the visual and somatosensory-motor cortices, respectively.

4. *Training effects may be lateralized when training input is lateralized, indicating that these effects do not arise from general hormonal or metabolic causes.* Rats trained on a complicated series of changing mazes with one eye occluded by an opaque contact lens exhibited increased dendritic branching in the visual cortex of the hemisphere predominantly receiving information from the eye that was open during training (Chang and Greenough, 1982). Similarly, in rats trained to reach for food with one forelimb, dendritic branching of the projection neurons was selectively incremented in the cerebral hemisphere governing the trained forelimb (Greenough et al., 1985); in other neuronal populations, change occurred bilaterally (Withers and Greenough, 1989). Even though not all effects are lateralized, the fact that some are rules out generally acting sources of the anatomical changes, such as a circulating growth factor.

5. *Similar structural changes occur in other plasticity-related paradigms.* For example, synapse formation has been reported to occur in hippocampal subfield CA1 (e.g., Chang and Greenough, 1984; Chang, Hawrylak, and Greenough, 1993; Lee, Schottler, Oliver, and Lynch, 1980) and in dentate gyrus (e.g., Geinisman, deToledo-Morrell, and Morrell, 1990; Geinisman et al., 1993) following long-term potentiation (LTP) and kindling.

6. *Synaptic structural changes occur across a wide range of species, in response to similar conditions.* Complex environment rearing phenomena similar to those in rats have been reported in cats (Beaulieu and Colonnier, 1987) and monkeys (Floeter and Greenough, 1979). Such changes have also been reported in association with imprinting and avoidance learning in birds

(Bateson, Rose, and Horn, 1973; Stewart, 1990) and with habituation and sensitization in mollusks (Bailey and Chen, 1989).

7. *These changes occur rapidly, on a time scale that may be compatible with that for the formation of stable long-term memories.* Synapses can form within minutes following the induction of LTP (Chang and Greenough, 1984). *Detectable* differences in dendritic field size, which presumably take some time to accumulate, in the form of individual instances of dendritic growth, are achieved within four days of postweaning exposure to a complex environment (Wallace et al., 1992).

8. *The structural changes have physiological correlates appropriate to the interpretation that they alter the functional organization of the brain region in which they occur.* In the visual cortex, a 30-day period of postweaning exposure to a complex environment increments visual cortical synapse to neuron ratios by 25% compared to individually cage-housed littermate rats. A correlate of this, the synchronous neuronal firing in response to afferent stimulation, is incremented by an even larger percentage, as reflected in the amplitude of the "population spike," an electrophysiological summation of the firing of individual neurons in the region of the recording electrode, in response to electrical stimulation of the subcortical white matter containing axons projecting to visual cortex (Wang and Greenough, 1993). Similarly, in the forelimb motor cortex, forelimb training to reach for food increments branching of pyramidal neurons in layers II–III of the motor cortex (Withers and Greenough, 1989). Motor cortex responses to somatosensory cortical electrical stimulation are incremented in these reach-trained animals (Yi and Greenough, 1994).

9. *Molecular changes that may underlie the structural changes are beginning to be identified.* For a structural change to occur in the right place in the synaptic network, there would appear to be at least three things that are needed: (a) one or more *orchestrators* to turn on all of the essential gene expression, (b) *effectors* that mediate the structural change, and (c) a *location marker* that "remembers" where in the network the change is to take place for long enough that the effectors can bring about the structural change. We are investigating some "model molecules" that can serve as exemplars of what might serve these purposes. As *orchestrators,* for example, *immediate early gene transcription factors,* which bind to DNA in the cell nucleus and regulate the expression of secondary genes that would instigate cellular change, are expressed in learning situations. ZENK, a DNA-binding protein previously identified as NGFI-A, Zif/268, Krox 24, and EGR-1 (e.g., Sheng and Greenberg, 1990), is elevated in complex environment–housed rats in regions of the brain that have been shown to be morphologically altered under the same circumstances (Wallace, Clayton, and Greenough, 1994). Similarly, expression of the transcription factor Fos is elevated in the motor cortex of rats learning a set of complex motor skills that also alters

the synaptic morphology of the motor cortex (Lussnig, Kleim, Schwarz, Comery, and Greenough, 1994; Schwarz, Kleim, Lussnig, Comery, and Greenough, 1994). As prototype *effectors,* we have been studying a set of microtubule proteins (DMAPS) first identified in *Drosophila* by Karr and colleagues (Srinivasan, Doe, and Karr, 1993). DMAP-45R is expressed in developing dendrites of rats and is upregulated by visual experience (Werner, Hawrylak, Comery, Karr, and Greenough, 1994) and post-developmentally in response to deafferentation (Armstrong et al., 1994). Its possible role in cytoskeletal plasticity, hinted at by these results, is a major target of our work. Finally, as a *location marker,* which would serve to identify synapses to be altered or dendritic locations of synaptogenesis pending effector arrival, we have recently worked out some of the pharmacology of *synaptically activated protein synthesis,* in which rapid postsynaptic polyribosomal aggregation and protein synthesis is triggered by activation of a metabotropic glutamate receptor (Weiler and Greenough, 1991, 1993).

10. *The structural correlates are associated with learning and not with mere neural activity.* In adult animals that learned a set of complex motor tasks, there was an increase in cerebellar paramedian lobule synapse numbers, while in controls that expended considerably more effort running on a treadmill or in a running wheel, there was an increase in blood vessel volume in this area but no change in synapse number (Black, Isaacs, Anderson, Alcantara, and Greenough, 1990). Both synapse number change and the expression of the immediate early transcription factor gene c-Fos in the motor cortex were similarly tied to learning and not to forced activity (Lussnig et al., 1994; Schwarz et al., 1994). These results strongly imply that learning drives synaptic change and that mere neural activity does not, even when the neural activity is sufficient to bring about other morphological changes in the same brain region. We will have more to say about these changes in the closing section of this chapter.

Taken together, these findings argue strongly that a substantial component of the brain memory process involves alterations in the functional pattern of connections among its neurons, in many cases via the physical pattern of their synapses. It is thus of interest to examine cases in which the seemingly "hard wired" character of a pattern of synaptic connections appears to be mitigated by other circumstances.

Hormonal Modulation

There are literally hundreds of reports that document the effects of gonadal and stress hormones on learning and memory. We would like to draw attention to a subset of these studies which are concerned with hormonal modulation of neuronal connectivity and physiology in the adult mammalian brain. In particular, we will focus on the hippocampus, a limbic structure that has been implicated in a variety of associative and nonassociative learning processes including motivation (Papez, 1937; Green and Arduini, 1954; Berry and Thompson, 1978; Berger, Berry, and Thompson, 1986; Berry and Swain, 1989), short-term or working memory (Olton, Becker, and Handelmann, 1979; Rawlins, 1985), recognition memory (Zola-Morgan and Squire, 1986), context discrimination (Hirsch, 1974; Hirsch, Holt, and Mosseri, 1978), and spatial learning (O'Keefe and Nadel, 1978).

Repeated daily acute stress has been variously shown to impair or facilitate behavioral conditioning and also hippocampal activity, the direction seeming to depend on the nature as well as the severity of the stress. Mild stress, for example that induced by 22 hours of water deprivation, has been found to significantly accelerate eyeblink classical conditioning in the rabbit (Berry and Swain, 1989) and contextual fear conditioning in the rat (Maren, DeCola, Swain, Fanselow, and Thompson, 1994). In both of these experiments, theta activity in the hippocampus was more pronounced. In the first study, hippocampal modeling of the behavioral response was more robust and started significantly earlier in water-deprived rabbits than in *ad libitum* controls. In the latter study, LTP of subfield CA1 was facilitated in the deprived rats. More severe stress, for example that induced by repeated shock, has also been found to expedite eyeblink classical conditioning in the rat (Shors, Weiss, and Thompson, 1992). Interestingly though, the same level of shock was found to impair induction of hippocampal LTP (Foy, Stanton, Levine, and Thompson, 1987; Shors, Foy, Levine, and Thompson, 1992; Shors and Thompson, 1992). Morphologically, recurrent daily stress, similar to that reported above, has been observed to induce atrophy of the apical dendritic arbor in rat hippocampal CA3 pyramids (Watanabe, Gould, and McEwen, 1992). These studies illustrate that stress, and by suggestion, stress-induced hormones, may have a profound impact on behavioral learning, neuronal signaling, and dendritic morphology. The observation that the effects on behavior and physiology are sometimes negatively correlated underscores our need for "dose-response" studies which evaluate the way in which stress, hormones, and learning may interact.

Gonadal hormones also impact behavioral and neuronal plasticity. Teresawa and Timiras (1968) initially showed that the dorsal hippocampus is more excitable during proestrus. Teyler and coworkers showed that the steady-state physiology of the hippocampal slice is subject to rapid change following hormone treatment *in vitro*: 17-beta-Estradiol enhanced field evoked responses (Foy and Teyler, 1983) and testosterone enhanced field evoked responses in diestrus females but decreased field evoked responses in proestrus females (Teyler, Vardaris, Lewis, and Rawitch, 1980). Structurally, the apical dendritic region of rat hippocampal CA1 pyramids was observed to exhibit a cyclic fluctuation of dendritic spine synaptic density across the estrous cycle. The fluctuation of the spiny dendrites across the estrous cycle was most pronounced (33% decrement) as the rats cycled from proestrus to estrus (Woolley and McEwen, 1992). A subsequent study by Woolley and McEwen (1993) showed that the time-course for the rapid increase of spine density during proestrus was due to the combined effect of the estrogen priming followed by the progesterone surge, whereas the decrease in spine density observed as the cycle moved from proestrus to estrus was due to the rapid drop in progesterone levels during this period.

Recently, we have found that hippocampal synaptic plasticity varies across the estrous cycle of the female rat as a function of the time of day. Proestrus, the phase during which prior studies indicate synapse number to be highest (Woolley and McEwen, 1992) was associated with the greatest LTP but only during afternoon hours. LTP induction during the morning hours did not vary across the estrous cycle. Interestingly, males also exhibited greater levels of LTP in the afternoon hours. These results suggest that gonadal hormones may interact with diurnal or circadian rhythms to produce transient changes in synaptic plasticity (Humphreys, Warren, Juraska, and Greenough, 1994). In general, extending these findings to account for aberrant memory is probably premature, but a speculative case might be made that hormonal conditions associated with stress or male/female cyclicity could modulate memory storage and behaviors dependent on working memory.

Song Learning in Birds

Gonadal hormone effects on learning and memory and CNS morphology may be even more extreme in some avian species. In many song-producing birds, song acquisition is accompanied by the production and incorporation of new neurons in areas related to vocal learning (Nottebohm and Arnold, 1976). Major regions of the avian brain that have been identified as essential for normal song learning or production include the higher vocal control center (HVc), the robust nucleus of the archistriatum (RA), the magnocellular nucleus of the anterior neostriatum (MAN), and Area X. Auditory information is relayed from HVc to Area X to MAN (via the medial portion of the dorsolateral nucleus of the thalamus) to RA (also substantially innervated by HVc). RA innervates the hypoglossal nuclei which regulate syringeal muscular contractions and hence the acoustic properties of song (reviewed by Konishi, 1989; DeVoogd, 1990). Lesions of either HVc or RA profoundly disturb song production in adult birds (Nottebohm, Stokes, and Leonard, 1976). MAN or Area X lesions disrupt juvenile song development but do not affect adulthood production of song when the lesion is performed after the period of initial song acquisition (Bottjer, Miesner, and Arnold, 1984). Thus, these four regions are likely sites for learning related plastic changes.

Steroid hormones are generally believed to exert their effects on behavior and brain morphology at either of two timepoints. Early in life, they may act to "organize" neural circuitry and the expression of certain behaviors in typical gender-specific patterns. In adulthood, their effects are viewed as largely "activational" insofar as they transiently turn on sex-specific behaviors laid down during development (Arnold and Breedlove, 1985). In songbirds, the mode of hormonal action appears to be species-dependent. For example, hormonal effects in the zebra finch appear to be largely organizational. Males (the singing gender) exhibit higher plasma levels of estradiol shortly after hatching than do females (Hutchison, Wingfield, and Hutchison, 1984). It has been proposed that this elevated level of estradiol masculinizes the male brain via neurogenesis in HVc and prevention of cell death in RA (Arnold, Bottjer, Brenowitz, Nordeen, and Nordeen, 1986), leading to larger song nuclei (3–5 times) in males than in females (Nottebohm and Arnold, 1976). Hormone manipulations have little effect in adult males (Arnold, 1980). Male patterns of brain morphology can be induced in the female if estradiol is administered shortly after hatching (Gurney and Konishi, 1980; Nordeen, Nordeen, and Arnold, 1987), but the females fail to sing much unless androgens are also administered (Gurney and Konishi, 1980). In contrast to the zebra finches, seasonal variations in androgen levels in adult male canaries as well as androgen administration in adult female canaries correlates highly with dramatic increases in HVc and RA volume and vocal behavior (Nottebohm, 1980, 1981). How long these effects last has not been determined.

Chronic Drug Administration

The effect of drug administration, particularly chronic alcohol exposure, on dendritic morphology has been extensively studied both in postmortem human tissue and in animal models. Reports of changes in dendritic spines following the administration of such drugs as ethanol, chloroform, and morphine have existed since the late nineteenth century (Monti, 1895; cf. Horner, 1993). Chronic ethanol administration in the adult organism is associated with a large number of degenerative changes within the brain (Walker, Hunter, and Abraham, 1981). Walker and colleagues report significant cell loss and deafferentation in both the hippocampus and cerebellum of rats and mice (Walker et al., 1981; Riley and Walker, 1978). Significant alterations in dendritic morphology and a 60% decrease in spine number is observed in the stratum radiatum of hippocampal field CA1 in mice after four months of alcohol consumption followed by two months of abstinence (Riley and Walker, 1978). In the rat cerebellar cortex, Tavares, Paula-Barbosa, and Gray (1983) report decreased Purkinje cell spine density and a concurrent three- to fourfold increase in length of remaining spines following long-term alcohol ingestion. The authors suggest that the elongation of remaining spines may constitute an effort to contact still viable parallel fibers following the alcohol-induced cell loss and deafferentation. Similar decreases in spine density and alteration in spine morphology have been reported in animals that received prenatal alcohol exposure (Galofre, Ferrer, Fabreques, and Lopez-Tejera, 1987; Miller, Chiaia, and Rhoades, 1990). Administration, either during development or in the adult, of a number of other drugs, including phenobarbital (Yanai et al., 1989), naloxone (Shepanek, Smith, Tyer, Royall, and Allen, 1989) and haloperidol (Klintzova, Uranova, Hashorst, and Schenk, 1990), has also been shown to alter both cell number and spine density. The relationship of such changes to behavioral or memorial defects has not been established, although memory deficits are associated with chronic exposure to many of these drugs.

Norepinephrine

The neurotransmitter norepinephrine (NE) exerts substantial impact on memory acquisition and retention (see McGaugh, Chapter 9 in this volume). Depletion impairs performance on various learning tasks (Bickford, Heron, Young, and Gerhardt, 1992; Cornwell-Jones, Palfai, Young, and Desai, 1990), while administration can facilitate performance on others (Roozendaal, Koolhaas, and Bohus, 1993). Kety (1970) proposed that NE selectively enhances firing in neurons receiving environmentally important information. Support for this view came from studies showing that NE depletion can disrupt visual cortical plasticity in kittens monocularly deprived during development (Kasamatsu and Pettigrew, 1976; but see Bear and Singer, 1986), NE release can be elicited in specific contexts (Sara, Grecksch, and Leviel, 1984), and NE infusion can facilitate performance on a learning task requiring attentional shifts (Devauges and Sara, 1990). Pharmacologically NE acts to reduce spontaneous neuronal background activity while potentiating both excitatory and inhibitory afferent activity (Freedman, Hoffer, Woodward, and Puro, 1977). NE may be involved in establishing patterns of neural connectivity appropriate to environmental input. For example, Loeb, Chang, and Greenough (1987) found that NE depletion by neonatal 6-OHDA injection in mice pups disrupted afferent-dependent dendritic field organization within whisker barrels of the somatosensory cortex.

Latent, Masked, Repressed, or Silent Synapses

A considerable number of reports have suggested that a general organizing feature of nervous system development may include a pool of nonactive or dormant synapses that can be recruited during activity or following disruption of traditional pathways (or conversely, that an active synapse may be deactivated under the appropriate circumstances). It is appealing to speculate that such a phenomenon might underlie memory acquisition or repression (or disturbances thereof) as well as any number of sensory/perceptual disturbances (e.g., phantom limb sensation). In the ensuing discussion, we will consider three disparate types of experiments that have examined the putative existence of pools of inactive synapses: (1) nerve-muscle regeneration in fish, (2) quantal profiles of fish and crustacean sensory and motor neurons, and (3) plasticity of neocortical sensorimotor maps in mammals. Our review of the literature indicates that the phrases "repressed synapses," "silent synapses," and "latent/masked synapses" are each almost exclusively associated with one type of experiment (1, 2, and 3 respectively). While the phrases may appear conceptually similar, we propose that they may indeed represent distinct phenomena. Furthermore, in at least two of the experiments (neuromuscular regeneration in fish and cortical map plasticity in mammals), the phrases may be misleading, describing a behavioral phenomenon rather than a synaptic event.

Nerve-Muscle Regeneration.   Recovery of function from specific nerve damage has been and continues to be an active area of scientific investigation. One issue that has arisen from this work is whether regenerating nerve fibers are selective concerning their target destination (for review see Landmesser, 1980; Mark, 1980; Grinnell and Herrera, 1981). Weiss (1955), for example, proposed that regenerating nerve fibers were nonselective in their target destination and that proper functional connections between nerve and muscle were attained through "myotypic modulation." Sperry and Arora (1965) tested this hypothesis in teleost fish by inserting terminals of oculomotor nerves into foreign muscle and found that myotypic respecification of the oculomotor nerves did not occur. Original patterns of electrical activity were maintained, and eye movement was abnormal. If regeneration of the original connection was then allowed to proceed, behavioral recovery was normal and contraction of the muscle via electrical stimulation of the foreign nerve was no longer demonstrable. Mark and colleagues (Marotte and Mark, 1970a, 1970b; Mark and Marotte, 1972; Mark, Marotte, and Mart, 1972) further demonstrated that the suppression of foreign input was rather abrupt in this preparation, occurring within two days of reinnervation by the original nerve. Electron microscopic examination of muscle indicated that terminals of the original and foreign nerves were indistinguishable, leading the authors to infer the presence of some unspecified molecular event that "represses" the synapse by reduction of presynaptic transmitter release, creation of a diffusion barrier, or alteration of postsynaptic receptivity.

Scott (1975, 1977), however, demonstrated electrophysiologically that both foreign and appropriate innervations are maintained and functional. The apparent "repression" of foreign input could only be observed at the behavioral level and occurred as a consequence of the foreign input also reinnervating its own original target. The two innervations produced opposite effects on eye rotation, resulting in behavioral but not physiological repression.

Quantal Profiles.   Quantal analyses of fish and crustacean sensory and motor neurons do indicate the presence of "silent" synapses. For example, Faber and colleagues (Faber, Lin, and Korn, 1991) have examined this phenomenon in the goldfish Mauthner cell preparation. The Mauthner cell is a large, easily identifiable neuron found in the teleost midbrain. Using simultaneous recordings of pre- and postsynaptic potentials, these researchers have characterized the quantal release properties of both inhibitory and excitatory afferents to the Mauthner cell. In the course of these investigations, they found numerous presynaptic neurons which failed to evoke a response in the Mauthner cell. Direct stimulation of inhibitory presynaptic neurons, though, if paired with stimulation of the eighth nerve (which projects to the inhibitory interneurons and produces an IPSP at the Mauthner cell), evokes a larger synaptic current than can be accounted for by stimulation of the eighth nerve alone. This finding led the authors to suggest that neurotransmitter is released from the "silent" synapse but that the corresponding postsynaptic receptors are unresponsive. The larger response to the paired stimulation would be due to diffusion of the transmitter to adjacent non-silent synaptic regions. Apparently, the responsivity of the postsynaptic receptors can be modulated by the second messenger cAMP. Weak stimulation of eighth nerve afferents which fails to produce any measurable inhibition in the Mauthner cell can do so following postsynaptic cAMP injection.

Quite a different picture has emerged for excitatory afferents (eighth nerve) to the Mauthner cell. The terminals of these cells contain both chemical synapses and gap junctions. Approximately 80% of the cells studied by Faber and colleagues were chemically silent. That is, presynaptic stimulation of the vast majority of cells produced electrotonic coupling potentials in the Mauthner cell lateral dendrite but no EPSP. Repetitive stimulation of eighth nerve fibers at frequencies that facilitated transmitter release at non-silent sites failed to unmask chemical transmission at the silent connections. Application of K^+ channel blockers such as Cs or 4-AP, however, increased the duration of the coupling potential and also produced an obvious chemical EPSP in the postsynaptic dendrite.

Atwood and colleagues have investigated the properties of "silent" synapses at the neuromuscular junction of crayfish claw opener muscles (Jahromi and Atwood, 1974; Wojtowicz and Atwood, 1986; Wojtowicz, Parnas, Parnas, and Atwood, 1988). Synapses at these junctions show activity-dependent alterations in transmission efficacy, both short-term and long-term facilitation. Brief bursts or single trains of stimulation induce increased transmitter release but only transiently. Longer-lasting trains produced longer-lasting increases in transmitter release. Multiple experiments have been conducted to identify the mechanism of this persistent change in transmission. It is believed that entry of Na^+ or Ca^{2+} leads to the induction of second messenger systems and protein phosphorylation. Protein phosphorylation, in turn, leads to recruitment of additional synapses. This recruitment has been postulated based on analyses of physiological studies which show that quantal events at this neuromuscular junction can be adequately described by the binomial model in which quantal content is the product of the number of synapses (n) and the mean probability of transmitter release per impulse at an active site (p). These data sets indicate that the binomial n usually increases during long-lasting potentiation, whereas only minor changes in the binomial p occur. Ultrastructural evidence, to date, supports the view that long-lasting enhancement of transmission is associated with synapse recruitment. Presynaptic dense bars increase during long-lasting potentiation.

Cortical Sensorimotor Maps.   The size and boundaries of cortical representation areas, or maps, in adult animals have been found to be remarkably malleable following peripheral or central manipulations (reviewed in Dykes and Ruest, 1986; Jenkins and Merzenich, 1987; Kaas, 1991), a phenomenon that may have human perceptual correlates (see next section). For example, transection of the facial nerves innervating the vibrissal musculature in adult rats causes an expansion of the forelimb representation area of the motor cortex such that movements of the forelimb or eye can be evoked by stimulating some parts of the former vibrissae representation area (Sanes, Suner, and Donoghue, 1990; Donoghue, Suner, and Sanes, 1990). Conceptually, the expansion of representation areas might be thought of as filling in the gaps created by the denervation. The expansion of cortical representation areas has been attributed to an "unmasking of latent pathways" (Dostrovsky, Millar, and Wall, 1976; Wall, 1977), resulting in the expansion of receptive fields into areas where they are not normally found to be responsive (at low thresholds) in electrophysiological and microstimulation studies. Alteration in the size of somatosensory representational areas occurs following amputation or nerve transection (e.g., Wall and Cusick, 1984; Kaas, Merzenich, and Killackey, 1983), peripheral stimulation (Recanzone, Allard, Jenkins, and Merzenich, 1990), behavioral training (Jenkins, Merzenich, Ochs, Allard, and Guic-Robles, 1990), cortical lesions (Jenkins and Merzenich, 1987; Doetsch, Johnston, and Hannan, 1990; Pons, Garraghty, and Mishkin, 1988; Pons, Garraghty, Friedman, and Mishkin, 1987), and repeated intracortical stimulation (Recanzone and Merzenich, 1988). A similar plasticity of cortical maps has been found in the auditory cortex (Recanzone, Schreiner, and Merzenich, 1993) and visual cortex (Kaas et al., 1990; Gilbert and Wiesel, 1992). For example, Gilbert and Wiesel (1992) have found that after retinal scotomas in monkeys, the zone normally responsive

to visual stimulation of the area occupied by the scotoma becomes responsive to visual stimulation of adjacent retinal areas. In other words, the scotoma area becomes "filled in" by remaining visual information.

Cortical map plasticity may be mediated by intracortical inhibitory neurons. Peripheral sensory deprivation via amputation or other methods
causes a marked reduction in GABAergic activity in neocortical areas associated with the affected periphery (Akhtar and Land, 1991; Garraghty, La-
Chica, and Kaas, 1991; Hendry and Jones, 1986). Jacobs and Donoghue
(1991) have found that localized ionotophoretic infusion of bicuculine (a
GABA receptor antagonist) into the forelimb area is followed by an ability to
elicit both vibrissae and forelimb movements from the otherwise exclusively
vibrissal representation area of rats (see also Dykes, Landry, Metherate, and
Hicks, 1984). These authors suggest that stimulation of one representation
area normally causes dual excitation and inhibition of adjacent cortical areas. That is, a neuron in the vibrissae area normally has excitatory connections with the dendrites of both excitatory and inhibitory neurons in the
forelimb area. The inhibitory interneurons have dominating contacts on the
soma and initial segment of the axon of nearby excitatory neurons so that
removal of this inhibition causes the "unmasking" of the activity of these
neurons. The activity of inhibitory interneurons may be of particular importance to the plastic map effects because glutamate and acetylcholine, although importantly involved in receptive field expression (Metherate, Tremblay, and Dykes, 1988), are not as strongly associated with map plasticity
(Jacobs and Donoghue, 1991). Map plasticity has been found to be dependent upon norepinephrine (NE) because NE depletion prevents cortical map
changes and this effect is reversed by localized infusion of NE (Levin, Craik,
and Hand, 1988; Kasamatsu, Pettigrew, and Ary, 1979).

Changes in representation areas occur within minutes (Calford and Tweedle, 1990) to hours (Donoghue et al., 1990; Sanes, Suner, Lando, and Donoghue, 1988) after peripheral manipulations. In the weeks to months there-
after, a remodeling of the maps has been found (Merzenich et al., 1983;
Sanes et al., 1990). Changes in somatosensory maps tend to be limited to
the extent of overlap, across areas, of pre-existing thalamocortical input
(e.g., Edelman and Finkle, 1984; Jenkins and Merzenich, 1987; Merzenich
et al., 1983), suggesting that immediate shifts in the representation areas
may be due to an unmasking of portions of pre-existing thalamocortical
connections. However, Pons and colleagues (1991) have found that the cortical map changes in monkeys 12 years after sensory deafferentation (i.e.,
monkeys from Taub, 1980) were approximately 10 times larger than normal
thalamocortical ramifications, which suggests a long-term reorganization of
cortical connectional patterns.

It is of considerable current debate whether cortical map plasticity generally
reflects an unmasking of pre-existing connections or can be attributed in part

to a growth and/or reorganization of cortical connections, as suggested by the findings of Pons and colleagues, 1991 (see, e.g., Lund, Sun, and Lamarre, 1994, and response by T. Pons). These two explanations need not be considered mutually exclusive as underlying processes. For example, it is conceivable that localized enhancement of excitatory activity, such as that suggested by Jacobs and Donoghue to underlie unmasking (1991; see also Allard, Clark, Jenkins, and Merzenich, 1991), could itself lead to reorganization and/or growth of connections, particularly if the altered activity is of sustained duration. In addition, many of the manipulations which have been found to lead to cortical map changes are remarkably similar to those which lead to synaptic and neural-structural reorganization, such as behavioral training (Greenough et al., 1979; Greenough et al., 1985; Withers and Greenough, 1989; see also Dunn-Meynell, Benowitz, and Levin, 1992) and cortical damage (Kolb and Gibb, 1993; Jones and Schallert, 1994). It is possible that these structural changes are reflected as changes in the extent of cortical maps.

Cortical Map Plasticity and Human Perceptual Phenomena

Direct evidence of cortical map plasticity in humans has recently been reported by Mogilner and colleagues (1993). Using magnetoencephalography (MEG) to map the somatosensory cortical representation, control subjects were found to have discrete topographical arrangement of the fingers of the hand representation area. Patients with syndactyly (webbed fingers) showed no distinct topology in the hand area, but when examined within weeks following surgical separation, distinct and separate cortical representations of the fingers emerge. In a related experiment, Yang and colleagues (Yang, Gallen, Ramachandran, Cobb, and Bloom, 1993) used MEG to map the arm representation of a patient who had received an amputation of the distal forearm 10 years earlier. Although a normal map of the hand could be found in the hemisphere opposite the patient's intact limb, a map of the hand was not discernible in the hemisphere opposite the amputation. Using the intact hemisphere as a guide to the location of the former hand representation area in the affected side, they found that activity in this area could be induced by stimulation of either the upper forearm or the lower face on the side of the amputation. The latter finding bears remarkable resemblance to the electrophysiological data of Pons and colleagues (1991) showing an expansion of the lower face representation into that of the forelimb area of macaques 12 years after sensory deafferentation of the limb.

Ramachandran and colleagues have hypothesized that expansion of cortical representation areas in humans may be linked to behavioral and perceptual phenomena (reviewed in Ramachandran, 1993), including the filling in of visual scotomas and phantom sensation following amputation. For example, these investigators find that in humans with amputation of one arm, stimulation of facial regions causes the perception of stimulation of the missing hand and arm simultaneous with the facial sensation. These human data may be considered a perceptual correlate of the plastic map phenomena. The perception is topologically ordered and modality-specific. For example, in patients who experience phantom limb sensation upon stimulation of the face, touching individual regions of the face causes the perception of touch on individual digits of the missing hand. Patients also perceive phantom sensations of warm or cold water, vibration, or simple touch depending on the type of stimulation applied to the face. As a striking example, Ramachandran reports that a drop of warm water trickled down a patient's face was perceived as warm water trickling down the phantom arm. Finally, humans with retinal scotomas do not have a visual perception of the scotoma; rather the region of the scotoma becomes, perceptually, filled in by surrounding areas (Ramachandran and Gregory, 1991). This phenomenon may be a perceptual correlate of the "filling in" by adjacent receptive fields of visual cortical areas affected by lesions or scotomas of the retina of cats (Kaas et al., 1990) and monkeys (Gilbert and Wiesel, 1992). It is interesting to speculate that the confabulation seen in amnestic patients represents an extension of this natural tendency of the nervous system to "fill in" where gaps exist. The apparent neural "need" for an intact and organized pattern of representation could lead to fabrication of "memories" that best fit in with the information available.

Conclusions

Taken together, these studies certainly indicate that there are a number of ways in which the fidelity of a seemingly hardwired system may be altered, through progressive function-induced change over time, through altered suppressive or occlusive interactions among neurons, or through trophic/antitrophic effects of hormones and exogenous substances. Whether these potential sources of memory disruption are in any way related to the distortion and reconstruction in memory upon which this volume is focused remains to be determined. Most of the effects we have described would appear to be rather nonsystematic in their distorting effects, but as the sensory reorganization experiments show, the brain seems poised to superimpose an integrated reorganization upon a disorganized neural system, and if there is distortion at the outset, this seems likely to lead to distortions in the reorganized system.

The Future: Synapses Are Only Part of the Story

It has recently become quite clear that plasticity of the brain in response to experience extends beyond synapses. As noted above, cerebellar blood vessels proliferate in response to physical exercise in the absence of any change in synapse numbers (Black et al., 1990). More generally, our research is beginning to point to the importance of an orchestrated set of changes in all of the major components that make up brain tissue—glia, blood vessels, neurons, and their synapses—in response to experience. To describe this array of changes with a term like "memory" does not seem appropriate, although we must be aware that changes in nonneural tissue components can affect neural function, and that a myriad of ways have been proposed in which the activity of astrocytes could modulate neuronal actions and interactions. While this may not be appropriate to a volume so tightly focused upon memory distortion, we propose in closing that the term "brain adaptation" might be considered as a general process, including vascular and glial as well as neuronal changes, and that "memory" might be considered a special case that may be more psychologically than physiologically identifiable.

References

Akhtar, N. D., and Land, P. W. (1991). Activity-dependent regulation of glutamic acid decarboxylase in the rat barrel cortex: Effects of neonatal versus adult sensory deprivation. *Journal of Comparative Neurology, 307,* 200–213.

Allard, T., Clark, S. A., Jenkins, W. M., and Merzenich, M. M. (1991). Reorganization of somatosensory area 3b representations in adult owl monkeys after digital syndactyly. *Journal of Neurophysiology, 66,* 1048–1058.

Armstrong, K. E., Comery, T. A., Jones, T. A., Bates, K. E., Karr, T. L., and Greenough, W. T. (1994). Enhanced expression of a novel microtubule-associated protein in the denervated dentate gyrus following entorhinal cortex lesions. *Society for Neuroscience Abstracts, 20,* 1321.

Arnold, A. P. (1980). Effects of androgens on volumes of sexually dimorphic brain regions in the zebra finch. *Brain Research, 185,* 441–444.

Arnold, A. P., Bottjer, S. W., Brenowitz, E. A., Nordeen, E. J., and Nordeen, K. W. (1986). Sexual dimorphisms in the neural vocal control system in song: Ontogeny and phylogeny. *Brain, Behavior and Evolution, 28,* 22–31.

Arnold, A. P., and Breedlove, S. M. (1985). Organizational and activational effects of sex steroid hormones on vertebrate brain and behavior: A re-analysis. *Hormones and Behavior, 19,* 469–498.

Bailey, C. H., and Chen, M. (1989). Time course of structural changes at identified sensory neuron synapses during long-term sensitization in Aplysia. *Journal of Neuroscience, 9,* 1774–1780.

Bateson, P. P. G., Rose, S. P. R., and Horn, G. (1973). Imprinting: Lasting effects on uracil incorporation into chick brain. *Science, 181,* 576–578.

Bear, M. F., and Singer, W. (1986). Modulation of visual cortical plasticity by acetylcholine and noradrenaline. *Nature, 320,* 172–176.

Beaulieu, C., and Colonnier, M. (1987). Effect of the richness of the environment on the cat visual cortex. *Journal of Comparative Neurology, 266,* 478–494.

Berger, T. W., Berry, S. D., and Thompson, R. F. (1986). Role of the hippocampus in classical conditioning of aversive and appetitive behaviors. In R. L. Isaacson and K. H. Pribram (Eds.), *The hippocampus, Vol. 4.* New York: Plenum Press.

Berry, S. D., and Swain, R. A. (1989). Water deprivation optimizes hippocampal activity and facilitates nictitating membrane conditioning. *Behavioral Neuroscience, 103,* 71–76.

Berry, S. D., and Thompson, R. F. (1978). Prediction of learning rate from the hippocampal electroencephalogram. *Science, 200,* 1298–1300.

Bhide, P. G., and Bedi, D. S. (1984). The effects of a lengthy period of environmental diversity on well fed and previously undernourished rats. II. Synapse to neuron ratios. *Journal of Comparative Neurology, 227,* 305–310.

Bickford, P. C., Heron, C., Young, D. A., and Gerhardt, G. A. (1992). Impaired acquisition of novel locomotor tasks in aged and norepinephrine depleted F344 rats. *Neurobiology of Aging, 13,* 475–481.

Black, J. E., Isaacs, K. R., Anderson, B. J., Alcantara, A. A., and Greenough, W. T. (1990). Learning causes synaptogenesis, whereas motor activity causes angiogenesis, in cerebellar cortex of adult rats. *Proceedings of the National Academy of Sciences (USA), 87,* 5568–5572.

Bottjer, S. W., Miesner, E. A., and Arnold, A. P. (1984). Forebrain lesions disrupt development but not maintenance of song in passerine birds. *Science, 224,* 901–903.

Calford, M. B., and Tweedle, R. (1990). Interhemispheric transfer of plasticity in the cerebral cortex. *Science, 249,* 805–807.

Chang, F.-L. F., and Greenough, W. T. (1982). Lateralized effects of monocular training on dendritic branching in adult split-brain rats. *Brain Research, 232,* 283–292.

Chang, F.-L. F., and Greenough, W. T. (1984). Transient and enduring morphological correlates of synaptic activity and efficacy change in the rat hippocampal slice. *Brain Research, 309,* 35–46.

Chang, F.-L. F., Hawrylak, N., and Greenough, W. T. (1993). Astrocytic and synaptic response to kindling in hippocampal subfield CA1. I. Synaptogenesis in response to kindling *in vitro. Brain Research, 603,* 302–308.

Cornwell-Jones, C. A., Palfai, T., Young, T., and Desai, J. (1990). Impaired hoarding and olfactory learning in DSP-4 treated rats and control cagemates. *Pharmacology, Biochemistry and Behavior, 36,* 707–711.

Devauges, V., and Sara, S. J. (1990). Activation of the noradrenergic system facilitates an attentional shift in the rat. *Behavioral Brain Research, 39,* 19–28.

DeVoogd, T. J. (1990). Recent findings on the development of dimorphic anatomy in the avian song system. *The Journal of Experimental Zoology, Supplement 4,* 183–186.

Doetsch, G. S., Johnston, K. W., and Hannan, C. J. (1990). Physiological changes in the somatosensory forepaw cerebral cortex of adult raccoons following lesions of a single cortical digit representation. *Experimental Neurology, 108,* 162–175.

Donoghue, J. P., Suner, S., and Sanes, J. N. (1990). Dynamic organization of primary motor cortex output to target muscles in adult rats. II. Rapid reorganization following motor nerve lesions. *Experimental Brain Research, 79,* 492–503.

Dostrovsky, J. O., Millar, J., and Wall, P. D. (1976). The immediate shift of afferent drive of dorsal column nucleus cells following deafferentation: A comparison of acute and chronic deafferentation in gracile nucleus and spinal cord. *Experimental Neurology, 52,* 480–495.

Dunn-Meynell, A. A., Benowitz, L. I., and Levin, B. E. (1992). Vibrissectomy induced changes in GAP-43 immunoreactivity in the adult rat barrel cortex. *Journal of Comparative Neurology, 315,* 160–170.

Dykes, R. W., Landry, P., Metherate, R., and Hicks, T. P. (1984). The functional role of GABA in cat primary somatosensory cortex: Shaping the receptive field of cortical neurons. *Journal of Neurophysiology, 52,* 1066–1093.

Dykes, R. W., and Ruest, A. (1986). What makes a map in the somatosensory cortex? In E. G. Jones and A. Peters (Eds.), *Cerebral cortex, Vol. 5.* New York: Plenum Press.

Edelman, G. M., and Finkel, L. H. (1984). Neuronal group selection in the cerebral cortex. In G. M. Edelman, W. M. Cowan, and W. E. Gall (Eds.), *Dynamic aspects of neocortical function.* New York: Wiley.

Faber, D. S., Lin, J.-W., and Korn, H. (1991). Silent synaptic connections and their modifiability. In J. R. Wolpaw, J. T. Schmidt, and T. M. Vaughn (Eds.), Activity-driven CNS changes in learning and development. *Annals of the New York Academy of Sciences, 627,* 231–247.

Floeter, M. K., and Greenough, W. T. (1979). Cerebellar plasticity: Modification of Purkinje cell structure by differential rearing in monkeys. *Science, 206,* 227–229.

Foy, M. R., Stanton, M. E., Levine, S., and Thompson, R. F. (1987). Behavioral stress impairs long-term potentiation in rodent hippocampus. *Behavioral and Neural Biology, 48,* 138–149.

Foy, M. R., and Teyler, T. J. (1983). 17-α-Estradiol and 17-β-estradiol in hippocampus. *Brain Research Bulletin, 10,* 735–739.

Freedman, R., Hoffer, B. J., Woodward, D. J., and Puro, D. (1977). Interaction of norepinephrine with cerebellar activity evoked by mossy and climbing fibers. *Experimental Neurology, 55,* 269–288.

Fuchs, J. L., Montemayor, M., and Greenough, W. T. (1990). Effect of environmental complexity on size of the superior colliculus. *Behavioral and Neural Biology, 54,* 198–203.

Galofre, E., Ferrer, I., Fabreques, I., and Lopez-Tejero, D. (1987). Effects of prenatal alcohol exposure on dendritic spines of layer V pyramidal neurons of the rat's somatosensory cortex. A qualitative and quantitative study with the Golgi method. *Journal fur Hirnforschung, 28,* 653–659.

Garraghty, P. E., LaChica, E. A., and Kaas, J. H. (1991). Injury-induced reorganization of somatosensory cortex is accompanied by reductions in GABA staining. *Somatosensory and Motor Research, 8,* 347–354.

Geinisman, Y., deToledo-Morrell, L., and Morrell, F. (1990). The brain's record of experience: Kindling-induced enlargement of the active zone in hippocampal perforated synapses. *Brain Research, 513,* 175–179.

Geinisman, Y., deToledo-Morrell, L., Morrell, F., Heller, R. E., Rossi, M., and Parshall, R. F. (1993). Structural synaptic correlate of long-term potentiation: Formation of axospinous synapses with multiple, completely partitioned transmission zones. *Hippocampus, 3*, 435–446.

Gilbert, C. D., and Wiesel, T. N. (1992). Receptive field dynamics in adult primary visual cortex. *Nature, 356*, 150–152.

Globus, A., Rosenzweig, M. R., Bennett, E. L., and Diamond, M. C. (1973). Effects of differential experience on dendritic spine counts in rat cerebral cortex. *Journal of Comparative and Physiological Psychology, 82*, 175–181.

Green, E. J., Greenough, W. T., and Schlumpf, B. E. (1983). Effects of complex or isolated environments on cortical dendrites of middle-aged rats. *Brain Research, 264*, 233–240.

Green, J. D., and Arduini, A. A. (1954). Hippocampal electrical activity in arousal. *Journal of Neurophysiology, 17*, 533–557.

Greenough, W. T., Juraska, J. M., and Volkmar, F. R. (1979). Training effects on dendritic branching in occipital cortex of adult rats. *Behavioral and Neural Biology, 26*, 287–297.

Greenough, W. T., Larson, J. R., and Withers, G. S. (1985). Effects of unilateral and bilateral training in a reaching task on dendritic branching of neurons in the rat motor-sensory forelimb cortex. *Behavioral and Neural Biology, 44*, 301–314.

Greenough, W. T., McDonald, J. W., Parnisari, R. M., and Camel, J. E. (1986). Environmental conditions modulate degeneration and new dendrite growth in cerebellum of senescent rats. *Brain Research, 380*, 136–143.

Greenough, W. T., Volkmar, F. R., and Juraska, J. M. (1973). Effects of rearing complexity on dendritic branching in frontolateral and temporal cortex of the rat. *Experimental Neurology, 41*, 371–378.

Grinnell, A. D., and Herrera, A. A. (1981). Specificity and plasticity of neuromuscular connections: Long-term regulation of motoneuron function. *Progress in Neurobiology, 17*, 203–282.

Gurney, M., and Konishi, M. (1980). Hormone induced sexual differentiation of brain and behavior in zebra finches. *Science, 208*, 1380–1382.

Hebb, D. O. (1949). *The organization of behavior.* New York: Wiley.

Hendry, S. H. C., and Jones, E. G. (1986). Reduction in number of immunostained GABAergic neurones in deprived-eye dominance columns of monkey area 17. *Nature, 320*, 750–753.

Hirsch, R. (1974). The hippocampus and contextual retrieval of information from memory: A theory. *Behavioural Biology, 12*, 421–444.

Hirsch, R., Holt, L., and Mosseri, A. (1978). Hippocampal mossy fibers, motivational states, and contextual retrieval. *Experimental Neurology, 62*, 68–79.

Horner, C. H. (1993). Plasticity of the dendritic spine. *Progress in Neurobiology, 41*, 281–321.

Humphreys, A. G., Warren, S. G., Juraska, J. M., and Greenough, W. T. (1994). Estrous cycle regulates synaptic plasticity: Enhanced LTP sensitivity in proestrous rats. *Society for Neuroscience Abstracts, 20*, 802.

Hutchison, J. B., Wingfield, J. C., and Hutchison, R. E. (1984). Sex differences in plasma concentrations of steroids during the sensitive period for brain differentiation in the zebra finch. *Journal of Endocrinology, 103*, 363–369.

Hwang, H.-M., and Greenough, W. T. (1986). Synaptic plasticity in adult rat occipital cortex following short-term, long-term, and reversal of differential housing environment complexity. *Society for Neuroscience Abstracts, 12,* 1284.

Jacobs, K. M., and Donoghue, J. P. (1991). Reshaping the cortical motor map by unmasking latent intracortical connections. *Science, 251,* 944–947.

Jahromi, S. S., and Atwood, H. L. (1974). Three-dimensional ultrastructure of the crayfish neuromuscular apparatus. *Journal of Cell Biology, 63,* 599–613.

Jenkins, W. M., and Merzenich, M. M. (1987). Reorganization of neocortical representations after brain injury: A neurophysiological model of the bases of recovery from stroke. *Progress in Brain Research, 71,* 249–266.

Jenkins, W. M., Merzenich, M. M., Ochs, M. T., Allard, T., and Guic-Robles, E. (1990). Functional reorganization of primary somatosensory cortex in adult owl monkeys after behaviorally controlled tactile stimulation. *Journal of Neurophysiology, 63,* 82–104.

Jones, T. A., and Schallert, T. (1994). Use-dependent growth of pyramidal neurons after neocortical damage. *Journal of Neuroscience, 14,* 2140–2152.

Juraska, J. M., Greenough, W. T., Elliott, C., Mack, K. J., and Berkowitz, R. (1980). Plasticity in adult rat visual cortex: An examination of several cell populations after differential rearing. *Behavioral and Neural Biology, 29,* 157–167.

Juraska, J. M. (1984). Sex differences in dendritic response to differential experience in the rat visual cortex. *Brain Research, 295,* 27–34.

Kaas, J. H. (1991). Plasticity of sensory and motor maps in adult mammals. *Annual Review of Neuroscience, 14,* 137–167.

Kaas, J. H., Krubitzer, L. A., Chino, Y. M., Langston, A. L., Polley, E. H., and Blair, N. (1990). Reorganization of retinotopic cortical maps in adult mammals after lesions of the retina. *Science, 248,* 229–231.

Kaas, J. H., Merzenich, M. M., and Killackey, H. P. (1983). The reorganization of somatosensory cortex following peripheral nerve damage in adult and developing mammals. *Annual Review of Neuroscience, 6,* 325–356.

Kasamatsu, T., and Pettigrew, J. D. (1976). Depletion of brain catecholamines: Failure of ocular dominance shift after monocular occlusion in kittens. *Science, 194,* 206–209.

Kasamatsu, T., Pettigrew, J. D., and Ary, M. (1979). Restitution of visual cortical plasticity by local microperfusion of norepinephrine. *Journal of Comparative Neurology, 185,* 163–182.

Kety, S. S. (1970). The biogenic amines in the central nervous system: Their possible roles in arousal, emotion and learning. In F. O. Schmitt (Ed.), *The neurosciences: Second study program.* New York: Rockefeller University Press.

Kilman, V. L., Sirevaag, A. M., and Greenough, W. T. (1991). Adult rats exposed to complex environments have a greater number of synapses per neuron than individually housed rats. *Society for Neuroscience Abstracts, 17,* 535.

Klintzova, A. J., Uranova, N. A., Hashorst, U., and Schenk, H. (1990). Synaptic plasticity in rat medial prefrontal cortex under chronic haloperidol treatment produced behavioural sensitisation. *Journal fur Hirnforschung, 31,* 175–179.

Kolb, B., and Gibb, R. (1993). Possible anatomical basis of recovery of function after neonatal frontal lesions in rats. *Behavioral Neuroscience, 107,* 799–811.

Konishi, M. (1989). Birdsong for neurobiologists. *Neuron, 3,* 541–549.

Landmesser, L. T. (1980). The generation of neuromuscular specificity. *Annual Review of Neuroscience, 3,* 279–302.

Lee, K. S., Schottler, F., Oliver, M., and Lynch, G. (1980). Brief bursts of high-frequency stimulation produce two types of structural change in rat hippocampus. *Journal of Neurophysiology, 44,* 247–258.

Levin, B. E., Craik, R. L., and Hand, P. J. (1988). The role of norepinephrine in adult rat somatosensory (SmI) cortical metabolism and plasticity. *Brain Research, 443,* 261–271.

Loeb, E. P., Chang, F.-L. F., and Greenough, W. T. (1987). Effects of neonatal 6-hydroxydopamine treatment upon morphological organization of the postero-medial barrel subfield in mouse somatosensory cortex. *Brain Research, 403,* 113–120.

Lund, J. P., Sun, G.-D., and Lamarre, Y. (1994). Cortical reorganization and deafferentation in adult macaques. *Science, 265,* 546–548.

Lussnig, E., Kleim, J. A., Schwarz, E. R., Comery, T. A., and Greenough, W. T. (1994). Synaptogenesis within the motor cortex of the rat following complex motor learning. *Society for Neuroscience Abstracts, 20,* 1435.

Maren, S., DeCola, J. P., Swain, R. A., Fanselow, M. S., and Thompson, R. F. (1994). Parallel augmentation of hippocampal long-term potentiation, theta-rhythm, and contextual fear conditioning in water-deprived rats. *Behavioral Neuroscience, 108,* 44–56.

Mark, R. F. (1980). Synaptic repression at neuromuscular junctions. *Physiological Reviews, 60,* 355–395.

Mark, R. F., and Marotte, L. R. (1972). The mechanism of selective reinnervation of fish eye muscles. III. Functional electrophysiological and anatomical analysis of recovery from section of the IIIrd and IVth nerves. *Brain Research, 46,* 131–148.

Mark, R. F., Marotte, L. R., and Mart, P. E. (1972). The mechanism of selective reinnervation of fish eye muscles. IV. Identification of repressed synapses. *Brain Research, 46,* 149–157.

Marotte, L. R., and Mark, R. F. (1970a). The mechanism of selective reinnervation of fish eye muscle. I. Evidence from muscle function during recovery. *Brain Research, 19,* 41–51.

Marotte, L. R., and Mark, R. F. (1970b). The mechanism of selective reinnervation of fish eye muscle. II. Evidence from electronmicroscopy of nerve endings. *Brain Research, 19,* 53–62.

Merzenich, M. M., Kaas, J. H., Wall, J. T., Sur, M., Nelson, R. J., and Felleman, D. J. (1983). Progression of change following median nerve section in the cortical representation of the hand in areas 3b and 1 in adult owl and squirrel monkeys. *Neuroscience, 10,* 639–665.

Metherate, R., Tremblay, N., and Dykes, R. W. (1988). The effects of acetylcholine on response properties of cat somatosensory cortical neurons. *Journal of Neurophysiology, 59,* 1231–1252.

Miller, M. W., Chiaia, N. L., and Rhoades, R. W. (1990). Intracellular recording and injection study of corticospinal neurons in rat somatosensory cortex: Effect of prenatal exposure to ethanol. *Journal of Comparative Neurology, 297,* 91–105.

Mogilner, A., Grossman, J. A. I., Ribary, U., Joliot, M., Volkmann, J., Rapaport, D., Beasley, R. W., and Llinás, R. R. (1993). Somatosensory cortical plasticity in adult humans revealed by magnetoencephalography. *Proceedings of the National Academy of Sciences (USA), 90,* 3593–3597.

Monti, A. (1895). Sur les alterations du systeme nerveux dans l'inanition. *Archives Italiennes de Biologie, 24,* 347–360.

Nordeen, E. J., Nordeen, K. W., and Arnold, A. P. (1987). Sexual differentiation of androgen accumulation in the zebra finch brain through selective cell loss and addition. *Journal of Comparative Neurology, 259,* 393–399.

Nottebohm, F. (1980). Testosterone triggers growth of brain vocal control nuclei in adult female canaries. *Brain Research, 189,* 429–436.

Nottebohm, F. (1981). A brain for all seasons: Cyclic anatomical changes in song control nuclei of the canary brain. *Science, 214,* 1368–1370.

Nottebohm, F., and Arnold, A. P. (1976). Sexual dimorphism in vocal control areas of the songbird brain. *Science, 194,* 211–213.

Nottebohm, F., Stokes, T. M., and Leonard, C. M. (1976). Central control of song in the canary. *Journal of Comparative Neurology, 165,* 457–468.

O'Keefe, J., and Nadel, L. (1978). *The hippocampus as a cognitive map.* Oxford: Oxford University Press.

Olton, D. S., Becker, J. T., and Handelmann, G. E. (1979). Hippocampus, space, and memory. *Behavioral and Brain Sciences, 2,* 313–322.

Papez, J. W. (1937). A proposed mechanism of emotion. *Archives of Neurology and Psychiatry, 38,* 725–743.

Pons, T. P., Garraghty, P. E., Friedman, D. P., and Mishkin, M. (1987). Physiological evidence for serial processing in somatosensory cortex. *Science, 237,* 417–420.

Pons, T. P., Garraghty, P. E., and Mishkin, M. (1988). Lesion-induced plasticity in the second somatosensory cortex of adult macaques. *Proceedings of the National Academy of Sciences (USA), 85,* 5279–5281.

Pons, T. P., Garraghty, P. E., Ommaya, A. K., Kaas, J. H., Taub, E., and Mishkin, M. (1991). Massive cortical reorganization after sensory deafferentation in adult macaques. *Science, 252,* 1857–1860.

Pysh, J. J., and Weiss, M. (1979). Exercise during development induces an increase in Purkinje cell dendritic tree size. *Science, 206,* 230–232.

Ramachandran, V. S. (1993). Behavioral and magnetoencephalographic correlates of plasticity in the adult human brain. *Proceedings of the National Academy of Sciences (USA), 90,* 10413–10420.

Ramachandran, V. S., and Gregory, R. L. (1991). Perceptual filling in of artificial scotomas in human vision. *Nature, 350,* 699–702.

Rawlins, J. N. P. (1985). Associations across time: The hippocampus as a temporal memory store. *Behavioral and Brain Sciences, 8,* 479–496.

Recanzone, G. H., Allard, T. T., Jenkins, W., and Merzenich, M. M. (1990). Receptive field changes induced by peripheral nerve stimulation in S-I of adult cats. *Journal of Neurophysiology, 63,* 1213–1225.

Recanzone, G. H., and Merzenich, M. M. (1988). Intracortical microstimulation in somatosensory cortex in adult rats and owl monkeys results in a large expansion of the cortical zone of representation of a specific cortical receptive field. *Society for Neuroscience Abstracts, 14,* 223.

Recanzone, G. H., Schreiner, C. E., and Merzenich, M. M. (1993). Plasticity in the frequency representation of primary auditory cortex following discrimination training in adult owl monkeys. *Journal of Neuroscience, 13,* 87–103.

Riley, J. N., and Walker, D. W. (1978). Morphological alterations in the hippocampus after long-term alcohol consumption in mice. *Science, 201,* 646–648.

Roozendaal, B., Koolhaas, J. M., and Bohus, B. (1993). Posttraining norepinephrine infusion into the central amygdala differentially enhances later retention in Roman high-avoidance and low-avoidance rats. *Behavioral Neuroscience, 107,* 575–579.

Sanes, J. N., Suner, S., and Donoghue, J. P. (1990). Dynamic organization of primary motor cortex output to target muscles in adult rats. I. Long-term patterns of reorganization following motor or mixed peripheral nerve lesions. *Experimental Brain Research, 79,* 479–491.

Sanes, J. N., Suner, S., Lando, J. F., and Donoghue, J. P. (1988). Rapid reorganization of adult rat motor cortex somatic representation patterns after motor nerve injury. *Proceedings of the National Academy of Sciences (USA), 85,* 2003–2007.

Sara, S. J., Grecksch, G., and Leviel, V. (1984). Intracerebroventricular apomorphine alleviates spontaneous forgetting and increases cortical noradrenaline. *Behavioral Brain Research, 13,* 43–52.

Schwarz, E. R., Kleim, J. A., Lussnig, E., Comery, T. A., and Greenough, W. T. (1994). Fos expression in the motor cortex of the rat during the acquisition of a complex motor learning task. *Society for Neuroscience Abstracts, 20,* 1435.

Scott, S. A. (1977). Maintained function of foreign and appropriate junctions on reinnervated goldfish extraocular muscles. *Journal of Physiology, 268,* 87–109.

Scott, S. A. (1975). Persistence of foreign innervation on reinnervated goldfish extraocular muscles. *Science, 189,* 644–646.

Sheng, M., and Greenberg, M. E. (1990). The regulation and function of c-fos and other immediate early genes in the nervous system. *Neuron, 4,* 477–485.

Shepanek, N. A., Smith, R. F., Tyer, Z. E., Royall, G. D., and Allen, K. S. (1989). Behavioral and neuroanatomical sequelae of prenatal naloxone administration in the rat. *Neurotoxicology and Teratology, 11,* 441–446.

Shors, T. J., Foy, M. R., Levine, S., and Thompson, R. F. (1990). Unpredictable and uncontrollable stress impairs neuronal plasticity in the rat hippocampus. *Brain Research Bulletin, 24,* 663–667.

Shors, T. J., and Thompson, R. F. (1992). Acute stress impairs (or induces) synaptic long-term potentiation (LTP) but does not affect paired-pulse facilitation in the stratum radiatum of rat hippocampus. *Synapse, 11,* 262–265.

Shors, T. J., Weiss, C., and Thompson, R. F. (1992). Stress-induced facilitation of classical conditioning. *Science, 257,* 537–539.

Sperry, R. W., and Arora, H. L. (1965). Selectivity in regeneration of the oculomotor nerve in the cichlid fish, *Astronotus ocellatus. Journal of Embryology and Experimental Morphology, 14,* 307–317.

Srinivasan, S., Doe, C. O., and Karr, T. L. (1993). Characterization of three novel microtubule-associated proteins expressed in *Drosophila melanogaster* embryos and rat brain. *Society for Neuroscience Abstracts, 19,* 1083.

Stewart, M. G. (1990). Morphological correlates of long-term memory in the chick forebrain consequent on passive avoidance learning. In L. R. Squire and E. Lindenlaub (Eds.), *The biology of memory.* New York: Verlag.

Taub, E. (1980). Somatosensory deafferentation in research with monkeys: Implications for rehabilitation medicine. In L. P. Ince (Ed.), *Behavioral psychology and rehabilitation medicine.* Baltimore: Williams and Wilkins.

Tavares, M. A., Paula-Barbosa, M. M., and Gray, E. G. (1983). Dendritic spine plasticity and chronic alcoholism in rats. *Neuroscience Letters, 42,* 235–238.

Teresawa, E., and Timiras, P. S. (1968). Electrical activity during the estrous cycle of the rat: Cyclic changes in limbic structures. *Endocrinology, 83,* 207–216.

Teyler, T. J., Vardaris, R. M., Lewis, D., and Rawitch, A. B. (1980). Gonadal steroids: Effects on excitability of hippocampal pyramidal cells. *Science, 209,* 1017–1019.

Turner, A. M., and Greenough, W. T. (1983). Synapses per neuron and synaptic dimensions in occipital cortex of rats reared in complex, social, or isolation housing. *Acta Stereologica, 2,* 239–244.

Turner, A. M., and Greenough, W. T. (1985). Differential rearing effects on rat visual cortex synapses. I. Synaptic and neuronal density and synapses per neuron. *Brain Research, 329,* 195–203.

Volkmar, F. R., and Greenough, W. T. (1972). Rearing complexity affects branching of dendrites in the visual cortex of the rat. *Science, 176,* 1445–1447.

Walker, D. W., Hunter, B. E., and Abraham, W. C. (1981). Neuroanatomical and functional deficits subsequent to chronic ethanol administration. *Alcoholism: Clinical and Experimental Research, 5,* 267–282.

Wall, J. T., and Cusick, C. G. (1984). Cutaneous responsiveness in primary somatosensory (S-I) hindpaw cortex before and after partial hindpaw deafferentation in adult rats. *Journal of Neuroscience, 4,* 1499–1518.

Wall, P. D. (1977). The presence of ineffective synapses and the circumstances that unmask them. *Philosophical Transactions of the Royal Society, London (Series B), 278,* 361–372.

Wallace, C. S., Clayton, D. F., and Greenough, W. T. (1994). Differential expression of the transcription factor ZENK in response to environmental complexity and handling. *Society for Neuroscience Abstracts, 20,* 1431.

Wallace, C. S., Kilman, V. L., Withers, G. S., and Greenough, W. T. (1992). Increases in dendritic length in occipital cortex after four days of differential housing in weanling rats. *Behavioral and Neural Biology, 58,* 64–68.

Wang, X., and Greenough, W. T. (1993). Altered NMDA glutamate receptor response in the visual cortex *in vivo* of rats reared in complex environments. *Society for Neuroscience Abstracts, 19,* 164.

Watanabe, Y., Gould, E., and McEwen, B. S. (1992). Stress induces atrophy of hippocampal CA3 pyramidal neurons. *Brain Research, 588,* 341–345.

Weiler, I. J., and Greenough, W. T. (1991). Potassium ion stimulation triggers protein translation in synaptoneurosomal polyribosomes. *Molecular and Cellular Neurosciences, 2,* 305–314.

Weiler, I. J., and Greenough, W. T. (1993). Metabotropic glutamate receptors trigger postsynaptic protein synthesis. *Proceedings of the National Academy of Sciences (USA), 90,* 7168–7171.

Weiss, P. A. (1955). Nervous system (Neurogenesis). In B. H. Willier, P. Weiss, and V. Hamburger (Eds.), *Analysis of development*. Philadelphia: Saunders.

Werner, D., Hawrylak, N., Comery, T. A., Karr, T. L., and Greenough, W. T. (1994). Expression of a novel microtubule protein in rat visual cortex is modulated by visual experience. *Society for Neuroscience Abstracts, 20,* 1321.

Withers, G. S., and Greenough, W. T. (1989). Reach training selectively alters dendritic branching in subpopulations of layer II-III pyramids in rat motor-somatosensory forelimb cortex. *Neuropsychologia, 27,* 61–69.

Wojtowicz, J. M., and Atwood, H. L. (1986). Long-term facilitation alters transmitter releasing properties at the crayfish neuromuscular junction. *Journal of Neurophysiology, 55,* 484–498.

Wojtowicz, J. M., Parnas, I., Parnas, H., and Atwood, H. L. (1988). Long-term facilitation of synaptic transmission demonstrated with macro-patch recording at the crayfish neuromuscular junction. *Neuroscience Letters, 90,* 152–158.

Woolley, C. S., and McEwen, B. S. (1992). Estradiol mediates fluctuation in hippocampal synapse density during the estrous cycle in the adult rat. *Journal of Neuroscience, 12,* 2549–2554.

Woolley, C. S., and McEwen, B. S. (1993). Roles of estradiol and progesterone in regulation of hippocampal dendritic spine density during the estrous cycle in the rat. *Journal of Comparative Neurology, 336,* 293–306.

Yanai, J., Fares, F., Gavish, M., Greenfeld, Z., Katz, Y., Marcovici, G., Pick, C. G., Rogel-Fuchs, T., and Weizman, A. (1989). Neural alterations after early exposure to phenobarbital. *Neurotoxicology, 10,* 543–554.

Yang, T. T., Gallen, C., Ramachandran, V., Cobb, S., and Bloom, F. (1993). Noninvasive study of neural plasticity in adult human somatosensory system. *Society for Neuroscience Abstracts, 19,* 162.

Yi, L., and Greenough, W. T. (1994). Enhancement of synaptic transmission induced by behavioral learning in rat motor cortex. *Society for Neuroscience Abstracts, 20,* 800.

Zola-Morgan, S., and Squire, L. R. (1986). Memory impairment in monkeys following lesions limited to the hippocampus. *Behavioral Neuroscience, 100,* 155–160.

Steps Toward a Molecular Definition of Memory Consolidation

11

Ted Abel
Cristina Alberini
Mirella Ghirardi
Yan-You Huang
Peter Nguyen
Eric R. Kandel

Memory, the retention of information acquired through learning, can be divided into at least two temporally distinct processes, short-term memory and long-term memory. Short-term memory lasts from minutes to hours, whereas long-term memory lasts days, weeks, or even years. The switch from short- to long-term memory is characterized by a consolidation period, during which memory is changed from a labile form that is sensitive to disruption to a stable, self-maintained form.

It has become possible to define an elementary consolidation period on the level of individual nerve cells for both implicit and explicit memory storage. Studies of implicit memory storage in the gill- and siphon-withdrawal reflex of *Aplysia* and of explicit memory storage in the mammalian hippocampus suggest that this cellular representation parallels the behavioral consolidation phase. In each case the consolidation period is manifest as a strengthening of synaptic connections that requires new protein synthesis and gene expression. These findings allow an examination of consolidation on the molecular level, and raise two questions relative to the modulation and distortion of memory, which we shall consider here: (1) What genes are expressed during the consolidation phase, and how do they lead to a stable self-maintained memory storage? (2) Why is there a consolidation phase? We will primarily address the first question and illustrate that it is now possible to define consolidation for both implicit and explicit memory in molecular terms. In the context of memory distortion, we also consider the second question and discuss, in a more speculative manner, the importance of this phase of storage for the strength, endurance, and accessibility of memory.

Introduction

A characteristic feature of long-term memory storage is that it does not become self-sustaining immediately after learning. Rather, a period of time is required for memory to become consolidated. A number of critical factors act during the consolidation period to initiate the self-sustaining process. As a result, the consolidation period serves as a regulatory checkpoint during which memory can be strengthened or weakened by various modulating influences capable of acting within the context of learning (see McGaugh, Chapter 9 of this volume). The consolidation period may therefore also be a period during which memory is susceptible to distortion.

Although memory consolidation is a characteristic of long-term memory found in almost all learning processes, it remains imperfectly understood despite almost a century of research (for review of the earlier literature, see Polster et al., 1991). This lack of understanding is due at least in part to two factors. First, there is a confusion of terminology. Consolidation was originally defined as the stabilization of long-term memory during the first few hours after learning. We therefore shall refer to this process as *initial consolidation*. The term, unfortunately, has subsequently also been used to refer to a very different phenomenon, the transformation of the memory trace over a period of several months to years (Squire et al., 1984). This transformation, which we shall refer to as *later transformation*, is postulated to reflect the transfer of the memory trace from one brain site, such as the hippocampus, to another, such as the neocortex. Clearly, the two processes are very different. Second, initial consolidation has been primarily studied in behavioral and pharmacological terms (for review, see McGaugh, this volume). Until recently, there have been few attempts to study it on the cellular level so as to determine whether there is an elementary representation of consolidation in the individual connections between the neurons involved in memory storage. If there were a cellular representation it might allow for a definition of consolidation in molecular terms and an understanding of the general mechanisms underlying the formation of long-term memory.

In this review, we consider initial consolidation from the perspective of cellular and molecular biology. We shall show that there is a representation of consolidation on the cellular level for both implicit and explicit learning. Analysis of this cellular representation for each of the two forms of learning reveals that both share a similar set of mechanisms for transforming a labile short-term process into a stable, self-maintained long-term process. This molecular analysis reveals that the consolidation period is highly regulated. This regulation could explain components of infantile amnesia on the one hand, and the regression, distortion, and partially accurate recall of repressed memories on the other.

Initial Consolidation Is a General Feature
of Memory Storage

Initial consolidation was first discovered while studying the transition from short-term to long-term memory for verbal learning in humans (Müller and Pilzecker, 1900; McGaugh, 1989). In the initial Müller and Pilzecker experiments, subjects were asked to learn a list of nonsense syllables. The subjects remembered the list well when tested 24 hours later, but they failed to remember the first list 24 hours later when also required to learn a second, different list of nonsense syllables within the first hour or two after learning the first list. By contrast, subjects who learned the second list three or more hours after learning the first had no difficulty in remembering the first list. This disruption (called *retroactive interference*) suggests that long-term memory was still sensitive to disruption even after the initial list had been placed into long-term memory, presumably because a certain amount of time was required for it to become consolidated. Once long-term memory is consolidated, it seems to be stored in a stable form that is not readily disrupted.

This distinction between an early, labile period of memory storage and a later, more stable form was supported by clinical observations of the *retrograde amnesia* following head trauma or epileptic convulsions (for review, see Russell, 1971). These produce a selective memory loss for events that occurred one to two hours before the trauma. These clinical observations were extended by Duncan (1949), who demonstrated retrograde amnesia in experimental animals. He found that long-term memory for a newly learned task in rats (tested 24 hours later) was disrupted when an electroconvulsive seizure was produced one to two hours after training. By contrast, seizures produced three hours or more after training had little or no effect on the ability to recall the learned event.

The first step toward a biochemical understanding of initial consolidation was provided by the observation that long-term memory storage requires new protein and RNA synthesis (Agranoff et al., 1967; Daniels, 1971; Flexner et al., 1983; Davis and Squire, 1984; Montarolo et al., 1986; Castellucci et al., 1989; Crow and Forrester, 1990; see also McGaugh, Chapter 9 of this volume). As with other agents that interfere with consolidation, inhibitors of translation and transcription only disrupt long-term memory when applied during and immediately after behavioral training. These findings first suggested that the consolidation period is a critical period during which genes are induced that give rise to proteins essential for the stable state of memory (Goelet et al., 1986).

What are these genes and proteins? How do they produce a stable memory trace? To understand which molecular mechanisms contribute to memory storage, it was necessary to examine the representation of the memory trace on its most elementary level—that of individual nerve cells and the synaptic connections between them. Studies of various implicit and explicit forms of learning have suggested that, even though memory storage is a complex distributed process involving a number of parallel pathways, there is a cellular representation of short- and long-term memory. What is perhaps even more surprising is that there is an elementary cellular representation of the consolidation process which appears to be similar in *Aplysia, Drosophila,* and mice. Given the distributed nature of memory storage and its complexity, it is reassuring for the future development of a molecular biology of cognition that the molecular nature of the consolidation switch for different types of learning processes is remarkably conserved.

We begin our examination of the cellular representation of consolidation with two examples of implicit learning—sensitization of the gill-withdrawal reflex of *Aplysia* and classical conditioning of odor avoidance in *Drosophila.*

Consolidation and Implicit Forms of Learning: The Gill-Withdrawal Reflex of *Aplysia*

The simple nervous system of the invertebrate *Aplysia* provides a useful model system for studying the mechanisms of consolidation on the molecular level. It contains only 20,000 neurons, many of which are large and identifiable, so that they can be recognized in every member of the species. These cells are collected into ten clusters called *ganglia,* each of which contain about 2,000 cells. It has been possible to identify major components of the neuronal circuits involved in its behavioral responses, and to specify at the cellular and molecular levels the sites and mechanisms used to store memory-related representations. The gill- and siphon-withdrawal reflex is perhaps one of the simplest behaviors of *Aplysia.* This defensive reflex can be modified by several forms of implicit learning: habituation, sensitization, classical conditioning, and operant conditioning. Each of these forms of learning gives rise to both a short-term and a long-term form dependent on the number of training trials.

Cellular Basis of Long-Term Facilitation

Of these several forms of learning, sensitization has been most extensively characterized. Sensitization is a nonassociative form of implicit learning in which an animal (or a human being) learns to alter its behavior after receiving a noxious stimulus. When an *Aplysia* receives a noxious stimulus to the tail, it recognizes the stimulus as aversive and rapidly learns to enhance its various defensive responses, including gill withdrawal to siphon stimulation. The duration of the ensuing memory for the noxious stimulus is a graded function of the number of training trials—the number of noxious stimuli

applied to the tail. Following a single noxious stimulus there is an enhancement of the gill-withdrawal reflex that lasts for minutes. This short-term
memory for sensitization does not require new protein synthesis. By contrast, repeated (four or five) noxious stimuli, each separated by a brief interval (20 minutes), produce a long-term memory that lasts one or more days
and requires protein synthesis during its consolidation phase.

Many of the cells that produce this reflex have been identified. Storage
of even this simple memory is distributed and is evident at several sites (Frost
et al., 1985; Frost et al., 1988). One site that is involved in the storage of
both the short- and the long-term forms of sensitization is a monosynaptic
component comprising the siphon sensory neurons and the gill motor neurons (Montarolo et al., 1986; Schacher et al., 1988; Bailey and Chen, 1983;
Frost et al., 1985; Bailey et al., 1992). This monosynaptic component has
a representation of both short- and long-term memory for sensitization. In
each case that representation is manifest by an enhancement of synaptic
effectiveness. This strengthening, mediated *in vivo* by facilitatory interneurons, is due to presynaptic facilitation—an enhanced transmitter release at
the synapse made by the sensory neuron on the motor neuron. Whereas
short-term facilitation involves an increase in transmitter release from preexisting synaptic terminals, long-term facilitation involves the growth of
new synaptic terminals. Thus, on the cellular level the switch from short-
term to long-term facilitation is a switch from a process-based memory to
a structural-based memory.

One of the advantages of the monosynaptic component of the gill- and
siphon-withdrawal reflex for studying learning is that it can be reconstituted
in vitro by coculturing individual siphon sensory and gill motor neurons.
This *in vitro* reconstituted circuit undergoes presynaptic facilitation when
serotonin (5-HT), a neurotransmitter released *in vivo* during the training
for sensitization, is applied to the culture (Clark and Kandel, 1984; Frost
et al., 1985; Montarolo et al., 1986; Rayport and Schacher, 1986; Glanzman
et al., 1989). As seen for behavioral sensitization, the duration of the facilitation in the *in vitro* reconstituted circuit is a function of the number of applications of 5-HT. A single pulse of 5-HT produces a short-term facilitation
of transmitter release lasting minutes; four or five pulses of 5-HT separated
by 20-minute intervals (or continuous prolonged exposure to 5-HT) elicit
a long-term facilitation lasting more than 24 hours. Moreover, as with behavioral sensitization, this cellular representation has a consolidation phase.
Long-term facilitation, as evident in dissociated cell cultures, requires RNA
and protein synthesis during the period of 5-HT application. One hour after
the last of five 5-HT applications, long-term facilitation is no longer disrupted by RNA or protein synthesis inhibitors (Montarolo et al., 1986).
Thus the transition from short- to long-term memory, the period that corresponds to the initial consolidation phase, is characterized on the cellular
level much as it is in the behavior of the organism, by its sensitivity to inhibi-

tors of macromolecular synthesis. This allows one to ask: What accounts for this consolidation phase? What is its molecular basis?

cAMP Acts as a Second Messenger Mediating Long-Term Facilitation

Serotonin, released *in vivo* during sensitization or applied directly to cultured neurons, regulates transmitter release. Serotonin binds to a cell surface receptor on the sensory neurons that activates the enzyme adenylyl cyclase. This enzyme converts ATP to the diffusible second messenger adenosine 3′,5′-cyclic monophosphate (cAMP). The increase in cAMP produced by the serotonin via adenylyl cyclase activates the cAMP-dependent protein kinase A. cAMP-dependent protein kinase A is made up of four subunits, two catalytic subunits that serve as the active enzyme and two regulatory subunits that interact with and inhibit the catalytic subunit. Binding of the second messenger cAMP to the regulatory subunit frees the active catalytic subunit of cAMP-dependent protein kinase A. Protein kinase A, like other kinases, is an enzyme that adds phosphate groups to target proteins, thereby altering the activity of the target protein.

cAMP-dependent protein kinase A plays a role in both short- and long-term facilitation. Indeed, cAMP can evoke both short- and long-term facilitation, and inhibitors of cAMP-dependent protein kinase A block both forms of facilitation (Ghirardi et al., 1992; Montarolo et al., 1986). How cAMP-dependent protein kinase A participates in the short- and long-term process was illustrated by an experiment carried out by Bacskai et al. (1993). They measured the increase in the free cAMP-dependent protein kinase A catalytic subunit and found that a single pulse of 5-HT, which produces short-term facilitation, increased the amount of catalytic subunit primarily in the presynaptic terminal of the sensory neurons (Figure 11.1A). In the presynaptic terminals of the sensory cells, cAMP-dependent protein kinase A phosphorylates target proteins leading to a transient enhancement of transmitter release (Siegelbaum et al., 1982; Shuster et al., 1985; Braha et al., 1990). In long-term facilitation, induced by repeated applications of 5-HT, the free cAMP-dependent protein kinase A catalytic subunit translocates to the cell body and enters the nucleus where it leads to the activation of specific genes that are important for the growth of new synaptic connections (Dash et al., 1990; Bacskai et al., 1993; Kaang et al., 1993; Figure 11.1B).

cAMP-Dependent Gene Expression Is Required for the Consolidation of Long-Term Facilitation

How does cAMP-dependent protein kinase A activate genes, and how does gene activation lead to stable memory storage?

A

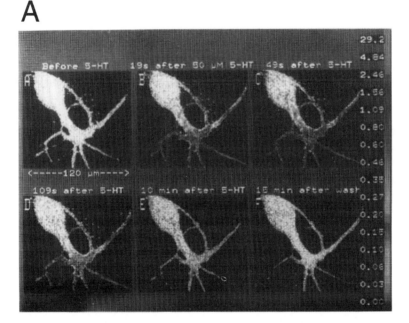

Before 5-HT | 19s after 50 μM 5-HT | 49s after 5-HT

29.2
4.84
2.46
1.66
1.09
0.80
0.60
0.46
0.35

109s after 5-HT | 10 min after 5-HT | 15 min after wash

<----120 μm---->

0.27
0.20
0.15
0.10
0.06
0.03
0.00

B

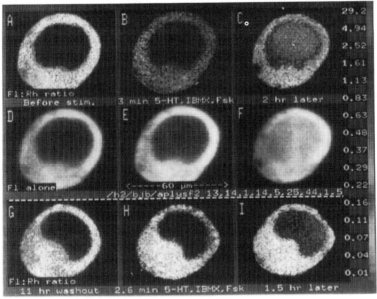

Fl:Rh ratio
Before stim. | 3 min 5-HT,IBMX,Fsk | 2 hr later

29.2
4.94
2.52
1.61
1.13
0.83
0.63
0.48
0.37
0.29
0.22

Fl alone | <----60 μm----> | /h2/bjb/aplusf2.13.14.1.19.5.25.4d.1.5

0.16

Fl:Rh ratio
11 hr washout | 2.6 min 5-HT,IBMX,Fsk | 1.5 hr later

0.11
0.07
0.04
0.01

Genes are made up of two contiguous DNA regions. There is a coding region, which is copied into mRNA by RNA polymerase and translated into protein. In addition, there is a control region, usually located upstream of the coding region, which determines when and to what levels the gene is expressed. The control region (also called a promoter) is made up of small (six to ten base pair) subregions called *DNA response elements*. These response elements bind different control proteins called *transcription factors*, which regulate the activity of RNA polymerase. It is the binding of these different transcription factors to the response elements contained within the control regions that switches genes on or off.

In mammalian cells, cAMP-dependent protein kinase A activates gene expression by the phosphorylation of transcription factors that bind to the cAMP-responsive element (CRE) (Montminy et al., 1990). A major target of this phosphorylation is a protein called CRE-binding protein (CREB), which functions as a transcriptional activator only after it is phosphorylated by cAMP-dependent protein kinase A. During long-term facilitation in *Aplysia* neurons, cAMP-dependent protein kinase A seems to activate gene expression via an *Aplysia* homologue of CREB (Dash et al., 1990). If this activation of CREB is essential for long-term facilitation, then blocking the binding of CREB to its DNA response element should selectively eliminate the long-term process. Dash et al. (1990) tested this idea by microinjecting

Figure 11.1 (*opposite*) A: Gradient in [cAMP] in *Aplysia* sensory neurons after uniform application of 5-HT. A single, cultured *Aplysia* sensory neuron was microinjected with cAMP-dependent kinase labeled with both fluorescein and rhodamine (FiCRhR). The image was pseudocolored from blues to reds, which correspond to low to high ratios and low to high concentrations of free cAMP (scale on right in μM cAMP). (A) Prior to 5-HT treatment. (B) A striking gradient of [cAMP] develops between the cell body and the distal processes after the application of 50 μM 5-HT. The increase in [cAMP] persisted in the continued presence of 5-HT (C through E), but after 5-HT was washed away (F), [cAMP] returned to control levels (A).

B: Nuclear translocation of the catalytic subunit of cAMP-dependent protein kinase. The nucleus excluded the labeled protein and was therefore not fluorescent; the cytoplasm, however, was very bright and exhibited negligible concentrations of cAMP. (B) Soon after application of 25 μM forskolin, 0.1 mM isobutylmethylxanthine (IBMX), and 20 μM 5-HT to raise [cAMP], the fluorescence ratio increased in the cytoplasm, although the nucleus remained dim. (C) The nucleus became brightly fluorescent 2 hours later. (D through F) Single-wavelength images of fluorescein fluorescence (distribution of C subunit) from the corresponding images of (A) through (C). (G) The same cell was washed and allowed to recover overnight. The emission in the cytoplasm fell to low levels, indicating reconstitution of holoenzyme, and the nucleus was again relatively devoid of fluorescence. (H) After treatment with 25 μM forskolin and 0.5 mM IBMX, the fluorescence ratio increased, showing that, after more than 12 hours in a cell, much of the FICRhR was still responsive to changes in [cAMP]. (I) Nuclear translocation could be observed again after an additional 1.5 hours of stimulation. From Bacskai et al. (1993).

oligonucleotides containing the CRE into sensory neurons cultured with motor neurons. This oligonucleotide inhibits the function of CREB by binding to the CREB protein within the cell, thereby preventing it from recognizing sites within the genome and activating gene expression. They found that injection of the CRE blocks long-term facilitation but has no effect on the short-term process (Figure 11.2A).

Does facilitation by 5-HT involve the phosphorylation of CREB? Is this phosphorylation mediated by cAMP-dependent protein kinase A? To address these questions and to explore further the mechanisms of CREB activation, Kaang et al. (1993) microinjected two constructs into *Aplysia* sensory neurons: an expression plasmid containing a chimeric transacting factor made by fusing the GAL4 DNA binding domain to the mammalian CREB activation domain and a reporter plasmid containing the chloramphenicol acetyltransferase (CAT) gene under the control of GAL4 binding sites (Figure 11.2B). This chimeric transcription factor binds to GAL4 sites, but only activates transcription when the CREB activation domain is phosphorylated by cAMP-dependent protein kinase. Since the yeast GAL4-binding site is not recognized by *Aplysia* transcription factors, the transcription of the CAT reporter gene will be induced when the activation domain of the GAL4-CREB hybrid protein is appropriately phosphorylated. Following coinjection of these two plasmids into sensory neurons, exposure to 5-HT produced a tenfold stimulation of CAT expression (Figure 11.2B). Thus, a CREB-related transcription factor that is activated by cAMP-dependent protein kinase A is required for long-term facilitation.

The Switch for Consolidation of Long-Term Facilitation Requires the Induction of ApC/EBP

The activation of adenylyl cyclase, the generation of cAMP, the activation of cAMP-dependent protein kinase A, the translocation of the catalytic subunit to the nucleus, and the phosphorylation of CREB are all unaffected by inhibitors of protein synthesis. Where then does the protein synthesis–dependent step that characterizes the consolidation phase appear? Clearly, it must require an additional step—the activation of genes by CREB. To address this question, Alberini et al. (1994) began to focus on cAMP-regulated transcription factors and particularly on the genes expressed during consolidation.

In searching for regulatory genes that might act on target genes important for stable long-term facilitation of a cascade downstream of CREB, Alberini et al. (1994) focused on the CCAAT enhancer binding protein (C/EBP) family of transcription factors. C/EBP family members contain a characteristic basic region–leucine zipper (bZIP) domain that mediates DNA binding and dimerization (Landschulz et al., 1989). Some members of the C/EBP family

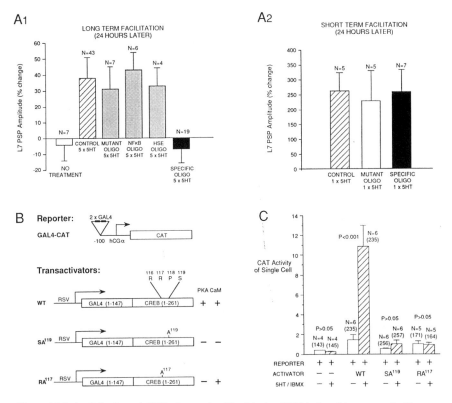

Figure 11.2 A$_1$: Injection of CRE oligonucleotides blocks 5-HT-induced long-term facilitation. Summary of the blockade of the 5-HT-induced increase in long-term facilitation by CRE injection. The height of each bar is the percentage change in the EPSP amplitude ± SEM retested 24 hr after treatment. A$_2$: Summary of the pooled data for short-term facilitation 24 hr after injection. From Dash et al. (1990).
B: 5-HT/IBMX lead to activation of CREB through the phosphorylation of cAMP-dependent protein kinase A. DNA constructs used for transactivation experiments. DNA-binding domain of yeast GAL4 transcription factor (amino acids 1-147) fused to wild-type or mutated forms of the mammalian CREB transactivation domain (amino acids 1-2610). Wild-type and mutated phosphorylation consensus sequences are indicated in single letter amino acid code above constructs.
C: Quantitative analysis of 5-HT-regulated CREB transactivation. The wild-type (WT) GAL4-CREB transactivator enhances 5-HT/IBMX-mediated expression of CAT, whereas mutant (SA[119] and RA[117]) GAL4-CREB show no enhancement. From Kaang et al. (1993).

are activated by cAMP (Metz and Ziff, 1991) or bind to CREs in the regulatory region of several genes (Park et al., 1990; Kageyama et al., 1991; Liu et al., 1991; Vallejo et al., 1993). C/EBP regulates the expression of the *c-fos* gene by binding the enhancer response element (ERE) in the *c-fos* promoter (Metz and Ziff, 1991). Alberini et al. (1994) used this element to screen an *Aplysia* cDNA expression library in order to isolate cDNA clones encoding proteins that specifically bind this sequence. ApC/EBP, a 286 amino acid polypeptide with the characteristic bZIP domain at the C-terminus, was isolated in this screen. The bZIP domain of ApC/EBP is most similar to that of other C/EBP family members, and ApC/EBP displays specific binding activity toward C/EBP-binding elements.

ApC/EBP Is an Immediate-Early Gene Induced during the Consolidation Phase

Where is ApC/EBP expressed? How is it regulated? Does it have a role in learning-related processes? To begin to address these questions, Alberini et al. (1994) investigated whether 5-HT modulates the levels of ApC/EBP mRNA. Levels of ApC/EBP mRNA are very low in untreated neurons, but they rapidly increase after treatment with 5-HT (Figure 11.3). In addition, compounds that increase the intracellular concentration of cAMP also led to induction of ApC/EBP mRNA (Figure 11.3). This cAMP-dependent regulation of ApC/EBP expression may be mediated directly by CREB, since a (nonpalindromic) CRE site is found upstream of the ApC/EBP gene.

Transcription factors are commonly divided into *constitutive* and *inducible,* depending on whether they are always present (constitutive) or whether they need to be induced by activation of their genes. Inducible transcription factors are further divided into *early* and *late,* depending on when in time they are activated in response to a given stimulus. CREB is a constitutively expressed transcription factor. Early genes (also called *immediate-early*), described in studies of viral regulation, are activated by the phosphorylation of constitutive transcription factors. As a result, they are induced rapidly and transiently by mechanisms that are independent of protein synthesis (Sheng and Greenberg, 1990). ApC/EBP is induced as an immediate-early gene: after 15 minutes ApC/EBP mRNA is detectable, and its levels peak at two hours and then decrease (Figure 11.3). Moreover, it is induced in the presence of inhibitors of protein synthesis and emetine.

ApC/EBP Is Essential for Stable Long-Term Facilitation

To determine whether ApC/EBP is necessary for the induction and maintenance of long-term facilitation, Alberini et al. (1994) used three different approaches: First, they interfered with the binding of the transcription factor to its DNA binding element by injecting ERE oligonucleotides that compete for the binding activity of the endogenous ApC/EBP to its target sequence. Second, they blocked the synthesis of endogenous ApC/EBP by injecting ApC/EBP RNA antisense into the sensory cells. Third, they blocked the binding activity of ApC/EBP to its DNA target sites by injecting an antisera

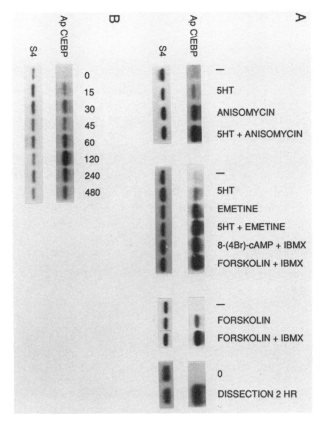

Figure 11.3 Induction of ApC/EBP mRNA.

A: ApC/EBP mRNA expression in CNS of untreated *Aplysia*, of *Aplysia* treated *in vivo* with the indicated drugs for 2 hr at 18°C, or dissected without treatment and kept at 18°C in culture medium. Four independent experiments are shown, in which 10 μg of total RNA extracted from CNS of untreated (−) or treated *Aplysia*, as indicated, were electrophoresed, blotted, and hybridized with ³²P-labeled ApC/EBP (top) or S4 (bottom) probes. The latter encodes the *Aplysia* homologue of S4 ribosomal protein (Thomas et al., 1987), which is constitutively expressed and used as a loading control. 0 indicates RNA extracted immediately after dissection of *Aplysia* CNS. Two hr dissection represents RNA extracted from *Aplysia* CNS dissected and incubated in culture medium for 2 hr at 18°C.

B: Time course of ApC/EBP mRNA induction following 5-HT treatment. Times of treatment are indicated. Five μg of total RNA extracted from total CNS of *in vivo* treated *Aplysia* were analyzed as described in (A). From Alberini et al. (1994).

specific for ApC/EBP into the sensory cells. All of these blocked long-term facilitation but had no effect on short-term facilitation (Figure 11.4).

Stable Long-Term Facilitation Is Associated with the Synthesis of "Late" as well as "Early" Proteins and with the Laying Down of New Synaptic Connections

In addition to ApC/EBP, a number of other proteins are altered in the sensory neurons of the gill-withdrawal reflex after exposure to 5-HT or behavioral training (Castellucci et al., 1988; Barzilai et al., 1989). One of the early effector genes is ubiquitin hydrolase, which may play a role in the cleavage of the regulatory subunit of cAMP-dependent protein kinase A, resulting in persistent kinase activation (Bergold et al., 1990, 1992; Hedge et al., 1993).

The stable phase of long-term facilitation involves the growth of new synaptic connections. Thus, as we have emphasized before, the stability of memory seems to be achieved by changing the nature of memory storage from a process-based memory system to a structural-based one. In dissociated cell culture 5-HT and cAMP lead to a 50% increase in the number of presynaptic contacts. This growth requires new protein synthesis and is paralleled by the increased expression of late effector genes, which included BiP, calreticulin, and clathrin (Bailey and Kandel, 1993; Hu et al., 1993;

Figure 11.4 (opposite) A: Injection of ERE oligonucleotides blocks 5-HT-induced long-term but not short-term facilitation in sensory motor synapses. A_1: Examples of EPSPs recorded in motoneuron L7 after stimulation of the sensory neuron before (0 hr) and 24 hr after 5-HT treatment. Injection of the ERE oligonucleotide but not of the corresponding mutant (ERE mutant) blocks the 5-HT-induced increase in EPSP amplitude at 24 hr. A_2: Bar graph representing the effects of oligonucleotide injections in long-term facilitation. A_3: Bar graph representing the mean EPSP amplitude percentage change $\pm$ SEM of short-term facilitated cells injected with ERE oligonucleotides or with ApCRE, or with buffer.
B: Injection of ApC/EBP antisense RNA blocks 5-HT-induced long-term but not short-term facilitation in the sensory motor synapses. B_1: Examples of EPSPs recorded in motoneuron L7 after stimulation of the sensory neuron before (0 hr) and 24 hr after the 5-HT treatment. Injection of the ApC/EBP antisense RNA but not of the corresponding sense RNA prevents the 5-HT-induced increase in EPSP amplitude at 24 hr. B_2: Bar graph representing the effects of RNA injections in long-term facilitation. B_3: Bar graph representing short-term facilitation of cells injected with ApC/EBP antisense or sense RNA.
C: Injection of antiserum anti-ApC/EBP (BCA) blocks 5-HT-induced long-term but not short-term facilitation in the sensory motor synapses. C_1: Examples of EPSPs recorded in motoneuron L7 after stimulation of the sensory neuron before (0 hr) and 24 hr after 5-HT treatment. Injection of the antiserum BCA, but not of the preimmune serum (PRE) blocks the 5-HT-induced increase in EPSP amplitude at 24 hr. C_2: Bar graph representing the effects of injection of the antiserum BCA or the preimmune serum on long-term facilitation. C_3: Bar graph representing short-term facilitation of cells injected with BCA antiserum or preimmune serum. From Alberini et al. (1994).

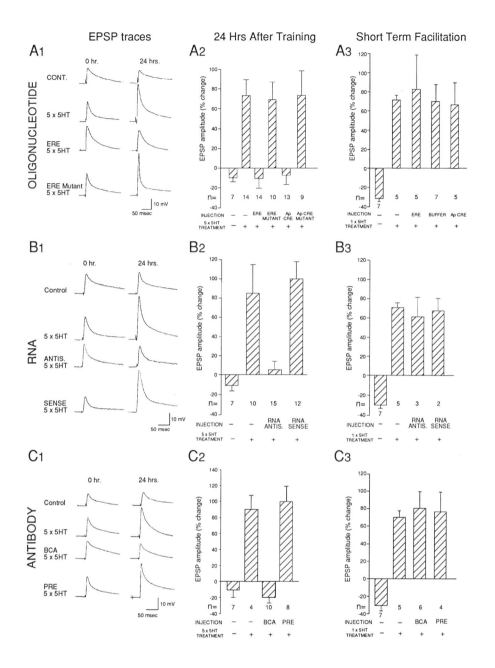

Kennedy et al., 1992; Kuhl et al., 1992). In addition, there are four proteins whose levels decrease following 5-HT treatment. These four proteins encode different isoforms of immunoglobulin-related cell adhesion molecules, termed apCAM, the *Aplysia* homologue of the vertebrate neural cell adhesion molecule, NCAM. Down-regulation is achieved by activation of the endosomal pathway leading to the internalization of apCAM (Bailey et al., 1992). The modulation of cell adhesion molecules by 5-HT may be an early step required for initiating the learning-related growth of synaptic connections that is the hallmark of the initial consolidation step in many long-term processes (Bailey and Kandel, 1993).

Long-Term Memory in *Drosophila* Involves the Activation of cAMP-Inducible Genes by CREB

We have so far only considered a simple form of implicit learning in *Aplysia*. There is, however, reason to believe that a similar mechanism for memory consolidation is operative in implicit forms of learning in *Drosophila*. *Drosophila* can be classically conditioned to discriminate odors, and several mutations have been generated in individual genes that effect this conditioning. The two mutations that have been best characterized, *dunce* and *rutabaga,* involve steps in the cAMP cascade (Dudai, 1988). Moreover, *Drosophila* also shows long-term memory lasting several days following training. This long-term memory process has a consolidation period that requires new protein synthesis and is specifically blocked by expressing a dominant negative transgene that inhibits CREB (Tully et al., 1994; Yin et al., 1994). Thus, in *Drosophila* as in *Aplysia,* the switch from short- to long-term memory requires the activation of cAMP-inducible genes by CREB.

A Critical Period of Transcription Is Required for Explicit Forms of Learning in Mammals: Induction of a Late Phase of Long-Term Potentiation in the Mammalian Hippocampus

In mammals, the hippocampus is essential for an initial consolidation of explicit (or declarative) memory (Squire, 1992). Explicit memory is the memory of facts and events, in contrast to implicit memory, which includes simple conditioning and the learning of skills and habits. To what degree are the molecular mechanisms for consolidation that we encountered for implicit forms of learning in *Aplysia* and *Drosophila* conserved in explicit forms?

Long-term potentiation is a persistent, activity-dependent form of synaptic modification that can be induced by brief, high-frequency stimulation of hippocampal neurons (Bliss and Collingridge, 1993). Because LTP can last

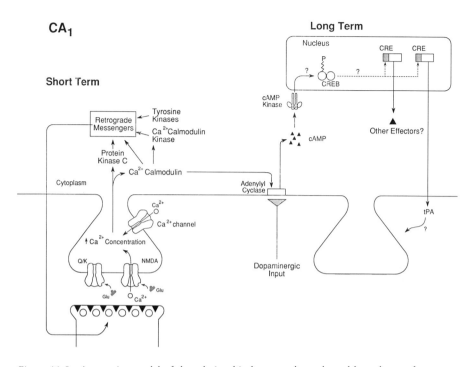

Figure 11.5   A tentative model of the relationship between the early and late phases of LTP in hippocampal area CA1. Activation of the postsynaptic cell by glutamate during LTP leads to an influx of CA^{2+} that activates two processes, a short-term process and a long-term process. The short-term process involves CaM kinase II, protein kinase C, and tyrosine kinases, and leads to the activation of a retrograde messenger that is thought to enhance transmitter release from the presynaptic terminals. This short-term process does not require new protein synthesis or transcription. By contrast, the long-term process is initiated by the Ca^{2+} stimulation of adenylyl cyclase, leading to an increase in cAMP and an activation of cAMP-inducible genes, perhaps via phosphorylation of transcription factors like CREB, the cAMP-dependent protein kinase.

for days to weeks in the intact animal, it is an attractive model for certain types of long-term memory in the mammalian brain. We have recently found that LTP in the CA1 and CA3 regions of hippocampal slices has distinct temporal phases (Figure 11.5) (Frey et al., 1993; Huang and Kandel, 1994; Nguyen et al., 1994). An early phase beginning immediately after tetanic stimulation and lasting one to three hours is induced by a single high-frequency train and does not require protein synthesis. A late phase (L-LTP) persists for at least eight hours in slices, requires three or more high-frequency trains for its induction, and is blocked by inhibitors of protein synthesis or inhibitors of cAMP-dependent protein kinase A.

Using two different RNA synthesis inhibitors, Nguyen et al. (1994) found that L-LTP requires RNA synthesis. The induction of L-LTP produced either by tetanic stimulation or by application of the cAMP analogues Sp-cAMPS was selectively prevented when transcription was blocked immediately after tetanization or during application of cAMP. As is the case with behavioral memory, this requirement for transcription had a critical time window. Thus, the late phase of LTP in the CA1 region requires transcription during a critical period immediately following tetanization, perhaps because cAMP-inducible genes must be expressed during this period.

Since NMDA receptor-dependent LTP in the Schaffer collateral pathway has early and late stages, Huang et al. (1994) explored whether NMDA-independent LTP in the mossy fiber pathway has a similar consolidation process and similar mechanisms for this phase. They found here, as in CA1, that one tetanus produces only transient LTP. By contrast, three tetani produce potentiation that lasts more than six hours. Bath application of forskolin, an activator of adenylyl cyclase that simulates the early phase, also simulates the late phase. Consistent with a consolidation phase, the late but not the early phase of mossy fiber LTP and forskolin-induced potentiation are both blocked by anisomycin and actinomycin-D. These findings further suggest that, although the early phases of NMDA-dependent and NMDA-independent LTP are different, the consolidation phases of LTP seem to involve a similar program of cAMP-induced gene activation.

Consolidation Can Now Begin to Be Defined in Molecular Terms

The data from *Aplysia, Drosophila,* and hippocampal LTP indicate that the consolidation phase has a cellular representation and can now be analyzed on the molecular level. On the molecular level, consolidation represents the period during which a gene cascade activated by learning switches on the self-perpetuating transcriptional events essential for long-term memory.

A schematic representation of the molecular events in *Aplysia* that consolidate short-term into long-term facilitation is shown in Figure 11.6. Serotonin binding to its receptor present on the surface of sensory neurons activates adenylyl cyclase, which catalyzes the synthesis of cAMP. Newly synthesized cAMP binds to the regulatory subunit of cAMP-dependent protein kinase A, leading to its dissociation from the catalytic subunit, which now becomes activated. cAMP-dependent protein kinase A acts on at least two mechanisms involved in the facilitation of the neurotransmitter release. It phosphorylates K^+ channels, which leads to a reduction of the outward K^+ current. This produces an increase of Ca^{2+} influx into the presynaptic neuron by delaying membrane repolarization. In addition, cAMP-dependent protein kinase A acts on other substrates that seem to be part of the exocytotic machinery involved in neurotransmitter release. These modifications in the

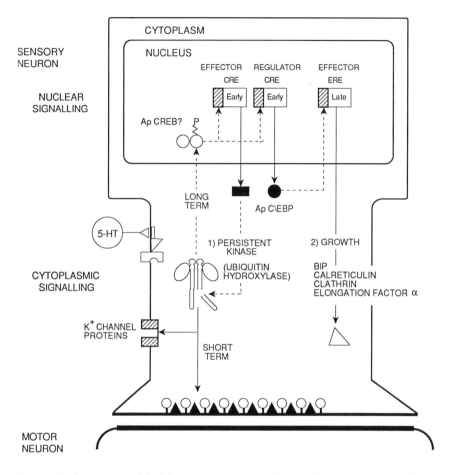

Figure 11.6 Schematic model of the activation pathways involved in *Aplysia* short- and long-term sensitization.

presynaptic terminals lead to short-term facilitation. When repeated stimulations are applied that give rise to long-term facilitation, the activation of cAMP-dependent protein kinase A lasts longer and the cAMP-dependent protein kinase A catalytic subunit translocates to the nucleus.

Nuclear target substrates of cAMP-dependent protein kinase A-dependent phosphorylation seem to include the transcription factors of the CREB family. In fact, the activity of CRE-binding proteins is necessary for long-term facilitation, and repeated HT stimulation, but not a single pulse, activates the transcription of microinjected reporter genes placed under the control of the CRE.

Transcription is the key event leading to consolidation of synaptic strengthening and the associated synaptic structural changes. During transcription-dependent consolidation there is a rapid induction of the transcription factor ApC/EBP. This suggests that consolidation involves a cascade of gene activation with constitutively expressed proteins (such as CREB) regulating the expression of immediate-early genes (such as ApC/EBP), which control the expression of late effector genes whose actions are self-maintaining. The activation of self-maintaining mechanisms explains why the characteristic protein synthesis–dependent consolidation phase is brief: the induction of regulatory factors is the limiting step that allows the expression of later events.

The consolidation of facilitation is characterized by morphological changes of the synapses that contribute to storage of the information. Among the late proteins, structural effectors such as BiP, calreticulin, and clathrin have been identified (Kennedy et al., 1992; Kuhl et al., 1992), and morphological studies have shown that structural changes appear within one hour after 5-HT or tail shock training and persist for days or weeks. Moreover, the decay of these structural changes parallels the decay of behavioral memory (Bailey and Chen, 1989; Bailey and Kandel, 1993). Thus, initial consolidation seems to achieve at least part of its stability from the fact that within the same cell it involves a switch from a process-based memory system to a structurally based one.

Common Steps Seem to Be Involved in the Consolidation of Explicit and Implicit Learning

The finding that LTP in the hippocampus also has an early and a late phase, and that the consolidation phase requires macromolecular synthesis and is mediated by cAMP, suggests that even though explicit and implicit memory utilize different circuity and recruit conscious awareness to very different degrees, they nevertheless seem to share a common molecular logic for initial consolidation. The apparent conservation of steps in the molecular mechanisms for consolidation may in turn reflect the fact that long-term memory storage commonly involves structural changes (Bailey and Kandel, 1993).

Finally, the finding that the cAMP pathway is necessary for neuronal changes related to long-term memory storage does not exclude the participation of other second-messenger pathways. Indeed, the CREB proteins, the nuclear targets of cAMP-dependent protein kinase A, are not only targets for the cAMP pathway. CREB is a multifunctional transcription factor that can also be activated by CaM kinase II as well as by various neurotrophins such as NGF and BDNF (Sheng et al., 1991; Dash et al., 1991; Ginty et al., 1994). It therefore will be interesting to see whether these neurotrophins can modulate the last phase of LTP and whether this modulation contributes to the growth of new synaptic connections following learning.

The Consolidation Period of Long-Term Memory Resembles the Commitment Period of Terminal Differentiation

Neurons are known to be maintained in a terminally differentiated state throughout their life and to respond to environmental stimuli by modifying their connections. Our data suggest that external stimuli may induce the activation of genetic programs that provide a key point for regulation of self-sustained long-lasting processes, similar to the genetic cascade of gene activation turned on during developmental lineage commitment.

Critical time windows, comparable to the consolidation period, are not unique to memory storage, but have been described as part of certain developmental sequences in other cells of the body. In mammals, blood cell types develop from an early multipotent hemopoietic stem cell, which generates several terminally differentiated derivatives. Hemopoietic growth factors such as colony-stimulating factors expand distinct sublineages and cause cells to commit to a particular cell lineage irreversibly (Metcalf, 1989).

In *Drosophila*, one of the most precise, temporally coordinated cascades of gene expression is evident in the waves of puffing activity in the polytene chromosomes of salivary glands. This puffing response is evoked by the action of the steroid hormone ecdysone at the onset of metamorphosis (reviewed in Ashburner, 1990). As with the viral infection cycle and our observation in *Aplysia* long-term facilitation, the induction of early puffs by ecdysone is rapid and protein synthesis independent, while the induction of "late" puffs is dependent on prior protein synthesis.

The similarity between critical periods in terminal differentiation and those in long-term memory suggests that the two processes may share a common molecular logic—a cascade of gene activation, with a critical time window in which the differentiated state is still labile and can be disrupted—and may perhaps even share similar molecules such as C/EBP. Indeed, the C/EBP family of proteins are associated characteristically with terminal cell differentiation in adipocytes, macrophages, and liver (Cao et al., 1991; Lin and Lane, 1992).

Recent studies (summarized in Blau and Baltimore, 1991; Lo et al., 1993) indicate that terminally differentiated states are not as stable as has long been thought, because cells are not locked into this state by passive repression. Rather, both the differentiated state and the repression are actively controlled. This principle is particularly evident in neurons. Although the withdrawal of neurons from the cell cycle is irreversible, neurons characteristically remain plastic throughout most of their life cycle and can grow and retract their connections with target cells in response to appropriate environmental stimuli. In fact, from this it appears that the reversibility of the terminally differentiated state is particularly developed in neurons and may underlie their ability to respond to environmental stimuli essential for learning and memory storage.

The Consolidation Period of Long-Term Memory May Be a Checkpoint for Regulating the Strength of Memory: Repression, Distortion, and the Return of Lost Memories

Why is there this relatively long time period, of several hours, during which long-term memory is sensitive to disruption? It seems likely that, as with terminal differentiation, the consolidation period is a checkpoint where a number of critical steps come together to initiate the induction of a self-sustained long-term memory process. This checkpoint could provide an opportunity for a variety of regulatory processes to modulate memory storage. Different regulatory processes might in turn give rise to *enhancement, distortion,* or *repression* of memory storage.

As discussed in McGaugh's contribution to this volume (Chapter 9), one important determinant of memory storage is the emotional context in which the acquisition of the learned information occurs. Emotionally charged stimuli exert powerful effects on storage and seem to do so in large part by modulating consolidation. Both McGaugh's extensive studies and our own, more preliminary data (Huang and Kandel, 1995) suggest that several key modulatory systems of the brain—the cholinergic, dopaminergic, noradrenergic, and serotonergic systems—act not only on the amygdala to affect the memory storage for the emotional component of the learned event, but also on the hippocampus to affect storage of the cognitive component. In the hippocampus these systems exert an effect on LTP by regulating the strength of consolidation.

For example, McGaugh and his colleagues and Michaela Gallagher and her collaborators have found that memories of fearful experiences are strengthened when norepinephrine is injected into the amygdala (McGaugh, 1989). Release of enkephalins weakens this type of storage. This modulation acts equally on the explicit and implicit memory components of fear. These findings suggest that a painful incident may lead to repression because endogenous opiates are released in response to the experience, and these in turn can interfere with the memory storing process. In rats, Gallagher found that blocking the action of endogenous opiates by naloxone at the time of consolidation enhances memory recall (Gallagher et al., 1985). Furthermore, injecting a stimulant drug like adrenaline can enhance weakly stored memories.

These studies give a biological context for considering how a traumatic memory might be suppressed in humans. This in turn raises the question: Once suppressed, how can the suppressed memory be retrieved? Clearly we do not know the answer to this question, but we now can begin to think about alternative possibilities in biological terms. To outline one possible mechanism (see Kandel and Kandel [1994] for details), suppose that a memory is stored weakly in the explicit system because endogenous opiates interfere with its consolidation. This storage might be so weak that the person has no conscious memory of the original painful event. The same event, though, might also be captured by the implicit system through characteristic physiological sensations or gestures. Perhaps later, the implicit system might provide clues such as physical sensations that might help stir the recall of weak explicit memories. People who say they were abused as children often do describe their memories returning first as bodily sensations. As reviewed by Krystal, Southwick, and Charney (Chapter 5), the release of noradrenaline in response to stress contributes to the powerful flashbacks of Vietnam veterans. Perhaps memories that survivors of abuse are normally not able to access are retrieved when their noradrenaline system is activated. As this discussion illustrates, it may soon be possible to study, at the molecular level, how different emotional experiences, acting through different modulatory systems, can lead to memory repression with subsequent recall (return of repressed memories) on the one hand, and to memory distortion on the other.

As these arguments make clear, one unanticipated consequence of the current debate on the reliability of memory—the discussion on repression, the return of repressed memories, and memory distortion—may be to increase the biologists' awareness that there are important problems here to be solved, problems with significant social consequences. Take the issue of repression. Whereas some psychologists question the existence of memory repression based on behavioral data alone, recent neurobiological studies of patients with brain damage suggest that some form of repression occurs. There also is evidence for a type of repression in infantile (amnesia) repression. To broaden the discussion of repression, we briefly consider these two sets of findings here.

Patients with a left hemiplegia following a stroke in the right hemisphere sometimes deny their paralysis, a syndrome called *anosognosia*. Ramachandran and his colleagues (1995) have found that these patients know, on some deeper level, that they are in fact paralyzed. Given a choice between a manual task that requires both hands or one that requires only one hand, these patients chose the two-handed task—tying their shoelaces—even though they were paralyzed on the left side. This clearly shows that they have no implicit knowledge of their paralysis. Moreover, the patients showed no recollection of their failed attempts, as if they had selectively repressed the memory of those attempts. To test whether the memory was

inaccessible or whether the patient had simply failed to store it, Ramachandran and his collaborators next irrigated the patient's left ear with ice water
(a procedure that, for unknown reasons, has been shown to lift the anosognosia transiently), and found that this produced a striking loss of the denial
of the syndrome. In parallel with the lifting of the denial, there was a return
of the repressed memories. Thus, on some deeper level, the patient apparently had knowledge of his paralysis, of his repeated attempts at tying the
shoelaces, and of his failure!

Infantile amnesia exists not only in humans (as first suggested by Freud);
it is also characteristic of mammalian learning. Young animals learn, but
do not recall that learned event well. Yet this recall can be enhanced by
various reminder stimuli, similar to the reminder stimuli thought to be important for later repression and amnestic recall. In attempts to cure infantile
amnesia, instances of learning during infancy have been spared from the
typical rapid forgetting by simple memory enhancers that introduce cues
periodically throughout the retention interval, or just prior to the retention
test (Campbell and Jaynes, 1966; Rohrbaugh and Riccio, 1970; Spear,
1978). These treatments do not alleviate infantile amnesia in any specific
manner; they enhance adult memory as well. Treatments that alleviate infantile amnesia reduce forgetting by older animals (Spear, 1978). But these
treatments show that memory storage for veridical events can be modified
so as to lift at least partially the repression of infant amnesia.

The clinical and the psychological evidence presented in several chapters of this volume, as well as the experiences of everyday life, indicate that
memory can under some circumstances be robust and veridical, whereas,
under other circumstances, it can be fragile, distorted, repressed, and re-
remembered. These modifications speak for biological modulation of memory storage. Our data in turn suggest that this modulation may involve consolidation to an important degree. As the current social debate on memory
distortion makes clear, without independent verification, the accuracy of
memory cannot be evaluated. Thus, a better understanding of the biological
underpinnings of memory consolidation and its modulation will not only
be of interest scientifically, but it may also, in the long run, prove important
for a more rational psychotherapy and a less politicized legal policy for evaluating the accuracy of memory. Much as DNA fingerprinting allows for a
more reliable identification of people, so a coherent biology of memory may
allow a more reliable evaluation of memory recall.

References

Agranoff, B. W., R. E. Davis, L. Casola, and R. Lin. 1967. "Actinomycin D blocks
    formation of memory of shock-avoidance in goldfish." *Science* 158:1600–1601.
Alberini, C. M., M. Ghirardi, R. Metz, and E. R. Kandel. 1994. "C/EBP is an

immediate-early gene required for the consolidation of long-term facilitation in *Aplysia*." *Cell* 76:1099–1114.

Ashburner, M. 1990. "Puffs, genes and hormones revisited." *Cell* 61:1–3.

Bacskai, B. J., B. Hochner, M. Mahaut-Smith, S. R. Adams, B.-K. Kaang, E. R. Kandel, and R. Y. Tsien. 1993. "Spatially resolved dynamics of cAMP and protein kinase A subunits in *Aplysia* sensory neurons." *Science* 260:222–226.

Bailey, C. H., and M. Chen. 1983. "Morphological basis of long-term habituation and sensitization in *Aplysia*." *Science* 220:91–93.

Bailey, C. H., and M. Chen. 1989. "Time course of structural changes at identified sensory neuron synapses during long-term sensitization in *Aplysia*." *Journal of Neuroscience* 9:1774–1780.

Bailey, C. H., and E. R. Kandel. 1993. "Structural changes accompanying memory storage." *Annual Review of Physiology* 55:397–426.

Bailey, C. H., P. Montarolo, M. Chen, E. R. Kandel, and S. Schacher. 1992. "Inhibitors of protein and RNA synthesis block structural changes that accompany long-term heterosynaptic plasticity in *Aplysia*." *Neuron* 9:749–758.

Barzilai, A., T. E. Kennedy, J. D. Sweatt, and E. R. Kandel. 1989. "5-HT modulates protein synthesis and the expression of specific proteins during long-term facilitation in *Aplysia* sensory neurons." *Neuron* 2:1577–1586.

Bergold, P. J., J. D. Sweatt, I. Winicov, K. R. Weiss, E. R. Kandel, and J. H. Schwartz. 1990. "Protein synthesis during acquisition of long-term facilitation is needed for the persistent loss of regulatory subunits of the *Aplysia* cAMP-dependent protein kinase." *Proceedings of the National Academy of Sciences (USA)* 87:3788–3791.

Bergold, P. J., S. A. Beushausen, T. C. Sacktor, S. Cheley, H. Bayley, J. H. Schwartz. 1992. "A regulatory subunit of the cAMP-dependent protein kinase down-regulated in *Aplysia* sensory neurons during long-term sensitization." *Neuron* 8:387–397.

Blau, H. M., and D. Baltimore. 1991. "Differentiation requires continuous regulation." *Journal of Cell Biology* 112:781–783.

Bliss, T. V., and G. L. Collingridge. 1993. "A synaptic model of memory: Long-term potentiation in the hippocampus." *Nature* 361:31–39.

Braha, O., N. Dale, B. Hochner, M. Klein, T. W. Abrams, and E. R. Kandel. 1990. "Second messengers involved in the two processes of presynaptic facilitation that contribute to sensitization and dishabituation in *Aplysia* sensory neurons." *Proceedings of the National Academy of Sciences (USA)* 87:2040–2044.

Campbell, B. A., and J. Jaynes. 1966. "Reinstatement." *Psychological Review* 73:478–480.

Cao, Z., R. M. Umek, and S. L. McKnight. 1991. "Regulated expression of three C/EBP isoforms during adipose conversion of 3T3-L1 cells." *Genes and Development* 5:1539–1552.

Castellucci, V. F., T. E. Kennedy, E. R. Kandel, and P. Goelet. 1988. "A quantitative analysis of 2-D gels identifies proteins in which labeling is increased following long-term sensitization in *Aplysia*." *Neuron* 1:321–328.

Castellucci, V. F., H. Blumenfeld, P. Goelet, and E. R. Kandel. 1989. "Inhibitor of protein synthesis blocks long-term behavioral sensitization in the isolated gill-withdrawal reflex of *Aplysia*." *Journal of Neurobiology* 20:1–9.

Clark, G. A., and E. R. Kandel. 1984. "Branch-specific heterosynaptic facilitation in

Aplysia siphon sensory cells." *Proceedings of the National Academy of Sciences (USA)* 81:2577–2581.

Crow, T., and J. Forrester. 1990. "Inhibition of protein synthesis blocks long-term enhancement of generator potentials produced by one-trial *in vivo* conditioning in Hermissenda." *Proceedings of the National Academy of Sciences (USA)* 87:4490–4494.

Daniels, D. 1971. "Effects of actinomycin D on memory and brain RNA synthesis in an appetitive learning task." *Nature* 231:395–397.

Dash, P. K., B. Hochner, and E. R. Kandel. 1990. "Injection of the cAMP-responsive element into the nucleus of *Aplysia* sensory neurons blocks long-term facilitation." *Nature* 345:718–721.

Dash, P. K., K. A. Karl, M. A. Colicos, R. Prywes, and E. R. Kandel. 1991. "cAMP response element-binding protein is activated by Ca^{2+}/calmodulin- as well as cAMP-dependent protein kinase." *Proceedings of the National Academy of Sciences (USA)* 88:5061–5065.

Davis, H. P., and L. R. Squire. 1984. "Protein synthesis and memory. A review." *Psychological Bulletin* 96:518–559.

Dudai, Y. 1988. "Neurogenetic dissection of learning and short-term memory in Drosophila." *Annual Review of Neuroscience* 11:537–563.

Duncan, C. P. 1949. "The retroactive effect of electroshock on learning." *Journal of Comparative Physiology and Psychology* 42:32–44.

Flexner, J. B., L. B. Flexner, and E. Stellar. 1983. "Memory in mice is affected by intracerebral puromycin." *Science* 141:57–59.

Frey, U., Y.-Y. Huang, and E. R. Kandel. 1993. "Effects of cAMP simulate a late stage of LTP in hippocampal CA1 neurons." *Science* 260:1661–1664.

Frost, W. N., V. F. Castellucci, R. D. Hawkins, and E. R. Kandel. 1985. "Monosynaptic connections from the sensory neurons of the gill- and siphon-withdrawal reflex in *Aplysia* participate in the storage of long-term memory for sensitization." *Proceedings of the National Academy of Sciences (USA)* 82:8266–8269.

Frost, W. N., G. A. Clark, and E. R. Kandel. 1988. "Parallel processing of short-term memory for sensitization in *Aplysia*." *Journal of Neurobiology* 19:297–334.

Gallagher, M., P. R. Rapp, and R. J. Fanelli. 1985. "Opiate antagonist facilitation of time-dependent memory processes: Dependence upon intact norepinephrine function." *Brain Research* 347:284–290.

Ghirardi, M., O. Braha, B. Hochner, P. G. Montarolo, E. R. Kandel, and N. Dale. 1992. "Roles of PKA and PKC in facilitation of evoked and spontaneous transmitter release at depressed and nondepressed synapses in *Aplysia* sensory neurons." *Neuron* 9:479–489.

Ginty, D., A. Bonni, and M. E. Greenberg. 1994. "Nerve growth factor activates a Ras-dependent protein kinase that stimulates *c-fos* transcription via phosphorylation of CREB." *Cell* 77:713–728.

Glanzman, D. L., S. L. Mackey, R. D. Hawkins, A. Dyke, P. E. Lloyd, and E. R. Kandel. 1989. "Depletion of serotonin in the nervous system of *Aplysia* reduces the behavioral enhancement of gill withdrawal as well as the heterosynaptic facilitation produced by tail shock." *Journal of Neuroscience* 9:4200–4213.

Goelet, P., V. F. Castellucci, S. Schacher, and E. R. Kandel. 1986. "The long and the short of long-term memory—a molecular framework." *Nature* 322:419–422.

Hegde, A. N., A. L. Goldberg, and J. H. Schwartz. 1993. "Regulatory subunits of cAMP-dependent protein kinases are degraded after conjugation to ubiquitin: A molecular mechanism underlying long-term synaptic plasticity." *Proceedings of the National Academy of Sciences (USA)* 90:7436–7440.

Hu, Y., A. Barzilai, M. Chen, C. H. Bailey, and E. R. Kandel. 1993. "5-HT and cAMP induce the formation of coated pits and vesicles and increase the expression of clathrin light chain in sensory neurons of *Aplysia*." *Neuron* 10:921–929.

Huang, Y.-Y., and E. R. Kandel. 1994. "Recruitment of long-lasting and protein kinase A-dependent long-term potentiation in the CA1 region of hippocampus requires repeated tetanization." *Learning & Memory* 1:74–82.

Huang, Y.-Y., and E. R. Kandel. 1995. "D1/D5 receptor agonists induce a protein synthesis-dependent late potentiation in the CA1 region of the hippocampus." *Proceedings of the National Academy of Sciences (USA)*, submitted.

Huang, Y.-Y., X.-C. Li, and E. R. Kandel. 1994. "cAMP contributes to mossy fiber LTP by initiating both a covalently-mediated early phase and a macromolecular synthesis-dependent late phase." *Cell* 79:69–79.

Kaang, B.-K., E. R. Kandel, and S. G. N. Grant. 1993. "Activation of cAMP-responsive genes by stimuli that produce long-term facilitation in *Aplysia* sensory neurons." *Neuron* 10:427–435.

Kageyama, R., Y. Sasai, and S. Nakanishi. 1991. "Molecular characterization of transcription factors that bind to the cAMP responsive region of the substance P precursor gene." *Journal of Biological Chemistry* 266:15525–15531.

Kandel, M., and E. R. Kandel. 1994. "Flights of memory." *Discover* 15(5):32–38.

Kennedy, T. E., D. Kuhl, A. Barzilai, J. D. Sweatt, and E. R. Kandel. 1992. "Long-term sensitization training in *Aplysia* leads to the increase in calreticulin, a major presynaptic calcium-binding protein." *Neuron* 9:1013–1024.

Kuhl, D., T. E. Kennedy, A. Barzilai, and E. R. Kandel. 1992. "Long-term sensitization training in *Aplysia* leads to an increase in the expression of BiP, the major protein chaperon of the ER." *Journal of Cell Biology* 119:1069–1076.

Landschulz, W. H., P. F. Johnson, and S. L. McKnight. 1989. "The DNA binding domain of the rat liver nuclear protein C/EBP is bipartite." *Science* 243:1681–1688.

Lin, F., and M. D. Lane. 1992. "Antisense CCAAT/enhancer-binding protein RNA suppresses coordinate gene expression and triglyceride accumulation during differentiation of 3T3-L1 preadipocytes." *Genes and Development* 6:533–544.

Liu, J., E. A. Park, A. L. Gurney, W. J. Roesler, and R. W. Hanson. 1991. "Cyclic AMP induction of phosphoenolpyruvate carboxykinase (GTP) gene transcription is mediated by multiple promoter elements." *Journal of Biological Chemistry* 266:19095–19102.

Lo, D. C., F. Allen, and J. P. Brockes. 1993. "Reversal of muscle differentiation during urodele limb regeneration." *Proceedings of the National Academy of Sciences (USA)* 90:7230–7234.

McGaugh, J. L. 1989. "Involvement of hormonal and neuromodulatory systems in the regulation of memory storage." *Annual Review of Neuroscience* 12:255–287.

Metcalf, D. 1989. "Hemopoietic regulators." *Trends in Biochemical Sciences* 17:286–289.

Metz, R., and E. Ziff. 1991. "cAMP stimulates the C/EBP-related transcription factor RNFIL-6 to translocate to the nucleus and induce *c-fos* transcription gene." *Genes and Development* 5:1754–1766.

Montarolo, P. G., P. Goelet, V. F. Castellucci, J. Morgan, E. R. Kandel, and S. Schacher. 1986. "A critical period for macromolecular synthesis in long-term heterosynaptic facilitation in *Aplysia*." *Science* 234:1249–1254.

Montminy, M. R., G. A. Gonzalez, and K. K. Yamamoto. 1990. "Regulation of cAMP-inducible genes by CREB." *Trends in Neurosciences* 13:184–188.

Müller, G. E., and A. Pilzecker. 1900. "Experimentelle beitrage zur lehre vom gedachtnis." *Zeitschrift fur Psychologie und Physiologie der Sinnesorgane Erganzungsband* 1:1–300.

Nguyen, P. V., T. Abel, and E. R. Kandel. 1994. "Requirement of a critical period of transcription for induction of a late phase of LTP." *Science* 265:1104–1107.

Park, E. A., W. J. Roesler, J. Liu, D. J. Klemm, A. L. Gourney, J. D. Thatcher, J. Shuman, A. Friedman, and R. W. Hanson. 1990. "The role of the CCAAT/enhancer binding protein in the transcriptional regulation of the gene for phosphoenolpyruvate carboxykinase (GTP)." *Molecular and Cellular Biology* 10:6264–6272.

Polster, M. R., L. Nadel, and D. L. Schacter. 1991. "Cognitive neuroscience. Analysis of memory: A historical perspective." *Journal of Cognitive Neuroscience* 3:95–116.

Ramachandran, V. S. 1995. "Anosognosia in parietal lobe syndrome." *Consciousness and Cognition* 4:22–51.

Rayport, S. G., and S. Schacher. 1986. "Synaptic plasticity *in vitro*: Cell culture of identified *Aplysia* neurons mediating short-term habituation and sensitization." *Journal of Neuroscience* 6:759–763.

Rohrbaugh, M., and D. C. Riccio. 1970. "Paradoxical enhancement of learned fear." *Journal of Abnormal Psychology* 75:210–216.

Russell, W. R. 1971. *The Traumatic Amnesias*. New York: Oxford University Press.

Schacher, S., V. F. Castellucci, and E. R. Kandel. 1988. "cAMP evokes long-term facilitation in *Aplysia* sensory neurons that requires new protein synthesis." *Science* 240:1667–1669.

Sheng, M., and M. E. Greenberg. 1990. "The regulation and function of c-*fos* and other immediate early genes in the nervous system." *Neuron* 4:477–485.

Sheng, M., M. A. Thompson, and M. E. Greenberg. 1991. "A Ca^{2+} regulated transcription factor phosphorylated by calmodulin-dependent kinase." *Science* 252:1427–1430.

Shuster, M. J., J. S. Camardo, S. A. Siegelbaum, and E. R. Kandel. 1985. "Cyclic-AMP-dependent protein kinase closes the serotonin-sensitive K^+ channels of *Aplysia* sensory neurones in cell-free membrane patches." *Nature* 313:392–395.

Siegelbaum, S., J. S. Camardo, and E. R. Kandel. 1982. "Serotonin and cAMP close single K^+ channels in *Aplysia* sensory neurones." *Nature* 299:413–417.

Spear, N. E. 1978. *Processing Memories. Forgetting and Retention.* Hillsdale, N.J.: Erlbaum.

Squire, L. R. 1992. "Memory and the hippocampus: A synthesis from findings with rats, monkeys and humans." *Psychological Review* 99:195–231.

Squire, L. R., N. J. Cohen, and L. Nadel. 1984. "The medial temporal region and memory consolidation: A new hypothesis." In *Memory Consolidation: Psychobiology and Cognition,* H. Weingartner and E. S. Parker (eds.). Hillsdale, N.J.: Erlbaum, pp. 185–210.

Tully, T., T. Preat, S. C. Boynton, and M. Del Vecchio. 1994. "Genetic dissection of consolidated memory in *Drosophila melanogaster.*" *Cell* 79:35–47.

Vallejo, M., D. Ron, C. P. Miller, and J. F. Habener. 1993. "C/ATF, a member of the activating transcription factor family of DNA-binding proteins, dimerizes with CAAT/enhancer-binding proteins and directs their binding to cAMP response elements." *Proceedings of the National Academy of Sciences (USA)* 90:4679–4683.

Yin, J. C. P., J. S. Wallach, M. Del Vecchio, E. L. Wilder, H. Zhuo, W. G. Quinn, and T. Tully. 1994. "Induction of a dominant-negative CREB transgene specifically blocks long-term memory in *Drosophila.*" *Cell* 79:49–58.

Acknowledgments

This work was supported by Howard Hughes Medical Institute, NIMH Program Project.

Sociocultural Perspectives

V

Some Patterns and Meanings of Memory Distortion in American History

12

Michael Kammen

Within less than a decade, beginning late in the 1980s, a distinctive body of writing began to appear that is concerned with aspects of collective memory in the history and culture of the United States. Comparable works have also been generated for France, Germany, Great Britain, Israel, and, to a lesser degree, Russia, Japan, and diverse developing nations or constituent social groups within those nations, such as tribes and sects. Much of this literature emphasizes the socially constructed nature of memory and its political or cultural uses.

Although memory distortion per se has not commonly been a defining focus in this literature, it does emerge as an implicit theme, and sometimes rather prominently. Its appearance thus far more nearly resembles the highly visible vein patterns of a leaf rather than the exoskeleton of shellfish. That is, an interest in memory distortion has become noticeable without being a mobile, weight-bearing structure. It offers important patterns but rarely an architectural framework that gives explanatory shape to evidence or data. It suggests lines of interpretation rather than firm connecting links. Combined with material found in many older works, however, it enables us to speculate about a configuration of reasons why collective memory in the United States has been subject to distortion and alteration.

When the literature does touch upon distortions of collective memory, it routinely tends to do so in a cynical manner, ascribing manipulative motives or the maintenance of hegemonic control by dominant social groups. I find, however, that memory distortion, viewed in historical context, has occurred under diverse circumstances and for variable reasons. Some are quite properly regarded with a cynical eye, and may be considered, for convenience, negative (i.e., self-serving) instances of memory distortion. Others, however,

might be regarded as positive, either because they have a democratizing outcome or else because they bring about a necessary readjustment of values
or value systems that are out of synch—anomalous—in a particular time
and place. If the adjustment helps to make the overall value system more
coherent and functional, memory distortion may very well serve a benign
purpose.

On still other occasions, memories are altered for reasons that are neither
positive nor negative. Alteration may be a side effect of nationalism, or the
desire for religious freedom, or the imperatives of domestic politics. In such
instances, description and explanation serve us in more satisfactory ways
than cynicism about bad faith or evil intent on the part of dominant elites.

In the chapter that follows I want to examine three categories of memory
distortion and alteration: first, social and cultural causes; second, nationalism and the *problematique* of American memory; and third, partisan politics
and the uses (or misuses) of memory by leaders in public affairs, mainly
American presidents. These categories are not watertight compartments, to
be sure. There are elements of overlap and a blurring of highly permeable
boundaries. Nevertheless, the range of illustrative situations that follows
should at least indicate the very broad spectrum of circumstances under
which collective memory undergoes distortion or alteration. If these situations supply less than a full-scale typology, they may at least serve to divert
us from the reductive inferences that tend to be derived from such phrases,
now virtually clichés, as "the invention of tradition" or "the heritage indus-
try," the latter referring, most often, to commercialization (or even the fabrication) of memories for a society whose thirst for nostalgia sometimes seems
unquenchable.

The distortion of memories can, indeed, serve as a panacea for an age of
anxiety. Yet I am persuaded that memory *and* amnesia have occurred in the
American experience for a more complex array of reasons. What follows is
designed to serve as an illustrative introduction to that complexity, at several
levels and with assorted stimuli, motives, and consequences taken into account.

Social and Cultural Causes of Memory Distortion

Memory distortion has occurred in important instances because of a profound desire for social or religious autonomy; or because the force of public
opinion requires more logical coherence between disparate elements in a
civic value system; or because of the desire for social accommodation or
assimilation among newcomers in a nation of immigrants. Let's look at concrete instances of each situation.

During the 1620s and early 1630s, when Puritan dissenters in England
suffered persecution at the hands of King Charles I and the Church of

England, an anguished debate occurred among the Puritan dissenters: what was the most appropriate course of action for them? What did God expect of his saints? Should they emigrate to the New World, or did they have an obligation to stay, tough it out, and seek to reform a morally corrupt society from within? A majority actually chose the latter option and stayed, but a minority migrated to the Massachusetts Bay Colony with this rationale: because the Church was hopelessly unreformed, they were obliged to leave in order to save their souls. But their mission would most likely not result in a permanent transplantation. The New Jerusalem that they expected to create would be so successful, such a model community in covenant with the Almighty, that they would eventually be recalled "in glory" to recreate their New Jerusalem at home (Delbanco, 1984; Delbanco, 1989; Bremer, 1989, chaps. 2–6; S. Foster, 1991; Anderson, 1991, chap. 1).

When the Civil War broke out in 1642 between the Royalists and the Calvinists (Cavaliers and Roundheads), the Puritans who had gone to New England should, in the name of consistency, have returned to the motherland to join their fellow dissenters in fighting the good fight. An opportunity to create the New Jerusalem at home was at hand. Nevertheless, very few returned because they now enjoyed considerable autonomy—not only from the Crown, but from sectarian Independents and Presbyterians whose theology and ecclesiastical politics they did not altogether share. After 1647 and the triumph of Oliver Cromwell's New Model Army and the creation of a Puritan Commonwealth, surely the self-exiled Puritans no longer had any excuse to remain overseas. According to their own explanations at the time of emigration, they should have returned to England to reinforce the new polity of Saints. The New Jerusalem was imminently at home. (See Miller, 1953, book I; Hall, 1972, chaps. 2–5; Morgan, 1963; and Collinson, 1989.)

Once again, however, the Puritan leadership in New England, both secular and clerical, ever mindful of theological differences that divided them from their brethren at home, chose to remain in the colonies of Massachusetts Bay, Connecticut, and ultra-dissident Rhode Island. They were not about to exchange their virtual autonomy in every sphere of life for Oliver Cromwell's iron-fisted control of a militant Commonwealth—or for the genuine risk of a royalist restoration. All of which required that memories of their own rhetoric during the 1620s and early 1630s be repressed or altered. Their mission to convert and Christianize heathen peoples in the New World suddenly seemed more imperative than ever. The need for a bulwark against Papist colonization in the Americas—France to the north and Spain to the south—also seemed greater than ever before.

So they stayed put and thereby provide us with an intriguing example, from the very onset of American history, that memories can readily, with scant embarrassment or challenge, be quietly repressed within a generation and replaced by alternative explanations, credible and defensible, for human impulses of the most elemental sort—such as relocating to a brave new world in quest of religious purity and autonomy.

For an illustration of memory distortion occurring because the sheer force of public opinion requires better coherence between the major components in a culture's value system, we need to "fast forward" two hundred years to the second quarter of the nineteenth century, when the political process and participation in public affairs began to be democratized during the so-called Age of Jackson. That new climate of opinion in American civic life required a major adjustment in the most fundamental assumptions about human nature and capacity for religious rebirth shared by most Americans ever since the early seventeenth century.

As Calvinists inspired by the Protestant Reformation, colonists had accepted the harsh doctrine of Predestination. God determined who would be saved and who would be damned even before an individual entered this world. Salvation and life everlasting derived from faith and faith alone. Good works kept the *social* covenant viable, but could not help an unregenerate soul become one of God's elect. It was an elitist system and, what was even more harsh, it was an inscrutably capricious system. The Almighty chose and disposed of souls for reasons that eluded human comprehension. Man's fate lay beyond his own control. (See Miller, 1956, pp. 48–98.)

The evangelical Protestantism that emerged from the Second Great Awakening during the early decades of the nineteenth century changed all of that, and consequently required theological and social acrobatics so that a value system that had endured for two centuries could be radically dismembered and disremembered. The concept of Predestination for a select few, derived from a long-standing interpretation of Original Sin, came to be supplanted by what is called the democratization of Christ's atonement. His death on the cross made possible the salvation of *all* rather than just a select group of pre-designated saints. Moreover, anyone could now make "a decision for Christ," undergo conversion, and be born again (Miller, 1956, pp. 184–203; Miller, 1967, pp. 90–120).

Christianity, like the polity, became more inclusive and more participatory. An Old Testament God of justice, inscrutable and judgmental, gave way to a New Testament God of love, more forgiving and compassionate. Members of that culture redefined the very nature of Divinity and what He (Prophetess Jemima Wilkinson said "She") expected or required of mortals. Memories of orthodox Calvinism, deeply ingrained after two centuries despite the Enlightenment, had to be repressed, rationalized away, and significantly reconfigured (Cross, 1950, chaps. 1, 4, 5; Mathews, 1977; Hatch, 1989). In this complicated transformation we tend to view the necessary distortion of collective memory as benign and beneficial, both because it served egalitarian ends and because it brought the dominant theological assumptions of American society into harmonic conjunction with emergent assumptions about political man and his capacities for civic participation and self-government.

Being a "nation of immigrants," as Franklin Delano Roosevelt described the United States to the assembled D.A.R. in 1937, makes it more problematic for a genuinely collective memory to exist and function. A highly pluralistic society shares in common concerns about the present and aspirations for the future. There is a politically constructed past, to be sure, transmitted by the schools, and an ethnic past frequently regarded as marginally useful to the individual seeking acceptance and prosperity. In fact, one's "un-American" past could be a hindrance. A guidebook prepared for immigrant Jews during the 1890s offered advice heard by many other newcomers as well: "Hold fast, this is most necessary in America. Forget your past, your customs, and your ideals" (Gutman, 1976, p. 69).

Dramatic narratives have come to light in recent decades illustrating the astonishing lengths that immigrants would go to in order to conceal potentially embarrassing episodes and memories from their children and grandchildren. The purpose of such repression or distortion was simply to avoid impeding the Americanization and assimilation of second- and third-generation hyphenated Americans (Gutman, 1987, chap. 12; for the same phenomenon in Canada, see Irwin-Zarecka, 1994, pp. 59–60). More often than not a revival of ethnic memory and culture had to wait until the fourth generation, when men and women, sufficiently secure about their American identity, could revive festivals, costumes, distinctive foods, and other Old World traditions. In doing so they frequently romanticized the past as a golden age—creating a mood of nostalgia that did not so much distort memories as fabricate them. Gazing at yellowed photographs and probing the recollections of ex-slaves and venerable forebears created myopic visions of the past—all the more deceptive because they seemed to be so empirically sound. Photographs and elderly relations surely don't lie. They are clear windows on the past, albeit dim and dangerously opaque, at times, in their revelations. With such feelings we enter the realm of self-deception rather than distortion, more often than not, although self-deception is obviously a mode of distortion and may readily be transmitted from one generation to the next (Kivisto and Blanck, 1990; Pederson, 1992; see also Terkel, 1970; Redford, 1988).

Nationalism and Problematic Distortions of Memory

Although conflict commonly emerges as a significant factor in American society and politics, it is demonstrable that the dominant pattern has been one of conflict within consensus. All across the spectrum we find historically a profound loyalty to the U.S. Constitution and its legal parameters. There is a normative desire for political stability; and the combination of loyalty and stability under the oldest written national constitution in the world has, indeed, been impressive. But stability is achieved at a price: a tendency to depoliticize the civic past by distorting the nation's memories of it—all in the name of national unity, stability, and state-building. (See Zelinsky, 1988; Kammen, 1991; Bodnar, 1992.)

The most significant example of this phenomenon, and the best documented perhaps, concerns the astonishing distortions of collective memory, by both North and South, during the two generations following the American Civil War. Individuals on both sides did not forget their personal losses, of course, nor the massive disruption of their lives. Southerners long remained bitter, both about their crushing defeat and about their treatment by northerners during Reconstruction. At that level, collective memories were vivid as well as reasonably veracious (Wilson, 1962; G. Foster, 1987).

Nevertheless, for about two decades there was an almost eerie silence in the press about the war and its causes. With some obvious exceptions, such as Walt Whitman, imaginative writers seemed to be too overwhelmed by the sheer enormity of the tragedy to compose significant works about it, despite the fact that a brothers' war ought to be the very stuff of great literature (Aaron, 1973). Healing the deep sectional scars and political wounds soon became imperative. Where had this impulse begun? In Abraham Lincoln's Gettysburg Address, no enemy is ever mentioned. Binding the nation together again—even redefining the nation as an imperishable federal State—swiftly became the order of the day. To achieve those goals, amnesia emerged as a bonding agent far preferable to memory. Picking at scabs would not advance the paramount goal of reconciliation.

Beginning in the mid- and later 1880s, however, the twenty-fifth anniversary of various catastrophic battles elicited a spate of vastly popular books and articles. At the Blue-Gray reunions, veterans from both sides shook hands and even embraced. According to orations, sermons, editorials, and essays, each and every partisan had been brave, valiant, and courageous. Both sides had fought for causes they believed to be just. The history of racial issues in general and the institution of slavery in particular virtually disappeared from mainstream public discourse.

Perpetuating the actual provocations to battle would only prolong animosities and impede sectional reconciliation. Partial amnesia became the order of the day—just when the legal and social barriers to full citizenship for African-Americans grew greater. This particular manifestation of memory distortion—repressing the racial issue as a major cause of the war—drew support from every section and social class. It persisted, moreover, for three-quarters of a century, reaching its apogee, perhaps, during the Golden Jubilee years of 1911 to 1915, but enjoying ongoing support from scholars as well as popular writers who explained the Civil War and Reconstruction to American students and the public at large. Not until the Civil Rights movement of the 1960s, and its aftermath, did the nation's greatest internal conflict begin to resemble in history what it had, in fact, been in reality (Kammen, 1991, chaps. 4 and 12; and see Pressly, 1954; Warren, 1961).

For a supplementary illustration of nationalism serving to alter collective memory, we might consider the immense influence of George Washington's Farewell Address, first published on September 17, 1796, as his second term moved toward closure. Writing during the chaos of Napoleonic upheaval overseas (with considerable assistance from Alexander Hamilton), Washington warned repeatedly against "foreign alliances, attachments, and intrigues."

> Why, by interweaving our destiny with that of any part of Europe, entangle our peace and prosperity in the toils of European ambition, rivalship, interest, humor, or caprice? It is our true policy to steer clear of permanent alliances with any portion of the foreign world. (Commager, ed., 1962, p. 174; Gilbert, 1961)

For more than a century that revered message provided a gyroscope for the conduct of American foreign policy, which remained more or less disentangled until the early twentieth century when presidents of both parties could not resist the temptation to intervene in politically unstable nations of Central America and the Caribbean. Despite broad support for such initiatives, Woodrow Wilson's opponents successfully defeated United States participation in the League of Nations during the post–World War I era by invoking memories of George Washington's wisdom and the enduring policy to which it gave rise (LaFeber, 1983, chaps. 1–2; LaFeber, 1989, chaps. 8–11).

Intervention in Central America meant expansion and control but not alliances. After 1945, however, when the United States emerged as the world's dominant superpower, it became necessary either to ignore Washington's Farewell Address or else give it a radically different interpretation than Washington had intended: first, that if the United States acted with restraint during the 1790s it would enjoy freedom *from* restraint subsequently; and then the Farewell Address could, with some sophistry, be claimed as a powerful rationale for the necessity of American freedom of action.

Be that as it may, one wonders how George Washington would have viewed partisan "intrigues" by the Central Intelligence Agency, for example, in Indonesia during the 1950s or in Cuba during the 1960s. Or, for that matter, permanent alliances and commitments that ranged from NATO to SEATO to South Korea. The anti-communist frenzy of the Cold War era made George Washington's advice anachronistic if not outright embarrassing. So the long-standing tradition of reading the entire Farewell Address out loud in the U.S. Senate on Washington's birthday quietly vanished. A tradition had to be disremembered because a customary perception of the national interest had been turned upside down. Sometimes symbols have a way of outliving the concept they are supposed to represent. In this instance policy imperatives quashed a legendary memory. The legend came to be minimized in little-noticed texts, whereas the policy came to be maximized in initiatives with pretexts.

It does need to be added, however, that the United States is hardly peculiar, or alone, in allowing nationalism to distort collective memory. In recent years the Japanese have rewritten their history textbooks more than once under governmental supervision, first to erase their heinous behavior in East Asia during the 1930s and 1940s, and then to make concessions when the Korean, Chinese, and Philippine governments demonstrated that Japanese history books were guilty of whitewash and cover-up tactics. On May 6, 1994, for example, a humiliated Japanese Minister of Justice publicly retracted his assertion that Japanese troops "were not aggressors in World War II, committed no atrocities in the Chinese city of Nanking, and behaved no worse toward Korean and Chinese women than did U.S. and British soldiers" (Radin, 1994; and see Hurst, 1982; Tanaka, 1993, pp. 228–283).

Domestic Politics, Partisanship, and the Uses of Memory

A plausible case could be made that the most successful (i.e., effective) American presidents have been the ones most likely to manipulate, "improve," or even distort their nation's collective memory. Take as an initial illustration the comparatively innocuous case of Thomas Jefferson as exemplified in his first inaugural address on March 4, 1801. The later 1790s had been absolutely tumultuous. Domestic politics have never been more virulent or venomous, and many citizens wondered whether a peaceful transition to a loyal opposition was even possible. It had not yet happened because only the Federalist Party had held power since the nation's inception in 1789 (Howe, 1967).

Understandably, then, Jefferson wanted to calm the fears of those who regarded him as a godless egalitarian, a Francophile and an Anglophobe, an advocate of state sovereignty, a wild-eyed civil libertarian with a mulatto mistress conceived from his father-in-law's loins. His first inaugural sought to minimize partisan differences, to draw a veil over the vicious hostilities of the 1790s. "Every difference of opinion," he declared, "is not a difference of principle. We have called by different names brethren of the same principle. We are all Republicans, we are all Federalists. If there be any among us who would wish to dissolve this Union or to change its republican form [such as Hamiltonian neo-monarchists], let them stand undisturbed as monuments of the safety with which error of opinion may be tolerated where reason is left free to combat it." To soothe those who feared that he might depart from George Washington's sage advice concerning foreign relations, Jefferson included language (little noticed ever since) that sounds more Washingtonian than the Father of His Country himself: "peace, commerce, and honest friendship with all nations, entangling alliances with none" (Commager, 1962, pp. 187, 188). Thomas Jefferson created the presidential precedent of stealing a page from his opponents' gospel. As we shall see, Jefferson's heir in terms of party lineage, Franklin D. Roosevelt, perfected that precedent (Kammen, 1993).

In between, however, such presidents as Andrew Jackson and Abraham Lincoln, along with major politicians like Daniel Webster and Henry Clay, had to deal with threats of southern state secession in a nation that itself had emerged in 1776 by invoking the right to revolution. The Declaration of Independence, the most sacred and best known of all American texts, had announced unequivocally:

> That whenever any Form of Government becomes destructive of these ends [Life, Liberty and the Pursuit of Happiness, i.e., governmental protection of private property], it is the Right of the People to alter or abolish it, and to institute new Government, laying its foundation on such principles and organizing its powers in such form, as to them shall seem most likely to effect their Safety and Happiness. (Commager, 1962, p. 100)

Both Andrew Jackson and especially Abraham Lincoln knew that text "cold" and fully understood that the United States had staked its own claim to independent nationhood upon Lockean principles of the right to revolution. How then could Jackson consistently deny South Carolina the right to secede in 1831, or Lincoln deny the Confederacy that right in 1861 (Potter, 1942; Freehling, 1966)? They did so by invoking a political fiction whose genesis is somewhat obscure: the notion of a "Perpetual Union." Exactly who invented that concept, and in what circumstances, is exceedingly hazy. What *is* clear is that for three decades following 1830 it became the ultimate line of defense for leaders who wished to deny a state (or states) the right to secede and be self-governing (Stampp, 1978).

The political fiction, moreover, required a monumental distortion of collective memory that seems to have troubled no one in the North and perplexed few people even in the South—perhaps because pro-Union sentiment there remained strong among many of those committed to the defense of slavery. In any event, the concept of "Perpetual Union" required an astonishing revision of historical reality in order to assert that the Union actually pre-existed the states. How could that possibly be? After all, the states declared their independence individually in 1776. Although most of them subscribed to a joint Declaration, that document did not create a government. Rather, eleven states composed brand new constitutions that created autonomous governments, while Connecticut and Rhode Island simply converted their colonial charters into frames of government adequate for statehood. The Articles of Confederation defined a loose and weak Confederation that left most sovereignty in the hands of the states. The Constitutional Convention did not meet in Philadelphia until 1787. The document it created was not ratified until the summer of 1788, and the new national government did not begin until the spring of 1789 when Congress first gathered and George Washington was inaugurated.

The advocates of "Perpetual Union," however, highlighted a different time line. The First Continental Congress, they observed, met on September 5, 1774, in Philadelphia, which is true, and little more than five weeks later, acting as a body, issued its Declaration and Resolves, a feisty assertion of grievances and rights. Then came the Second Continental Congress; then came the Confederation followed by the permanent federal government in 1789—all in a direct line of descent. Therefore the Union, being older than the states, was intended to be a perpetual union. Once a state joined, it did so irrevocably. The Union came first, the states second. The Union was superior, the states inferior. They simply could not legitimately secede (Commager, 1962, pp. 82–84; Stampp, 1978).

Although it may sound like a bizarre reconstruction of the political past, Abraham Lincoln relied upon that mystical, ahistorical formula during his remarkable pre-inaugural journey from Springfield to Washington, D.C., in February 1861, when he gave one speech after another conciliatory to the South, all the while insisting upon the inviolable character of a "Perpetual Union."

Although we hear rather little about "Perpetual Union" after 1865, no one ever repudiated the fictive concept. It had served a highly utilitarian purpose, it received credence, and like many memories that outlast their immediate usefulness, it slowly dissipated to be replaced by a redefinition of the political nation that first appeared in Lincoln's Gettysburg Address but was capped expansively by the Supreme Court's decision in *Texas v. White* (1869), which legitimized "Perpetual Union" by contextualizing it more comprehensibly. According to the opinion written by Chief Justice Salmon P. Chase, when Texas joined the United States,

> she entered into an indissoluble relation. All the obligations of perpetual union, and all the guaranties of republican government in the Union, attached at once to the State. The act which consummated her admission into the Union was something more than a compact; it was the incorporation of a new member into the political body. And it was final. The union between Texas and the other States was as complete, as perpetual, and as indissoluble as the union between the original States. (Commager, 1962, p. 511)

History had been supplanted by constitutional theory, while memory became a casualty of political expediency. Call it casuistry or sophistry, but not cynicism or hypocrisy. Those who rationalized the Union believed every word that they said and wrote.

Franklin D. Roosevelt provides us with a different kind of casuistry that was not merely expedient but cynical and manipulative as well. As a Democrat he fell heir to the party founded by Jefferson and Jackson. But as a superb coalition-builder and shrewd politician, he coveted the votes of African-Americans and certain immigrant groups that had traditionally voted Republican—the party associated with Abraham Lincoln. Beginning in 1935–1936, Roosevelt mentioned Lincoln at every possible opportunity in speeches and press conferences. Consequently, he succeeded in "reformulating" the memories of blacks and ethnic groups, who assumed that FDR must stand in a direct line of political descent from Lincoln! In 1936 they shifted their votes to FDR—partially for substantive reasons but partially because of image-manipulation—and provided him with a hefty margin of victory in subsequent elections. Roosevelt clearly "stole" Lincoln from the Republican Party, and in the process successfully managed to maneuver the political memories of a great many people (Lubell, 1952, chaps. 4 and 5; Jones, 1974).

More subtle and more complicated, of course, was FDR's need to honor Thomas Jefferson, the founder of his own party, while pursuing Hamiltonian policies that had defined the anti-Jeffersonian Federalist tradition, such as strong central government and management of the banking system to provide for economic growth (Peterson, 1960, chap. 7). Talk about a wolf in sheep's clothing! By the end of Roosevelt's second term, memories of America's contrapuntal political traditions had become conflated, blurred, and confused. Which statesmen had stood for what policies was anyone's guess. And no public forum, classroom, or journal provided much in the way of illumination on such matters.

More recently Ronald Reagan raised amnesia almost to the level of an art form with respect to "Irangate" and other policy initiatives that did not succeed. More to the point, however, even though they have all but vanished from memory in the civic culture, are the occasions when Reagan and his advisers deliberately (though not exactly deftly) attempted to distort public memory in order to advance an ideological agenda. Claiming that many New Deal administrators during the 1930s had been Socialists or Communists provides one example, and insisting that the United States fought the Vietnam War with "one hand tied behind our backs" supplies another (Kammen, 1991, pp. 658–662).

Even though news articles offering correctives appeared soon after each of these pronouncements, with formidable evidence from scholars and other authorities, the presidential "bully pulpit" exercised considerable and enduring influence on the collective memory. A fictive Rambo so favored by Reagan gradually became a blend of what some men did and many others might have done if only Gulliver hadn't been strapped down by small men of little brain and less courage (Wills, 1987, chaps. 38–41).

Conclusions and Comparisons

As I tried to suggest at the outset, the distortion or even the manipulation of collective memory does not always, or inevitably, occur for cynical or hypocritical reasons. That has certainly been the case on occasion, as we have seen; but memory distortion also occurs commonly in post-colonial situations where the creation of national identity is necessary for functional reasons of political and cultural cohesion. The United States alone provides abundant documentation on this point (see Lipset, 1963; Somkin, 1967; Kammen, 1978).

Moreover, even when leaders (political and spiritual) do engage in memory distortion or "practice" historical amnesia, we must recognize that members of the public at large are often likely to believe and internalize the rationalizations they receive. Frequently, as we have seen, the willful alteration of collective memory becomes a necessity for a viable, progressive society. How else can it coherently adapt to change, often desirable change, without being plagued by a sense of inconsistency or sham?

When our scope becomes more international, moreover, we find that the United States is not alone in presenting us with instances of memory distortion on account of diverse stimuli with variable consequences. Constructive, "positive," or harmless examples of memory reconstruction, as described at the end of the preceding paragraph, can be found in Mexico, Scandinavia, and France (Greenway, 1977; Agulhon, 1981; Florescano, 1994). A greater degree of distortion—yet still neither cynical nor harshly hegemonic—resulting from a sense of shame or the need to define national identity in more particular ways, can be found in Brazil, England, Germany, France, and Israel (Viotti da Costa, 1985, chap. 9; Mosse, 1990; Porter, 1992; Lebovics, 1992; and Zerubavel, 1994).

And then, undeniably, there are egregious instances of memory distortion whose sole or primary purpose is to legitimize a regime, empower a rising social class, or else reduce (or even eliminate) the stigma of war crimes or inhumane atrocities (Lewis, 1975; Hobsbawm and Ranger, 1983, chap. 7; Maier, 1988; Baram, 1991; Lipstadt, 1993).

Although space does not permit systematic consideration of memory distortion on the part of individuals, I want to conclude with the observation that here, too, motives range from benign to moralistic or didactic (the autobiographies of Benjamin Franklin and Henry Adams) to self-serving (the political memoirs of such presidents as Truman, Nixon, and Reagan) to utterly malicious (Ernest Hemingway's posthumous memoir, *A Moveable Feast*, 1964).

None of these instances or categories comes as any sort of revelation. More difficult to evaluate, however, are literary works derived from memory that nonetheless are more concerned with artistry than veracity, works such as Mark Twain's *Life on the Mississippi* (1883) or Anaïs Nin's *Diary* (7 vols., 1966–1980) or James Baldwin's *Notes of a Native Son* (1957), books that embroider autobiographical memories in varying degrees with diverse motives. Unlike the political memoirists, who would vigorously deny any deliberate act of memory distortion, creative writers have other objectives that, in their view, validate sins of omission or commission, inhibition or exhibition. As Anaïs Nin said, "The only person I do not lie to is my journal. Yet out of affection even for my journal I sometimes lie by omissions. There are still so many omissions!" (Nin, 1992, p. 110).

Most intriguing of all, however, at least in my view, are the would-be memoirists who set their projects aside because they recognize that their memories have become sieve-like and integrity compels them to avoid even inadvertent distortion—like the cultural critic Gilbert Seldes (1893–1970), or like the writer Allen Tate, who abandoned a projected memoir in the 1970s, some years after he had started it, for a cluster of reasons that illuminate the highly complex and subjective nature of remembrance in the face of fear—fear that the synapses may fail to connect, but even worse, fear that they might connect all too well, resulting in unwanted revelations about oneself and others. Tate explained this dilemma with immense charm in his Preface to *Memoirs and Opinions*:

> In 1966 I decided to write an entire book of memories, and I was persuaded by certain friends that my "prodigious memory" would make the task an easy one. After I had written, with considerable difficulty, "A Lost Traveller's Dream" and "Miss Toklas' American Cake," I decided to try something else— what, I couldn't then be sure. My memory became less and less prodigious: my account of my first year in Paris had to be "checked" twice for the exposure of seventeen errors of simple fact. But this is not the principal reason why I decided to halt the memoir.
>
> The "real" reason was that, unlike Ernest Hemingway in *A Moveable Feast*, I couldn't bring myself to tell what was wrong with my friends—or even mere acquaintances—without trying to tell what was wrong with myself. I am not sure even now, what was, or is, wrong with me, and I was unwilling to give the reader the chance to make up his own mind on this slippery matter. Then, too, I fell back on authority: I couldn't let myself indulge in the terrible fluidity of self-revelation. (Tate, 1975)

The immense irony, however, is that the circumstances of Tate's youth, early manhood, and family background were (and are) so deeply veiled in mystery, even to him, that he (and we) do not know where veracity ends and distortion begins. The first third of his life remains an enigma (Tate, 1960; Squires, 1971, chap. 1). So much for those who claim that compared to the empirical verifiability of personal memory, collective memory is a will-o'-the-wisp. I have found them equally elusive.

Perhaps it might be appropriate to close with some queries—I suppose we would call them rhetorical—jotted down by Bronson Alcott, the Massachusetts Transcendentalist, mystic, and sometime seer, a self-educated contemporary of Ralph Waldo Emerson. Four of his provocative queries give us pause.

> Which is the older, the memory, the thing remembered, or the person remembering?
> Can you remember when you did not remember?
> Which is predecessor, Time or the memory?
> Are moments born of the memory, or memory of the moments? (Quoted in Seldes, 1928, p. 224)

Giving pause gave meaning, if not memory, to Bronson Alcott's life. It could very well do the same for ours.

References

Aaron, Daniel. 1973. *The Unwritten War: American Writers and the Civil War.* New York: Alfred A. Knopf.

Agulhon, Maurice. 1981. *Marianne into Battle. Republican Imagery and Symbolism in France, 1789–1880.* Trans. Janet Lloyd. Cambridge: Cambridge University Press.

Anderson, Virginia D. 1991. *New England's Generation: The Great Migration and the Formation of Society and Culture in the Seventeenth Century.* New York: Cambridge University Press.

Baram, Amatzia. 1991. *Culture, History and Ideology in the Formation of Ba'thist Iraq, 1968-89.* New York: St. Martin's Press.

Bodnar, John. 1992. *Remaking America: Public Memory, Commemoration, and Patriotism in the Twentieth Century.* Princeton: Princeton University Press.

Bremer, Francis J. 1989. *Puritan Crisis: New England and the English Civil Wars, 1630-1670.* New York: Garland Publishing, Inc.

Collinson, Patrick. 1989. *The Puritan Character: Polemics and Polarities in Early Seventeenth-Century English Culture.* Los Angeles: William Andrews Clark Memorial Library.

Commager, Henry Steele, ed. 1962. *Documents of American History.* New York: Appleton-Century-Crofts.

Cross, Whitney R. 1950. *The Burned Over District: The Social and Intellectual History of Enthusiastic Religion in Western New York, 1800–1850.* Ithaca: Cornell University Press.

Delbanco, Andrew. 1984. "The Puritan Errand Re-viewed," *Journal of American Studies,* 18: 343–360.

Delbanco, Andrew. 1989. *The Puritan Ordeal.* Cambridge, Mass.: Harvard University Press.

Florescano, Enrique. 1994. *Memory, Myth, and Time in Mexico from the Aztecs to Independence.* Austin: University of Texas Press.

Foster, Gaines M. 1987. *Ghosts of the Confederacy: Defeat, the Lost Cause, and the Emergence of the New South, 1865 to 1913.* New York: Oxford University Press.

Foster, Stephen. 1991. *The Long Argument: English Puritanism and the Shaping of New England Culture, 1570–1700.* Chapel Hill: University of North Carolina Press.

Freehling, William W. 1966. *Prelude to Civil War: The Nullification Controversy in South Carolina, 1816–1836.* New York: Harper and Row.

Gilbert, Felix. 1961. *To the Farewell Address: Ideas of Early American Foreign Policy.* Princeton: Princeton University Press.

Greenway, John L. 1977. *The Golden Horns: Mythic Imagination and the Nordic Past.* Athens, Ga.: The University of Georgia Press.

Gutman, Herbert G. 1976. *Work, Culture, and Society in Industrializing America: Essays in American Working-Class and Social History.* New York: Alfred A. Knopf.

Gutman, Herbert G. 1987. *Power and Culture: Essays on the American Working Class.* New York: Pantheon.

Hall, David D. 1972. *The Faithful Shepherd. A History of the New England Ministry in the Seventeenth Century.* Chapel Hill: University of North Carolina Press.

Hatch, Nathan. 1989. *The Democratization of American Christianity.* New Haven: Yale University Press.

Hobsbawm, Eric, and Terence Ranger, eds. 1983. *The Invention of Tradition.* Cambridge: Cambridge University Press.

Howe, John R. 1967. "Republican Thought and the Political Violence of the 1790s," *American Quarterly,* 19: 147–165.

Hurst, G. Cameron, III. 1982. *Weaving the Emperor's New Clothes: The Japanese Textbook "Revision" Controversy.* Hanover, N.H.: Universities Field Staff International Reports, No. 46 (Asia).

Irwin-Zarecka, Iwona. 1994. *Frames of Remembrance: The Dynamics of Collective Memory.* New Brunswick, N.J.: Transaction Publishers.

Jones, Alfred Haworth. 1974. *Roosevelt's Image Brokers: Poets, Playwrights, and the Use of the Lincoln Symbol.* Port Washington, N.Y.: Kennikat Press.

Kammen, Michael. 1978. *A Season of Youth: The American Revolution and the Historical Imagination.* New York: Alfred A. Knopf.

———. 1991. *Mystic Chords of Memory: The Transformation of Tradition in American Culture.* New York: Alfred A. Knopf.

———. 1992. *Meadows of Memory: Images of Time and Tradition in American Art and Culture.* Austin: University of Texas Press.

———. 1993. "Changing Presidential Perspectives on the American Past," *Quarterly of the National Archives,* 25: 48–49.

Kivisto, Peter, and Dag Blanck, eds. 1990. *American Immigrants and Their Generations: Studies and Commentaries on the Hansen Thesis after Fifty Years.* Urbana, Ill.: University of Illinois Press.

LaFeber, Walter. 1983. *Inevitable Revolutions: The United States in Central America.* New York: W.W. Norton and Company.

LaFeber, Walter. 1989. *The American Age: United States Foreign Policy at Home and Abroad since 1750.* New York: W.W. Norton and Company.

Lebovics, Herman. 1992. *True France: The Wars Over Cultural Identity, 1900–1945.* Ithaca: Cornell University Press.

Lewis, Bernard. 1975. *History—Remembered, Recovered, Invented.* Princeton: Princeton University Press.

Lipset, Seymour Martin. 1963. *The First New Nation: The United States in Historical and Comparative Perspective.* New York: Basic Books.

Lipstadt, Deborah. 1993. *Denying the Holocaust: The Growing Assault on Truth and Memory.* New York: Free Press.

Lubell, Samuel. 1952. *The Future of American Politics.* New York: Harper and Row.

Maier, Charles S. 1988. *The Unmasterable Past: History, Holocaust, and German National Identity.* Cambridge, Mass.: Harvard University Press.

Mathews, Donald G. 1977. *Religion in the Old South.* Chicago: University of Chicago Press.

Miller, Perry. 1953. *The New England Mind from Colony to Province.* Cambridge, Mass.: Harvard University Press.

———. 1956. *Errand into the Wilderness.* Cambridge, Mass.: Harvard University Press. "The Marrow of Puritan Divinity," pp. 48–98, and "From Edwards to Emerson," pp. 184–203.

———. 1967. *Nature's Nation.* Cambridge, Mass.: Harvard University Press. "From the Covenant to the Revival," pp. 90–120.

Morgan, Edmund S. 1963. *Visible Saints: The History of a Puritan Idea.* New York: New York University Press.

Mosse, George L. 1990. *Fallen Soldiers: Reshaping the Memory of the World Wars.* New York: Oxford University Press.

Nin, Anaïs. 1992. *Incest: From a Journal of Love: The Unexpurgated Diary of Anaïs Nin, 1932–1934.* Intro. by Rupert Pole. New York: Harcourt, Brace, Jovanovich.

Pederson, Jane Marie. 1992. *Between Memory and Reality: Family and Community in Rural Wisconsin, 1870–1970.* Madison: The University of Wisconsin Press. Chap. 2, "Between Memory and Reality."

Peterson, Merrill D. 1960. *The Jefferson Image in the American Mind.* New York: Oxford University Press.

Porter, Roy, ed. 1992. *Myths of the English.* Cambridge, Eng.: Polity Press.

Potter, David M. 1942. *Lincoln and His Party in the Secession Crisis.* New Haven: Yale University Press.

Pressly, Thomas J. 1954. *Americans Interpret Their Civil War.* Princeton: Princeton University Press.

Radin, Charles A. 1994. "Japan Official Retracts Statements on WWII," *Boston Globe,* May 7, 1994, p. 2.

Redford, Dorothy Spruill. 1988. *Somerset Homecoming: Recovering a Lost Heritage.* New York: Doubleday.

Seldes, Gilbert. 1928. *The Stammering Century.* New York: John Day Company.

Somkin, Fred. 1967. *Memory and Desire in the Idea of American Freedom, 1815–1860.* Ithaca: Cornell University Press.

Squires, Radcliffe. 1971. *Allen Tate: A Literary Biography.* New York: Pegasus.

Stampp, Kenneth M. 1978. "The Concept of a Perpetual Union," *Journal of American History,* 65: 5–33.

Tanaka, Stefan, 1993. *Japan's Orient: Rendering Pasts into History.* Berkeley: University of California Press.

Tate, Allen. 1960. "A Southern Mode of the Imagination," in Joseph J. Kwiat and Mary C. Turpie, eds., *Studies in American Culture: Dominant Ideas and Images,* pp. 96–108, esp. p. 99. Minneapolis: University of Minnesota Press.

Tate, Allen. 1975. *Memoirs and Opinions.* Chicago: Swallow Press.

Terkel, Studs. 1970. *Hard Times: An Oral History of the Great Depression.* New York: Pantheon Books.

Viotti da Costa, Emilia. 1985. *The Brazilian Empire: Myths and Histories.* Chicago: University of Chicago Press.

Warren, Robert Penn. 1961. *The Legacy of the Civil War.* Cambridge, Mass.: Harvard University Press.

Wills, Garry. 1987. *Reagan's America: Innocents at Home.* Garden City, N.Y.: Doubleday.

Wills, Garry. 1992. *Lincoln at Gettysburg: The Words That Remade America.* New York: Simon and Schuster.

Wilson, Edmund. 1962. *Patriotic Gore: Studies in the Literature of the American Civil War.* New York: Oxford University Press.

Zelinsky, Wilbur. 1988. *Nation Into State. The Shifting Symbolic Foundations of American Nationalism.* Chapel Hill: University of North Carolina Press.

Zerubavel, Yael. 1994. "The Historic, the Legendary, and the Incredible: Invented Tradition and Collective Memory in Israel," in John R. Gillis, ed., *Commemorations: The Politics of National Identity,* pp. 105–123. Princeton: Princeton University Press.

Dynamics of Distortion in Collective Memory

13

Michael Schudson

The notion that memory can be "distorted" assumes that there is a standard by which we can judge or measure what a veridical memory must be. If this is difficult with individual memory, it is even more complex with collective memory, where the past event or experience remembered was truly a different event or experience for its different participants. Moreover, whereas we can accept with little question that biography or the lifetime is the appropriate or "natural" frame for individual memory, there is no such evident frame for cultural memories. Neither national boundaries nor linguistic ones are as self-evidently the right containers for collective memory as the person is for individual memory. If you recall the wars between the United States government and Native Americans as part of the history of nation-building, it is one story; if you recall it as part of a history of racism, it is another. If you see the skeletal remains of Native Americans from long ago as part of an impersonal history of the human species, the remains are valuable specimens for scientific research; if you understand them as the cherished property of their descendants, they deserve reverent treatment and should be reburied according to the customs of Native American groups (Roark, 1989).

I take the view that, in an important sense, there is no such thing as individual memory, and it is well for me to make this plain at the outset. Memory is social. It is social, first of all, because it is located in institutions rather than in individual human minds in the form of rules, laws, standardized procedures, and records, a whole set of cultural practices through which people recognize a debt to the past (including the notion of "debt" itself) or through which they express moral continuity with the past (tradition, identity, career, curriculum). These cultural forms store and transmit information that individuals make use of without themselves "memorizing" it. The individual's capacity to make use of the past piggybacks on the social and cultural practices of memory. I can move over great distances at a speed of 600 miles per hour without knowing the first thing about what keeps an airplane aloft. I benefit from a cultural storehouse of knowledge, very little of which I am obliged to have in my own head. Cultural memory, available for the use of an individual, is distributed across social institutions and cultural artifacts.

Second, memory is sometimes located in collectively created monuments and markers: books, holidays, statues, souvenirs. This is really a restatement of my first point except to say that these are *dedicated* memory forms, cultural artifacts explicitly and self-consciously designed to preserve memories and ordinarily intended to have general pedagogical influence. This is not the case with jet engines.

Third, where memory can be located in individual minds, it may characterize groups of individuals—generations or occupational groups. In these cases memory is an individual property but so widely shared as to be accurately termed social or collective (Mannheim, 1970; Schuman and Scott, 1989).

Fourth, even where memories are located idiosyncratically in individual minds, they remain social and cultural in that (a) they operate through the supra-individual cultural construction of language; (b) they generally come into play in response to social stimulation, rehearsal, or social cues—the act of remembering is itself interactive, prompted by cultural artifacts and social cues, employed for social purposes, and even enacted by cooperative activity; and (c) there are socially structured patterns of recall. This last point is well illustrated in the work of Robert Merton on the "Matthew effect" in science, where citations tend to credit the better-known scientist of jointly authored papers, even when the scientist is the junior author of the work (Merton, 1968, 1988). You can see this kind of social structure of recall operating in almost instantaneous fashion, as I did at a conference of well-known journalists and moderately well known academics. Two or three times in the space of several hours of discussion, a participant referred back to something that one of the academics had said earlier, remarking, "As Daniel Schorr told us earlier . . . ," attributing the statement to the most famous journalist in the group.

As soon as you recognize how collective memory, and even individual memory, is inextricable from social and historical processes, the notion of "distortion" becomes problematic. As the British historian Peter Burke writes, "Remembering the past and writing about it no longer seem the innocent activities they were once taken to be. Neither memories nor histories seem objective any longer. In both cases, this selection, interpretation and distortion is socially conditioned. It is not the work of individuals alone" (Burke, 1989, p. 98). Distortion is inevitable. Memory is distortion since memory is invariably and inevitably selective. A way of seeing is a way of not seeing, a way of remembering is a way of forgetting, too. If memory were only a kind of registration, a "true" memory might be possible. But memory is a process of encoding information, storing information, and strategically retrieving information, and there are social, psychological, and historical influences at each point.

This is not to say that there are no grounds for arriving at a degree of consensus about the past. People normally accept some sorts of standards of what counts as true distortion and what counts simply as the inevitable variability of perspectives of people looking at the same phenomenon from different values and viewpoints at different points in time. Leaving aside the question of what distortion is inevitable versus what distortion is open to remedy, I want to offer here a catalogue of forms of distortion in collective memory. There are at least four important and distinguishable processes of distortion in collective memory: distanciation, instrumentalization, narrativization, and conventionalization. I will devote some remarks to each of these, drawing on my own research on American memories of Watergate as well as on other materials.

The dynamics of distortion operate in three different realms, all of which might be referred to as "social" or "collective" or "cultural" memory. I will not often need to distinguish among these types of social memory, but it may help clarify the subject to recognize the differences at the outset. First, collective memory may refer to the fact that individual memory is socially organized or socially mediated. Second, collective memory may refer not to socially organized memories in individuals who experienced the past but to the socially produced artifacts that are the memory repositories for it—libraries, museums, monuments, language itself in clichés and word coinages, place names, history books, and so forth. Third, collective memory may be the image of the past held by individuals who did not themselves experience it but learned of it through cultural artifacts. My remarks here concern all three domains of cultural memory—socially mediated individual memories, cultural forms for social mediation, and individual memories constructed from the cultural forms.

Distanciation: The Past Recedes

The simple passage of time reshapes memory, in at least two respects. First, there is a loss of detail. Memory grows more vague. Second, there tends to be a loss of emotional intensity. This is culturally variable, of course. Serbs, Croats, and Bosnians seem able to harbor ancient hurts in ways many other people cannot. Family attachments—and grievances—persist across generations; in China, vengeance may be sought for wounds inflicted well beyond living memory (Madsen, 1990). Cultural traditions may overcome the loss of individual memory over time, by no means always to the good.

Still, as a general rule, time heals all wounds. Constructing cultural objects as memoirs of the past may mitigate the ebbing of memory, but they battle an ultimately irresistible force. The mystery writer K. C. Constantine has one of his characters express it this way: "The surest way you know something's dead was when somebody started talking about preserving its memory. There wasn't a coffin around that could match a museum for saying something was croaked" (Constantine, 1993, p. 3). The novelist Robert Musil observed, "There is nothing in the world as invisible as a monument . . . Anything that endures over time sacrifices its ability to make an impression. Anything that constitutes the walls of our life, the backdrop of our consciousness, so to speak, forfeits its capacity to play a role in that consciousness" (Wieseltier, 1993, p. 19). If memory retains intensity, it sometimes does so at the cost of sentimentality of some sort. The recovery of ethnic origins and loyalties among third and fourth generations who retain little in the way of lived experience of ethnicity may be one example. The question of sentimentality we might think of as the Stephen Spielberg problem. If it is granted that human beings not only write poetry after Auschwitz but about it, what kind of poetry will that be? Is it doomed to demean, reduce, or sentimentalize the events it seeks to sanctify? Not everyone agrees that Spielberg failed in this with his film *Schindler's List,* but everyone recognizes that this was the sort of failure he risked.

There are gains as well as losses in distanciation. The major gain is perspective—distance can give people historical perspective on matters that may have been hard to grasp at the time they happened. With time, not only does emotional intensity diminish but individuals can increasingly view from multiple perspectives events they originally could see only from one. Sometimes this is because the past changes—and should change—with time. In an era of liberalization and the cultural enfranchisement of groups denied a voice in the past, a history told from the viewpoint of elite white males is rewritten from multiple viewpoints. Often new information becomes available about events experienced at the time through a veil of misinformation and ignorance. The past, at any rate the significance of the past, is not a constant. Judgments of the meaning of Richard Nixon's Watergate misdeeds in 1973 and 1974 when they became public knowledge were necessarily revised in 1975 when it became apparent—through congressional investigations that Watergate itself had prompted—that earlier presidents, including Lyndon Johnson and John F. Kennedy, had like Nixon engaged in extra-legal activities in both foreign and domestic policy. They approved the CIA's involvement in domestic surveillance in violation of its charter, illegal wiretaps on Martin Luther King, attempted assassinations of foreign leaders, and so forth. In a word, they abused the powers of office in ways not at all dissimilar from those in Article I of the articles of impeachment against Richard Nixon. Nixon's opponents in the Congress had taken pains to distinguish his misdeeds from those of past presidents. Their case, and public outrage at large, rested on the uniqueness of Nixon's errors. It turned out that, although some of his misdeeds were in fact novel, others were entirely in keeping with a degree of lawlessness in the White House that in the era of the Cold War had become nearly routine. In retrospect, some of the indignation turned toward Richard Nixon personally was misplaced. What people thought to be unique and unprecedented wrongdoing in 1974 we learned to be part of a continuing pattern in the modern presidency (Schudson, 1992).

To take another example, the Holocaust, though a central element in thousands of private memories, did not command public attention from the time of the Nuremberg trials until the Eichmann trial in 1963 and then, in a more sustained way, following the 1967 Six-Day War. Until then, the Holocaust was a matter held within the Jewish community but not paraded before a general public. What changed, it appears, was a new openness and pride on the part of Jews about their Jewishness, a reflected glory for European and American Jews from the valor and expertise of the Israeli military.

The moral character of memory is implicated in distanciation. As Iwona Irwin-Zarecka observes, distance in time is invoked as an argument both for and against attention to Nazi (and other) war crimes. On the one hand, people argue that "the sheer passage of time removes that past from the sphere of direct communal responsibility" and so justifies reducing attention. On the other hand, "with the passage of time, moral lessons acquire ever greater universal significance" and so justify increased focus on the past. "On both sides," Irwin-Zarecka adds, "the increasing distance in time appears to reframe remembrance, from that of concrete individual actions to one of general cultural background" (Irwin-Zarecka, 1994, pp. 94–95). It is no wonder that anniversaries or commemorations of events forty and fifty years in the past become especially significant, as the possibility of living memory fades and the only memories that remain are those culturally institutionalized.

The moral character of memory is asserted in a different fashion by the historian Carl Degler, who observed that historians are obliged to rewrite history as social values change. If historians did not change their minds about the past, he wrote, "their history would cease to be a living part of the culture and therefore incapable of illuminating the present with the light of the past." A historian of slavery who did not begin from the assumption that slavery is bad, he argues, would not be a historian but an antiquarian, someone for whom there is no vital connection between present values and telling the story of past events (Degler, 1976, p. 184). Our history, writes Stephen Macedo, is no more than the record of the past, but our "tradition," in contrast, "is a critical distillation of the past, a rendering that seeks to be true not to the past entire but to what is best in it, to what is most honourable and most worth carrying forward" (Macedo, 1990, p. 171). Tradition, not history, is imbued with moral purpose—and, Macedo obviously believes, rightly so.

One powerful counter to the usual diminished intensity of memory with the passage of time lies in trauma and various manifestations of post-traumatic stress disorder. "The traumatized person," writes Cathy Caruth, ". . . carries an impossible history within them, or they become themselves the symptoms of a history that they cannot entirely possess" (Caruth, 1991, p. 4). With trauma, whether in the experience of war veterans or Holocaust survivors or the survivors of other major disasters, or in the wider run of "normal traumatic events" like incest, child sexual abuse, and rape, including acquaintance-rape, there may be intrusive recollections of the traumatic event later in life, or recurrent dreams of it, or the sudden acting by the person as if the event were reoccurring, or more generalized responses to new phenomena with the frightful image of the past experience blotting out normal perceptions of the new. Traumatic bodily experience may have a special capacity to renew itself in memory without emotional or psychological distanciation.

Instrumentalization: The Past Is Put to Work

Memory selects and distorts in the service of present interests. The present interest may be narrowly defined—memory may be called up and shaped in an instrumental fashion to support some current strategic end. Or the present interest may be more a semiotic one than a strategic one. That is, the rememberer may be seeking not to conquer the world through the manipulation of the past but to understand the world—especially the present world—through the use of the past. Israelis recall Masada and Texans the Alamo not because these were triumphs that flatter the present but because they were tragedies that can help explain it (Schwartz et al., 1986).

Examples of instrumentalization are legion. Indeed, the problem may be to find cases of cultural memory that cannot be readily understood as the triumph of present interests over truth. The world of Orwell's *1984* is the extreme case. But it was not necessary to wait for twentieth-century totalitarianism for rulers to see instrumental value in manipulating the past. It was Louis XIV's censor who declared that changes in the political situation may "make it necessary to suppress or correct" information about the past (Burke, 1992, p. 126). Efforts at censorship and "cover-up" are all cases of instrumentalization. What Richard Nixon's aides, H. R. Haldeman and John Ehrlichman and Charles Colson, really remembered about Watergate, we don't know. What they said on the record was, "I don't recall," "I don't exactly remember," "I have no recollection." The way the military has re-membered the role of the media in Vietnam is a nice case of instrumentaliza-tion. By blaming media coverage of the war for the war's failure, the mili-tary, following the lead of the Nixon administration itself, drew attention away from its own failures of intelligence and strategy and training in Viet-nam, and justified subsequent curtailments of press freedom in Grenada and the Gulf War. George Bush self-consciously evoked the consensually pleas-ing, grand memory of World War II in leading the United States into the Gulf War, in an effort to prevent comparisons to the more recent and wounding Vietnam war (*New York Times,* 1991, p. A16).

On the fiftieth anniversary of D-Day in 1994, instrumentalization lay not in a particular version of what happened on the beaches of France in 1944 but in choosing this event rather than some others to commemorate so lav-ishly. The commemoration, *New York Times* reporter R. W. Apple ob-served, lacked "context." The British prominence at the commemoration was in some respects an act of nostalgia for a time when Britain was a world power on a par with the United States. The Russian absence from the cere-monies—Russian President Boris Yeltsin was not invited—is perhaps pecu-liar because, although Russian troops did not participate in D-Day, Soviet forces suffered many more casualties than the British or American armies and incurred many more losses to the Germans on the Eastern front than in all other engagements in the West, Italy, and North Africa (*New York Times,* June 5, 1994). The Russian absence reflected as much their unsettled international standing in 1994 as the historical reality of 1944.

Intellectuals are often the agents of instrumentalizing the past. Early nine-teenth-century European intellectuals, imbued with romantic nationalism, created the field of folklore and made use of folk culture to advance national-ist causes. This led to some remarkable fabrications, like the kilt and tartans of the Scottish Highlands (Trevor-Roper, 1984). The Kalevala, the purport-edly ancient Finnish epic poem, was in fact constructed of unrelated frag-ments of folk poetry by folklorist Elias Lonnrot and carefully cultivated by later scholars as Finland's ancient treasure, even when they knew better, as part of Finland's struggle for political independence (Wilson, 1976).

Instrumentalization is not necessarily calculated. A study of French bakers found that those who rose from apprentice to master tended to forget the humiliations of apprenticeship, while those who remained workers tended to recall them vividly (Debouzy, 1990, p. 60). Is there conscious or intentional distortion going on here? Not necessarily. Rationalization is a more complex process than that. This is related to the cognitive bias that Anthony Greenwald calls "beneffectance," the bias of recalling success more readily than failure or seeing the self as responsible for success and outside forces responsible for failure. These and other "ego biases" serve the ego but do not necessarily do so self-consciously (Greenwald, 1980, 1984). A kind of "beneffectance" may operate at a community or national level, too. Nineteenth-century Jacksonville, Illinois, town leaders shifted quickly from boosting their town as one with a glowing future to celebrating it as one with a glorious past when the legislature located the state university that Jacksonville had been counting on in Champaign-Urbana (Doyle, 1978, p. 265).

Some things that appear to be instrumentalization may be instances of cognitive bias not directly connected to self-interested motives. Michael Ross and Fiore Sicoly suggest that the tendency, in co-authored scientific papers, for each co-author to believe he or she made the larger contribution is not an obvious case of ideology serving self-interest. Instead, they suggest, it has to do with the "egocentric bias in availability of information in memory." Each co-author is better informed and more knowledgeable about the contribution he or she has made than about the work put in by the partner (Ross and Sicoly, 1982, pp. 180–189). Similarly, I suspect that in the organization of household chores between a husband and wife, the husband's belief that he has done his share is not necessarily patriarchal pig-headedness nor the wife's view that she has done the lion's share necessarily feminist protest. Both are more knowledgeable about and better able to recall the labor they themselves put in.

Repression is a special case of instrumentalization. Winners name the age. With Watergate, Senator Ervin's partisanship or Archibald Cox's Kennedy ties or the *Washington Post*'s long record of liberalism are typically repressed. In textbooks, the partisanship of Watergate evaporates altogether. One would never know that Richard Nixon was a Republican facing a Democratic-dominated Congress. The repression may be a form of censorship—liberal historians and journalists repressing something they do not want to remember or to face. Or it may be something less conscious than that, a repression in the name not of partisan triumph but of a drive for consensus or reconciliation. Community and town historians regularly repress past social conflict in the interest of present togetherness (Dykstra, 1968, pp. 361–367). French recollection of the Holocaust is shaped by a willful effort to avoid reliving conflicts that would tear contemporary French society apart, with resistance members and collaborators condemning each other (Miller, 1990, p. 141).

First-order instrumentalization promotes a particular version of the past to serve present interests. Second-order instrumentalization makes use of the past, and distorts it, without necessarily favoring a particular vision of the past. What is favored is any version of the past that can add fame or fortune to those charged with conveying it. So, for instance, journalists who tell the story of John F. Kennedy's assassination assimilate it to a larger myth about journalism itself. They typically recast an event that did not include them—reporters did not see Kennedy shot, after all—into an event in which they are heroes. Journalists' narratives typically emphasize Oswald's murder by Jack Ruby, which television crews did witness, and the President's funeral, where reporters served a ritual function in healing the nation. As Barbie Zelizer's studies suggest, journalistic accounts and retellings of the assassination hijacked the past for purposes of their own unconnected to the event narrated. That is, the journalists' interest was not to promote one or another version of the assassination but to "consolidate the authority" of the journalists themselves as narrators (Zelizer, 1990, p. 373; Zelizer, 1992).

Commercial culture offers many instances of second-order instrumentalization. It is not, for commercial developers, that a particular meaning of the past is sought but that meaningfulness can be made marketable. So the past is employed not to promote a particular view of it but to attract a ticket-buying crowd to a book, movie, or play. Thus an effort may be made to make an account of the past palatable to all tastes—hence, bland and uncontroversial—an effort that often characterizes the writing of textbooks to be sold to school districts throughout the country (Schudson, 1994). Or, at the opposite extreme, an account of the past may be sensationalized to attract adventurous or prurient tastes, as seems to be the case in the writing of some idol-bashing biographies.

The use of history, not as memorial to the past or promotion of a particular view of it, but as fodder for amusement attracted the indignation of many professional historians in the recently proposed "Disney's America" theme park. "We have so little left that's authentic and real. To replace what we have with plastic, contrived history, mechanical history is almost sacrilege," said historian David McCullough of the theme park plans (Rich, 1994).

Without doubting that commercial memorialization distorts and may diminish the past, it is worth observing that public, non-profit memorialization distorts as well. What possible relationship does a stately seated Lincoln inside a mammoth Greek temple have to the sixteenth president of the United States? Indeed, there was opposition to this Great Emancipator-as-Deity model when the Lincoln Memorial was designed and built in the 1920s. "Our national capital has Washington as a Roman general. Let us not add the more atrocious anachronism of Lincoln as Apollo," according to one contemporary critic. Some advocated a living memorial, like a national vocational school, or a parkway from Washington to Gettysburg as more fitting for the democratic Lincoln. But a memorial that may have been ill-suited to the living Lincoln represented very ably the reverence in which by the 1920s he had come to be held; the monument was a "virtual reality" in its own way that quickly came to be a fully consecrated, utterly uncontroversial sacred place (Peterson, 1994, pp. 206–217).

The controversy over the Lincoln Memorial is a fair indication that instrumentalization—like the other processes I am discussing here—operates on a social playing field. *1984* is the near-perfect case where the past is remade to serve present power, and no opposition dares raise a protest. But in liberal societies and in a porous international system where it is difficult or impossible to curtain one population from the next, instrumentalization is more often attempted than achieved. In Japan in 1994, Justice Minister Shigeto Nagano was forced to resign within days of a public statement denying Japanese atrocities in China and Korea during World War II. His comments "sparked outrage across Asia" and quickly sealed his political fate (*Boston Globe*, 1994). Powerful as the tendency to instrumentalization is, it is checked and countered so long as living memory, available written records, the integrity of journalists and historians, and a pluralistic world where different groups make competing claims on the past endure (Schudson, 1992, pp. 205–221).

Narrativization: The Past Gets Interesting

To pass on a version of the past, the past must be encapsulated into some sort of cultural form, and generally this is a narrative, a story, with a beginning, middle, and end; with an original state of equilibrium, a disruption, and a resolution; with a protagonist and obstacles in his or her way and efforts to overcome them. Reports of the past observe certain rules and conventions of narrative (White, 1973). An account of the past must choose a point to begin. This is not always easy or obvious; indeed, it is always to some degree arbitrary. When Russians commemorate the "Great Patriotic War," their beginning point is June 1941 when Germany invaded the Soviet Union. This enables Russians to pay homage to the 20 million war dead but at the same time conveniently helps them to overlook the 1939 Hitler-Stalin Non-Aggression Treaty that so significantly aided the build-up of the German military machine (Miller, 1990, p. 212; Tumarkin, 1987).

The usual telling of the story of Watergate begins with a burglary at the Democratic National Committee headquarters in Washington, D.C. Why? Because that was the point at which the set of events to which the term "Watergate" was ultimately attached first became known publicly. But that burglary was one of several, that particular flouting of the law one of many, and the cover-up that began days later that became a larger and more identifiable crime than the burglary itself was probably centered on concealing from public knowledge not White House involvement in the burglary but in other scurrilous deeds. To start the Watergate story on June 17, 1972, seems by no means inevitable.

Narrativization is an effort not only to report the past but to make it interesting. Narratives simplify. The most popular version of the Watergate story makes the journalists the central part of the story and nearly excludes the battles among the branches of government. Watergate has come down to us most prominently as a battle between a liberal, investigative press in the persons of Bob Woodward and Carl Bernstein of the *Washington Post,* and Richard Nixon and his cronies in the White House. The book by Woodward and Bernstein, *All the President's Men,* was published in 1974 even before Richard Nixon left office. When it appeared in May, it was the fastest-selling nonfiction hardcover book in the history of American publishing. A few months before, actor Robert Redford, who had acquired film rights to the book, asked screenwriter William Goldman if he had heard of Carl Bernstein and Bob Woodward. He had not, even at a time when people claimed that they had heard quite enough about Watergate. The film version of the book appeared in the spring of 1976 during the presidential primaries and became both a critical and commercial success. In the film, as in the book, Woodward and Bernstein are the protagonists, and a set of mysterious, shadowy figures in the White House and in the Committee to Re-Elect the President are the antagonists seeking to damage our heroes and protect the President from scrutiny.

The curious thing about the book and the film, in retrospect, is that they end in January 1973, six months after the Watergate break-in, with the second inauguration of Richard Nixon and a public backlash against the *Washington Post* for having published a (slightly) misleading story on the Watergate affair. Only then, as a coda to the film, does the viewer see a teletype machine printing out the indictments and guilty verdicts on Watergate conspirators and the notice of Nixon's resignation from office. The actual experience of Watergate, if I may speak of it that way, did not begin for most Americans until the Senate Watergate committee hearings in the summer of 1973, followed by the Saturday Night Massacre in October, the release of the White House tapes in April 1974, and the House Judiciary Committee hearings in June and July. All this is omitted from *All the President's Men,* a story of David and Goliath, this two-headed David young, innocent of politics, ever stumbling and learning—the book is a kind of novel of education—all in the effort to uncover a dark mystery. It is a tale of growing up, a mystery story, a true-crime drama, an update of the newspaper film of the 1930s, all rolled into one. On June 17, 1972, Woodward and Bernstein were freshmen in Washington politics; by January 1973, though most of Watergate had yet to happen, they were seniors ready to graduate.

Although the Woodward-Bernstein version of Watergate is the most familiar one, and the one that has most successfully reshaped the memory of Watergate for people who can personally recall the events, passing on a memory to a next generation may operate by different rules. Woodward and Bernstein fall out of the Watergate story in schoolbook renditions. These typically focus on the President, the Ervin committee, and the Supreme Court decision against Nixon on the question of executive privilege for the subpoenaed White House tapes. In textbook accounts of Watergate, there is little or no mention of the role played by the news media or by the special prosecutor. Why? I think that these actors fail to make an impression largely because "Watergate" is presented as a late-in-the-school-year reprise of lessons learned about the Constitution early on. The *dramatis personae* in the American history course are the executive, judicial, and legislative branches of government—adding a "fourth branch" of government, with the press, is messy. To discuss the special prosecutor, technically an agent of the executive but acting in the case of Archibald Cox out of a primary loyalty to the Congress, confuses the otherwise neat scenario of the separation of powers. In textbooks, Watergate is reorganized to fit into a larger narrative about constitutional government.

Successful narratives often foreground individual protagonists and antagonists rather than structures, trends, or social forces. Particular works of art or efforts at story-telling may live on in memory in ways that overwhelm less dramatic, less lucid, less epitomized, less narrativized ways of telling the past. Judith Miller offers two instances in her comparative study of how six nations recall the Holocaust—and their own involvement in it. She suggests that Austria, from early on portrayed worldwide as the first "victim" of Nazism, was in most respects an exceedingly willing, even enthusiastic, victim. Three-quarters of the guards at the Nazi concentration camps, for instance, were Austrians. Yet a combination of political expediency on the part of the Allies and the 1965 film *The Sound of Music* have left for Americans at least an image of the Austrians as noble folk resisting the Nazis (Miller, 1990, p. 62).

Similarly, the Dutch have wrapped themselves around a book by a thirteen-year-old girl, *The Diary of Anne Frank*, as proof to the ages of their national heroism in saving Dutch Jews from destruction. But the Dutch were in fact among the strongest collaborators with the Germans. And while their historical tradition demonstrates much less anti-Semitism than in Austria or France or many other countries in Europe, the widespread rule-following, order-obeying, well-mannered behavior of hundreds of thousands of Dutch citizens made the Netherlands perhaps the easiest of all occupied countries for the Germans to administer (Miller, 1990, pp. 95–98).

Narrativization, as I have discussed it so far, refers to telling a story about the past. But there is a second line of narrativization: telling a story about the past's relation to the present. In this larger narrative, understanding the past is often subjugated to an overarching story about how our own time fits into the passage of human history. For much of the past 200 years in the West, the grand narrative has been one of human progress or "Whig history." This was not always the case, of course, and in some fields and in some countries the overarching narrative line is a story of decline. The Romantics felt burdened by the "perfection of the past." John Keats worried that there was nothing original for a poet in the land of Shakespeare to achieve—Shakespeare had done it all (Bate, 1970, pp. 5, 82). For the past fifty years in the United States, both past and present have been understood in terms of the Cold War struggle with the Soviet Union, and other narratives of recent history have necessarily borrowed their structure or framework from this overarching narrative. After the Cold War, making sense of international affairs becomes more difficult.

Cognitivization and Conventionalization: The Past Becomes Knowable

In a well-known essay, "On Memory and Childhood Amnesia," Ernest Schachtel makes some telling observations about how adults remember, from their own lives, not what they experienced but what they learn they are conventionally supposed to have experienced. "Thus the memories of the majority of people come to resemble increasingly the stereotyped answers to a questionnaire, in which life consists of time and place of birth, religious denomination, residence, educational degrees, job, marriage, number and birthdates of children, income, sickness and death." A traveler remembers the road signs better than the landscape he or she has passed through, and the "average traveler through life remembers chiefly what the road map or the guide book says, what he is supposed to remember because it is exactly what everybody else remembers too" (Schachtel, 1982, pp. 193–194).

What Schachtel refers to as "the conventionalization of the adult memory" is a vital process in social or collective as well as in individual memory (Schachtel, 1982, p. 195). The past that comes to be known best or known at all is not only the one made into stories; it is the one *made* at all rather than the one experienced without being specifically constructed. John Dean certainly heard both his own words in conversations with President Nixon and the words of Nixon himself. One might even predict that he would recall Nixon's words better than his own—Nixon, after all, was the President of the United States, and Dean, his young counsel, might be expected to hang on his every word. But when Ulric Neisser compared John Dean's Watergate testimony to the record of the tape-recorded White House conversations, he discovered that Dean recalled his own remarks better than he did Nixon's. Neisser believes that this is because Dean prepared and rehearsed his own comments ahead of the meeting with Nixon and may very well have agonized over them afterwards, wondering if he had said the right thing or if he should have put his thoughts in a different way. The planning, preparing, and rehearsing, both before and after the "performance," enhanced Dean's recall for his own words (Neisser, 1982, p. 158).

Memories are prepared, planned, and rehearsed socially as well as individually. Experiences attended to by powerful social institutions are likely to be better preserved than experiences less favored by rich institutional rememberers. Recorded or archived materials are more likely to enter into public memory than materials that are never recorded or stored, or poorly recorded or stored. Oral histories may, with effort, be collected by professional historians; but people or institutions with their own tape recorders, minutes, file cabinets, and institutionalized, legally pertinent reasons for keeping records are more likely than others to produce materials that will one day be made part of a public record. Culturally valued and memorialized activities are more easily retrievable than culturally denigrated, repressed, or stigmatized activities. Whatever past is remembered or commemorated, it must be drawn from the available past; and availability of the past, to borrow a term from Amos Tversky and Daniel Kahneman (1974), is socially structured.

Within the public domain, not only the recording of the past but active re-working of the past is more likely to be transmitted if it happens in high-prestige, socially consensual institutions than if it happens at or beyond the edges of conventional organization. The retrospective narration of Watergate is conducted not only by historians with a relatively wide range of views or journalists of various stripes but also Congressmen who invariably represent centrist liberal and conservative positions. When they battled over the meaning of Watergate as they did in debating government ethics legislation for several years after Nixon's resignation, they did so with each other as chief antagonists, excluding any mention of viewpoints to the left or right of congressional representatives. They also seemed obliged by their legitimate political position to dignify Watergate's memory. They may think that Watergate proved the system worked (conservatives) or that it almost failed to work and so requires reform (liberals), but the very process of shaping post-Watergate legislation requires them all to take Watergate seriously as a constitutional crisis. More skeptical, subversive, or irreverent views have been proffered by intellectuals and political activists on the far left and far right, but these never had a hearing in the central political arena.

A special case of conventionalization is memorialization. Turning something into a monument or memorial changes the past in that very process. Memorialization moralizes the past, creates out of a chronicle a tradition. A commemorated event is one "invested with an extraordinary significance and assigned a qualitatively distinct place in our conception of the past." It is in a sense "a register of sacred history" (Schwartz, 1982, p. 377). Memorials—whether in monuments, holidays, or commemorative programs—tend to be audience-centered, and their creators worry about their rhetorical effect. Critics of the twenty-fifth anniversary celebration of Stonewall, the beginnings of the contemporary gay liberation movement, have objected to its commercialization, its corporate sponsorship, and the selling of T-shirts and other merchandise. But organizers of the celebration observe how expensive the Central Park rally would be (*New York Times,* May 6, 1994).

Frequently, memorialization evokes conflict even though it may be meant to pacify it. Efforts to name the campus library at the University of Massachusetts, Amherst, after black leader W. E. B. Du Bois (who was born nearby and whose papers are deposited in the library's special collections) evoked heated opposition from a conservative student newspaper (*Boston Globe,* May 8, 1994). Debates rage over how to preserve Auschwitz as a memorial to the Holocaust (*New York Times,* January 5, 1994). Efforts to create a national Martin Luther King, Jr., holiday and local attempts to rename streets or parks in King's honor evoked conflict (*New York Times,* January 18, 1987). The fortieth anniversary of the Warsaw ghetto uprising, sponsored by the Communist government in Poland, presumably in an effort to gain international support for a regime then operating under martial law, spawned protests by Jewish groups and by supporters of Solidarity. When a P.L.O. representative laid a wreath at the memorial to the Jewish resisters in the ghetto, the Israeli delegation was ordered home. What was to be a great public relations gesture became a political embarrassment (*New York Times,* April 17, 1983, p. 9 and April 22, 1983, p. A5). Protesters used the Communist government's official commemoration of Hungary's 1848 nationalist revolution in 1987 to protest and question the legitimacy of the regime (*New York Times,* March 16, 1987, p. 3).

Conclusion

In broad terms, collective memory is characterized by four general principles. First, memory is in fact social. People remember collectively, publicly, interactively. This is true even of individual memory that is sustained only by social interaction, by rehearsal, review, and the language people have by virtue of being social beings.

Second, memory is selective. Remembering one thing requires forgetting another.

Third, selection is driven by various processes, both willful and unconscious. Most often, students of a particular cultural memory seek to show the self-interested ways in which the memory has been shaped. The focus on self-interest may be the beginning but should not be the end of wisdom. Instrumentalization is one of the dynamics of memory construction, but it does not operate independently of other processes like narrativization, conventionalization, and distanciation. Nor is it necessarily the captain of this contingent of forces. Judging which processes of memory are most important depends on the particular case at hand.

Fourth, collective memory, at least in liberal pluralistic societies, is provisional, always open to contestation and often actually contested. In the American case, no icon is so sacred that its sanctity will not be challenged. Indeed, the more sacred the symbol is, the more potent it becomes as a focal point for protest. This makes legitimated historical markers, from school textbooks to monuments, apt targets for symbolic politics. The negotiations over the Vietnam Veterans Memorial are a case in point. So is the speech of Supreme Court Justice Thurgood Marshall on the 200th anniversary of the Constitution, attacking the Founding Fathers for leaving out of constitutional purview so many peoples, notably African-Americans (*New York Times,* May 7, 1987, p. 1).

The past, anthropologist Arjun Appadurai has suggested, is a "scarce resource," and conflict over its ownership is recurrent. Today, however, the past may be increasingly a superabundant resource, and conflict may emerge not from its scarcity but from its superfluity. Memory today has a thousand champions. We even memorialize memorialization. Spielberg's *Schindler's List* was a testimony to the Holocaust. The Jewish sector of Krakow, where the filming took place, has now become a tourist attraction, an actual site of Jewish suffering made famous as much for its filmic role as for the role the film commemorated (National Public Radio, Deidre Berger, reporter, July 7, 1994).

Contest, conflict, controversy—these are the hallmark of studies of collective memory, rather than the concept of distortion. Discovering the attitudes and interests of the present becomes of much greater concern than the legitimate claims of the past upon them. Still, a focus on distortion makes sense in studies of collective or cultural memory. Even the most ardently relativist scholars among us shiver with revulsion at certain versions of the past that cry out "distortion." The most famous example is the flourishing fringe group of Holocaust revisionists who deny that there was ever a plan to exterminate the Jews or that such a plan was ever set in place. The question of what content of the past is not or cannot or should not be subject to later-day reinterpretation haunts the papers at a 1990 conference at U.C.L.A. on "Nazism and the 'Final Solution': Probing the Limits of Representation" (Friedlander, 1992). The fascination with conflicting versions of the past and the excitement over legitimately revisionist interpretations of once settled and consensual accounts come precisely from the fact that even trained historians (or perhaps especially trained historians) retain strong beliefs in a veritable past. If interpretation were free-floating, entirely manipulable to serve present interests, altogether unanchored by a bedrock body of unshakable evidence, controversies over the past would ultimately be uninteresting. But in fact they are interesting. They are compelling. And they are gripping because people trust that a past we can to some extent know and can to some extent come to agreement about really happened.

References

Appadurai, Arjun. 1981. "The Past as a Scarce Resource." *Man* (N.S.) 16: 201–219.

Apple, R. W., Jr. 1991. "Defining the Issue." *New York Times,* Jan. 7: A16.

Apple, R. W., Jr. 1994. "The Longest Day Is Being Marked by Those with Shortened Memories." *New York Times,* June 5: E4.

Bate, W. Jackson. 1970. *The Burden of the Past and the English Poet.* Cambridge, Mass.: Harvard University Press.

Burke, Peter. 1989. "History as Social Memory," in Thomas Butler, ed., *Memory: History, Culture and the Mind.* Oxford: Basil Blackwell, pp. 97–113.

Burke, Peter. 1992. *The Fabrication of Louis XIV.* New Haven: Yale University Press, 1992.

Caruth, Cathy. 1991. "Introduction." *American Imago: Spec. Issue Psychoanalysis, Culture and Trauma* 48.

Chant, Cate. 1994. "UMass Paper Opposes Du Bois Honor." *Boston Globe,* May 8: 29.

Constantine, K. C. 1993. *Bottom Liner Blues.* New York: Mysterious Press.

Debouzy, Marianne. 1990. "In Search of Working-Class Memory: Some Questions and a Tentative Assessment," in Noelle Bourguet, Lucette Valensi, and Nathan Wachtel, eds., *Between Memory and History.* Chur, Switzerland: Harwood Academic Publishers, pp. 55–76.

Degler, Carl. 1976. "Why Historians Change Their Minds." *Pacific Historical Review* 45.

Doyle, Don H. 1978. *The Social Order of a Frontier Community.* Urbana: University of Illinois Press.

Dykstra, Robert R. 1968. *The Cattle Towns.* New York: Alfred A. Knopf.

Friedlander, Saul, ed. 1992. *Probing the Limits of Representation: Nazism and the "Final Solution."* Cambridge, Mass.: Harvard University Press.

Greenwald, Anthony. 1980. "The Totalitarian Ego: Fabrication and Revision of Personal History." *American Psychologist* 35: 603–618.

Greenwald, Anthony. 1984. "The Self," in Robert S. Wyer and Thomas K. Srull, eds., *Handbook of Social Cognition,* vol. 3. Hillsdale, N.J.: Lawrence Erlbaum, pp. 129–178.

Irwin-Zarecka, Iwona. 1994. *Frames of Remembrance.* New Brunswick, N.J.: Transaction.

Janofsky, Michael. 1994. "Learned Opposition to New Disney Park." *New York Times,* May 12: A8.

Kamm, Henry. 1987. "1,500 March Freely in Budapest for a New Democracy." *New York Times,* March 16: 3.

Kifner, John. 1983. "In Warsaw, Few Flowers at the Ghetto." *New York Times,* April 17: 9.

Kifner, John. 1983. "Some Jews Leave Polish Ceremony." *New York Times,* April 22: A5.

Macedo, Stephen. 1990. *Liberal Virtues.* Oxford: Clarendon Press.

Madsen, Richard. 1990. "The Politics of Revenge in Rural China during the Cultural Revolution," in Jonathan N. Lipman and Stevan Harrell, *Violence in China:*

Essays in Culture and Counterculture. Albany: State University of New York Press, pp. 175–201.

Mannheim, Karl. 1970. "The Problem of Generations." *Psychoanalytic Review* 57: 378–404.

Merton, Robert. 1968. "The Matthew Effect in Science." *Science* 159 (Jan. 5): 56–63.

Merton, Robert. 1988. "The Matthew Effect in Science, II." *Isis* 79: 606–623.

Miller, Judith. 1990. *One, by One, by One: Facing the Holocaust.* New York: Simon and Schuster.

Neisser, Ulric. 1982. "John Dean's Memory: A Case Study" in Ulric Neisser, ed., *Memory Observed.* San Francisco: W. H. Freeman, pp. 139–159.

New York Times, 1994. "Remember Stonewall! But How? Groups Ask." May 6: A13.

Perlez, Jane. 1994. "Decay of a 20th Century Relic: What's the Future of Auschwitz?" *New York Times,* Jan. 5: A4.

Peterson, Merrill. 1994. *Lincoln in American Memory.* New York: Oxford University Press, pp. 206–217.

Radin, Charles A. 1994. "Japanese Justice Minister Resigns." *Boston Globe,* May 8: 8.

Rich, Frank. 1994. "Disney's Bull Run." *New York Times,* May 22: E15.

Ross, Michael, and Fiore Sicoly. 1982. "Egocentric Biases in Availability and Attribution," in Daniel Kahneman, Paul Slovic, and Amos Tversky, eds. *Judgment Under Uncertainty: Heuristics and Biases.* Cambridge: Cambridge University Press, pp. 180–189.

Schachtel, Ernest G. 1982 (1947). "On Memory and Childhood Amnesia," in Ulric Neisser, ed., *Memory Observed.* San Francisco: W. H. Freeman, pp. 189–200. Originally published in *Psychiatry* 10: 1–26.

Schudson, Michael. 1992. *Watergate in American Memory: How We Remember, Forget, and Reconstruct the Past.* New York: Basic Books.

Schudson, Michael. 1994. "Textbook Politics." *Journal of Communication* 44: 43–51.

Schuman, Howard, and Jacqueline Scott. 1989. "Generations and Collective Memories." *American Sociological Review* 54: 513–536.

Schwartz, Barry. 1982. "The Social Context of Commemoration: A Study in Collective Memory." *Social Forces* 61: 374–402.

Schwartz, Barry, Yael Zerubavel, and Bernice M. Barnett. 1986. "The Recovery of Masada: A Study in Collective Memory." *Sociological Quarterly* 27: 147–164.

Taylor, Stuart. 1987. "Marshall Sounds Critical Note on Bicentennial." *New York Times,* May 7: 1.

Trevor-Roper, Hugh. 1983. "The Invention of Tradition: The Highland Tradition in Scotland," in Eric Hobsbawm and Terence Ranger, eds. *The Invention of Tradition.* Cambridge: Cambridge University Press, pp. 15–41.

Tumarkin, Nina. 1987. "Myth and Memory in Soviet Society." *Society* 24 (September/October): 69–72.

Tversky, Amos, and Daniel Kahneman. 1974. "Judgment Under Uncertainty: Heuristics and Biases." *Science* 185: 1124–1131.

White, Hayden. 1973. *Metahistory*. Baltimore: Johns Hopkins University Press.

Wieseltier, Leon. 1993. "After Memory." *New Republic*, May 3: 16–26.

Williams, Lena. 1987. "Most of U.S. Will Honor Dr. King, But Some Still Dispute the Holiday." *New York Times*, Jan. 18: 1.

Wilson, William A. 1976. *Folklore and Nationalism in Modern Finland*. Bloomington: Indiana University Press.

Zelizer, Barbie. 1990. "Achieving Journalistic Authority Through Narrative." *Critical Studies in Mass Communication* 7: 366–376.

Zelizer, Barbie. 1992. *Covering the Body*. Chicago: University of Chicago Press.

Ancient Egyptian Antijudaism: A Case of Distorted Memory

14

Jan Assmann

During the last two decades, our sensibility has been sharpened for the role of collective imagination in the construction of reality and the building up of the world we live in. Cornelius Castoriadis (1975) has analyzed the "imaginary institution of society"; Benedict Anderson (1983) has shown the nations of modern nationalism to be "imagined communities"; the French notion "imaginaire" has been made use of in a great variety of contexts and usually with great profit (Baczko, 1984). This chapter follows this line of research in elaborating on the imaginary side of historiography and in focusing on the image of the (religious and/or ethnic) other. The case that will be presented here sheds light on the question of how the image of "the" enemy is generated. It draws its general interest and relevance from the fact that the construction of the "Jew" as the religious enemy par excellence passed through and determined the course of Christian occidental history and culminated, in the context of German fascism, in genocide. It is important to know that Christian anti-Jewish propaganda inherited some of its central clichés from Egyptian paganism. It is even more important to realize that in Egypt these clichés can be traced back to a past which originally had nothing to do with the Jews but which, in the course of history, underwent such transformations and "distortions" in the collective memory of the Egyptians that it could eventually be cast into the Egyptian version of the exodus and fulfill the function of anti-Jewish propaganda. By retracing these transformations we get new insights into the workings of collective cultural memory but above all into the social construction of religious otherness.

It is a well-known fact that there is no absolute and objective truth in memory. Remembering is always transformation and reconstruction. This applies to collective as well as to individual memory. One could perhaps think that writing or other systems of codification should save information from getting lost or transformed in the way of transmission. But whatever advantages symbolic codification might provide over individual memory, they are more than balanced by the fact that writings and other forms of objectivization and codification are open to censorship, manipulation, and even annihilation. In a way, every memory is "distorted" memory, just as every tradition is an "invented tradition" (Hobsbawm and Ranger, 1983). The past has always to be reconstructed and tradition has always to be (re-)invented. But it is equally clear that there are differences, that some memories are more distorted than others and some traditions more invented than others. The kind of distortion that will be dealt with in the course of this chapter concerns not the reconstruction but the eradication of the past. It is this attitude toward the past that has been described so impressively by George Orwell in his novel *1984*. Applied to cultural theory, the notion "distorted memory" seems to presuppose that there is something like "undistorted memory." This, however, is not the case: remembering is always transformation and reconstruction. The past can never be preserved in a pure, complete, and authentic form but must always be reconstructed from the viewpoint and within the semantic frames of a changing present (Halbwachs, 1925, 1950).

If, therefore, every collective memory is, in a way, "distorted memory," there are, however, degrees of distortion. The most extreme case of distortion is the eradication of memory.

Umberto Eco (1987) has made the point that there is no "ars oblivionalis" corresponding to "ars memorativa." There are, however, forms of collective forgetting that correspond pretty well to forms of collective remembering. One is what ethnologists call "structural amnesia" (the term was coined by J. A. Barnes; see Schott, 1968, p. 184); this form consists in forgetting those elements of the past that are no longer in meaningful relation to the present and is typical of oral societies. Its counterpart in literal societies is the willful destruction of commemorative symbols (documents and monuments), including the burning of books, the destruction of inscriptions (*damnatio memoriae*), and the rewriting of history as described, for example, by Orwell in *1984*. There is (as far as I can see) no comprehensive term to denote these acts of intentional and violent cultural oblivion. They seem to correspond, on the individual level, to repression, whereas structural amnesia corresponds rather to forgetting. "Cultural repression" might therefore serve as a term for the various forms of annihilating cultural memory.

Two cases in point may serve to illustrate both structural amnesia and cultural repression. One is the Hyksos occupation of Egypt by Canaanitic invaders and its "inverted tradition" in Hebrew and Greek tradition; the other is the monotheistic revolution of Akhenaten and its non-tradition in Egypt.

My starting point is the extra-biblical tradition of Israel's exodus from Egypt as it is found in various works of Greek and Roman historiographers, from Hekataios of Abdera, who wrote his History of Egypt about 300 B.C.E., to Tacitus and later writers. (The sources have been collected by Stern, 1974–1984; see Yoyotte, 1963; Redford, 1986, pp. 276–296; Redford, 1992, pp. 408–422.) They relate the story in such different versions that they obviously base themselves on oral tradition rather than on written sources, let alone on the canonical version of the Bible. The homeland of these oral traditions (popular legends) is Egypt, and the versions of Egyptian historians are by far the most explicit. These versions are completely different from—even an inversion of—the biblical account. (Indeed, the difference from the biblical account is so striking that one might think of a polemical counter-statement by someone who perfectly knew and contradicted the biblical version. This is the opinion of Funkenstein [1993]. But I think that the Egyptian tradition is much older than their first encounter with the biblical exodus tradition.) But the most striking feature is the strong attitude of hatred, fear, and abomination which pervades these exodus stories (also the biblical one, but in the opposite direction). This affective coloring is what seems most problematic about this tradition. It brought on the Egyptians the reputation of being the first anti-Semites in world history (Gager, 1983; Kasher, 1985). Where does it come from?

By far the most explicit and apparently most bluntly anti-Jewish version of the story is to be found in Manetho, an Egyptian priest, who wrote his History of Egypt under Ptolemaios II in the first half of the third century B.C.E. (I am using the edition by W. G. Waddell, Loeb Classical Library, 1940.) We know his account from two excerpts by Josefus Flavius, a Jewish historiographer, who in his book *Contra Apionem* collected testimonies about the Jews from pagan authors. The first excerpt he adduces as proof for the high antiquity of the Jewish people, the second as an example of anti-Jewish calumny. The intention of quotation is, therefore, different in both cases. The first excerpt is offered as truth, the second as lie. The first excerpt deals with the Hyksos. They are said to have conquered Egypt without resistance and to have treated the population with the utmost cruelty. They reigned for more than 500 years, until finally the kings of Thebes made a rebellion against them and laid siege to their capital, Awaris. The Hyksos emigrated into Syria and settled finally in what is now called Iudaea.

The second excerpt opens the series of anti-Jewish calumnies which Josefus wants to refute. Here, Manetho is adduced not as a witness, but as an enemy. In the first version, Josefus tells us, Manetho follows the "sacred Scripture" *(ta hiera grammata)*; in the second, popular tales and legends *(mutheuomena kai legomena)*. It is this version which I propose for closer examination. Ninety years ago Eduard Meyer (1904, pp. 92–95) identified in this text a distant but quite unmistakable echo of the Amarna experience.

The Canadian egyptologist Donald B. Redford (1970; 1986, pp. 276–296; 1992, pp. 408–422) has recently confirmed this identification. On a different track, I came to the same conclusion. This story presents us with what survived, in the collective memory of Egypt, of the Amarna experience, and its "distortions" can easily be explained by the cultural repression of the same period.

This is Manetho's account: King Amenophis wanted to see the gods. The sage Amenophis, son of Hapu, tells him that he may see the gods if he cleanses the land of lepers. The king sends all lepers, among them priests, into the quarries in the eastern desert. Amenophis, the seer, predicts divine punishment for this inhuman treatment of the sick: they will receive help from outside, conquer Egypt, and reign for thirteen years. Not daring to tell the king this oracle in person, he writes everything down and commits suicide. The lepers are allowed to settle in Awaris, the ancient capital of the Hyksos. They choose as their leader Osarsiph, a Heliopolitan priest. He makes for them laws that prescribe all that is forbidden in Egypt and forbid all that is prescribed there. The first and foremost commandments are not to worship the gods, not to abstain from their forbidden food, and not to associate with people from outside. He then fortifies the city and invites the Hyksos who were driven out of Egypt some two or three hundred years earlier to join their revolt. The Hyksos return. King Amenophis remembers the prediction, declines to fight the rebels, hides the divine images, and emigrates with the sacred animals to Ethiopia. The lepers and the Hyksos rule Egypt for thirteen years in a way that lets the former Hyksos rule appear, in the memory of the Egyptians, like a Golden Age. For now not only are the towns and temples laid waste and the holy images destroyed, but the sanctuaries are turned into kitchens and the sacred animals roasted on fires. Osarsiph takes on the name "Moses." But finally, Amenophis and his grandson Ramses return from Nubia and drive out the lepers and their allies.

This is Manetho's version of the story, which I shall call version "A." It might be structured into five main episodes:

1. The original state of lack or distress from which the course of events takes its start: the invisibility of the gods, which prompts the wish of the king to see them.

2. The steps taken by the king to overcome the original situation: concentration and enslavement of the lepers in the quarries, then their ghettoization in Awaris.

3. The organization of the lepers under the leadership of Osarsiph and his legislation that inverts the laws and customs of Egypt, especially by forbidding the worship of the gods and consorting with other people.

4. The thirteen years of reign of terror by the Hyksos and the lepers and their war against the temples, cults, images, and animals.

5. The liberation of Egypt and the expulsion of the lepers and the Hyksos.

As stated earlier, the story circulates in many different versions among the ancient historiographers. It is therefore obvious that they not only copied from each other but used different (oral) material. Common to all these other versions including the biblical one is that they know only of one expulsion whereas Manetho knows two: first the expulsion of the Hyksos and then, two to three hundred years later, the expulsion of the lepers and their allies. The earliest author, who wrote one or two generations before Manetho, is Hekataios of Abdera. (Hekataios v. Abdera, Aigyptiaka, apud Diodor, Bibl. Hist. XL, 3. F. R. Walton, *Diodorus of Sicily* [Loeb Classical Library, 1967], p. 281; Redford, 1986, pp. 281f.) His version, which I will call version "B," is almost free from any anti-Jewish polemics. Here, the main episodes are reduced to three: 1. (original situation): The course of events starts from a situation of distress: a plague ravaging Egypt. The Egyptians interpret this as divine punishment for the presence of aliens and the introduction of alien rites and customs in Egypt. 2. (expulsion): The aliens are expelled. Some, under the leadership of Kadmos and Danaos, colonize Greece; others, under the leadership of Moses, colonize Palestine. 3. (legislation): Moses forbids the making of divine images, because all-encompassing heaven alone is god, who cannot be depicted in images. (See Stern, 1974–1984, pp. 20–44. Also Tacitus characterizes the Jewish concept of god as monotheistic and aniconic [Historiae, V, § 5.4; Stern, II, pp. 19 and 26].)

In version B, the positive content of the new religion is emphasized, namely monotheism, whereas in version A only its negative aspect is shown, namely iconoclasm and intolerance. The later versions (more than a dozen) do not adduce much more material. Sometimes, the name of the king appears as Bocchoris, not Amenophis (for example, Lysimachos, Aegyptiaca, apud Josephus, C. A. I, 304–311; Stern, 1974–1984, Nr. 158, I, 383–386; and Tacitus). Sometimes, the Egyptians are suffering from a plague or famine, sometimes the aliens/lepers, sometimes both. Sometimes their monotheism is emphasized, sometimes their iconoclasm and intolerant exclusiveness. The only original versions among these later treatments are Plutarch's and Strabo's. Plutarch tells the story in a completely mythologized form. The god Seth, the murderer of Osiris, is driven out of Egypt and spends seven days flying into Palestine. There he engenders his sons Hierosolyma and Juda (*De Iside* cap. 31). Strabo, on the contrary, gives a completely demythologized account of the story (Strabon of Amaseia, Geographica XVI, 2:34–46; Stern, 1974–1984, Nr. 115, I, 294–311). The plague-motif is missing. The events start with the decision of an Egyptian priest named Moses, who feels unsatisfied with Egyptian religion, to found a new religion and to emigrate with his followers into Palestine. His religion consists in the recognition of only one divine Being "who encompasses all of us, and earth and sea, whom we call heaven and earth and nature" and whom no image can represent. The only way to approach this god is to live in virtue and justice.

This version is interesting because it so closely corresponds to the very latest manifestation of this mythology, namely Sigmund Freud's book *Der Mann Moses und die monotheistische Religion* (1939/1964; see Yerushalmi, 1992). Both agree that monotheism is originally an Egyptian movement, which—being persecuted in Egypt—has been transferred to the Hebrews. But Freud knows what neither Manetho nor Strabo could know: that there was in fact such a movement in Egypt which actually ruled Egypt for some twenty years. These historical events have been exposed to a most radical and complete cultural repression. The monuments were not only dismantled but concealed in new buildings. The names of the kings were cancelled from official records. It was only archaeological investigation that brought these things to light at the end of the nineteenth century (Hornung, 1992, pp. 43–49). Eduard Meyer, and then Freud, were among the first to fill the void and to reintroduce the name of Akhenaten into this pseudo-historical tradition about a monotheistic revolution in Egypt and its final persecution and expulsion.

The story of the lepers can thus be explained as a most conspicuous case of distorted memory. In this tradition survive Egyptian recollections of Akhenaten's monotheistic revolution which, because of the banishment of the latter's name and monuments from cultural memory, became dislocated and exposed to all kinds of transformations and proliferations. This interpretation is based on the assumption that the Amarna experience must have left an extremely strong and even traumatic impression on the contemporary generation. The closure of the temples and the discontinuation of the cults must have been a shock for a mentality that sees the closest interdependence between cult and natural, social and individual prosperity. Ritual negligence interrupts the maintenance of cosmic and social order. The consciousness of a catastrophic and irreparable crime must have been quite general. Discontinuation of the cult also implied the cessation of festivals, and this must have been resented even more drastically than the desolation of the temples because this actually affected the whole population. The religious feast in ancient Egypt is the one occasion when the gods leave their temple and appear to the people at large, whereas they normally dwelt in complete darkness and seclusion inside the sanctuaries of their temples, inaccessible to all save to the priest in service. But on the occasion of a feast, these boundaries between secrecy and publicity, sacred and profane, inner and outer, were suspended. The gods appeared to the people outside the temple walls. Every major Egyptian religious feast was celebrated in the form of a procession (Assmann, 1991).

The Egyptian idea of the city is centered around and shaped by this festive situation (Assmann, 1984, pp. 25–35). The city is the place on earth where, on the occasion of the main processional feast, the divine presence can be sensed by everyone. The more important the feast, the more important the city. The feasts therefore procured not only religious participation but also social identification. The Egyptian conceived of himself as a member not of a "nation," but of a town or city. The city was the place where he belonged and where he wanted to be buried. Belonging to a city meant in the first place belonging to a deity as the lord or lady of that city, and this belonging to a god was formed and confirmed by participating in the feasts. The abolition of the feasts must have deprived the individual Egyptian of his sense of identity and, what is even more, of his hopes of immortality. For following the deity in her/his earthly feasts was held to be the first and most necessary step toward that worldly beatitude. I stress these facts because I am trying to reconstruct the frames of experience within which the Amarna period must have been lived through by a normal Egyptian. These are also the frames of recollection. It is only through such frames that an event becomes experienceable, communicable, and memorable. It seems to me quite clear that the Amarna period must have meant for the Egyptians the utmost sacrilege, destruction, and horror, a time of divine absence, of darkness and disease. Some intimations of this consciousness reverberate in the short allusions which Tutankhamen gives in his Restauration stela:

> The temples of the gods and goddesses were desolated from
> Elephantine as far as the marshes of the Delta . . .
> their holy places were about to disintegrate,
> having become rubbish heaps, overgrown with thistles.
> Their sanctuaries were as if they had never been,
> their houses were trodden roads.
> The land was in grave disease.
> The gods have forsaken this land.
> If an army was sent to Syria to extend the borders of Egypt,
> it had no success at all.
> If men prayed to a god for help,
> he did not come.
> If men besought a goddess likewise,
> she came not at all.
> Their hearts have grown weak in their bodies,
> because "they" had destroyed what has been created.
>
> (*Urk* IV 2025ff.)

In the Theban tomb of Pairi there is a graffito which the scribe Pawah wrote there in the time of Semenkhkare, the last of the Amarna-kings. It is a lamentation for the absent god and starts with the words: "My heart longs for seeing you!" Its theme is the nostalgia for the sight of Amun in his feast. We have every reason to imagine the Amarna experience as traumatic and the memories of Amarna among the contemporary generation as painful and problematic. The recollection of the Amarna experience became even more problematic because of the process of systematic suppression by deleting all the visible traces of that period and by removing the names of the kings from all official records. Not even as a heretic has Akhenaten survived in the memory of the Egyptians. His name and his teaching fell into complete oblivion. Only the imprint of the shock remained, the vague remembrance of something religiously unclean, hateful and disastrous to the extreme. It is this remembrance that gave rise to the legend of the lepers.

Let me recall some of the decisive features of the story. First and foremost, it is a religious conflict. This becomes most clear in the version of Manetho, who distinguished between the Hyksos and the lepers. The Hyksos invasion is reported as a political event without specific religious elements. The story of the lepers, on the other hand, is laden with religious motifs. It even starts with such a motif: the wish of the king to see the gods. We remember that this was exactly what Pawah longed for in his graffito. In the graffito we are to understand that divine absence is caused by the new religion. In Manetho's version it is clear that the presence of the lepers is the cause for the invisibility of the gods. The lepers can thus be identified as a transformation or distortion of the heretics. This becomes even more clear in the continuation of the story. The lepers are shown as religious revolutionaries. The king fears them as such because he makes his preparations by hiding the divine images and rescuing the sacred animals; and they confirm their image by destroying the temples, slashing the remaining idols, and roasting the rest of the sacred animals. The very first of their laws is a religious one: the prohibition to worship the gods. The story of the lepers is about religion. The religious conflict is its dominating feature in all the extant versions.

For the Egyptians, the Amarna religion was their first and—until their encounter with the Jews—also their only experience of an alien religion. They knew of course about alien deities, such as Baal, Anat, Astarte, Teschup, Marduk, Aschur, and so on, but not about structurally alien religions. The religions were felt to be much the same everywhere, and so were most of the gods because their names could be easily translated from one language and one religion into another. Some of these alien gods were even integrated into Egyptian mythology. It is quite impossible that this kind of religious confrontation and conflict which is so prominent in the story of the lepers could have ever occurred in Egypt outside the Amarna age and before the Late period. Very probably the Amarna age was generally the first confrontation of different religious systems in the history of mankind. To the Egyptians it must have meant the confrontation with extreme alterity, even more so than the Hyksos. It is therefore quite understandable that in later retrospect the Amarna reminiscences were projected onto the Hyksos and conflated with their tradition in historiography and romance.

This conflation seems to start already some seventy or eighty years afterward, when we read in a Ramesside novel that Apophis, the Hyksos king, practiced a monolatric religion:

> king Apophis chose for his lord the god Seth.
> He did not worship any other deity in the whole land
>   except Seth.
> (Sallier I, 1.2–3, ed. Gardiner 1932)

Presumably already in this time, other memories and experiences invade the void in the collective memory which has been created both by trauma and by the annihilation of traces and turn the Hyksos conflict into a religious conflict. This process of distortion continues through the centuries as events occur that fit into the story of religious otherness and its dangerous semantics of abomination and persecution. It is in the course of this process that Seth gradually begins to incorporate these traits of religious otherness and to assume the characteristics of both a devil and an Asiatic. In Plutarch's version he is openly equated with Israel, and in other late sources he appears as god of the Jews. The Assyrian and Persian invasion of Egypt enriched the story with new details. The void which had been created by the cultural repression of the Amarna period tended always to get filled by new experiences which in their turn were already formed by the semantic frame of this mythology.

But instead of pursuing this process through all its stages of transformation and proliferation I would like to bring into focus a third version of the exodus story: the biblical account. The biblical text is a very complex and multi-layered structure which contains much more material than is relevant in our present context, but some of its elements seem directly connected with our tradition and appear to form just another version of the same events. These are:

1. Concentration and enslavement, with forced labor and oppression, provoking divine wrath, as in Manetho's version.

2. A plague, enforcing Egypt's separation from the "aliens," as in Hekataios' version. This motif appears here multiplied by 10.

3. The separation, here realized in the form of a finally and reluctantly conceded emigration and not as expulsion, and the exodus under the leadership of Moses.

4. The legislation of Moses, with the prohibition of worshipping (other) gods as the most prominent commandment.

The most striking common denominator of Manetho's version and the biblical version is the strong affective stamp of the narrative. Both are dictated by mutual hatred and abomination. In the biblical version, the Egyptians are shown as torturers and oppressors, idolators and magicians; in the Egyptian version, the "Jews" are shown as lepers, impure people, atheists, misanthropes, iconoclasts, vandals, and sacrilegious criminals. But equally striking are the differences between the two versions, because they relate to each other in the form of an exact inversion. All the extrabiblical versions agree that the aliens or impure ones are driven out of Egypt. In the Bible, the Hebrews are retained in Egypt against their will and only allowed to emigrate after divine interventions in the form of the plagues. But even in this version the report of the emigration contains elements of expulsion.

It would of course be most instructive to confront these different versions with what could count for historical evidence. But there is next to nothing. The only historical event that is both archaeologically provable and semantically comparable with the content of these different versions of the expulsion/emigration story is the sojourn of the Hyksos in Egypt. I completely agree with Donald B. Redford, who in various publications held that the Hyksos' sojourn in and withdrawal from Egypt was all that happened in terms of historical fact and that different memories of these events lived on in the traditions of Canaan and Egypt. The Hebrews only fell heir to the Canaanite part of these memories. If we accept this theory, we are in a position to evaluate the stages of transformation and to recognize its direction. The Hyksos stayed in Egypt, not as slaves but as rulers. They withdrew from Egypt not as finally released slaves, but as expulsed enemies. The inversions which the Hebrew tradition effected to the historical facts find their explanation in the semantic frame of the covenant-and-election theology. This is a semantics of small beginnings and great promises. Within this frame the withdrawal from Egypt could not be understood otherwise than as a rise from nothingness to identity, from bondage to freedom, from impurity to purity, and from forlornness to alliance. In the context of oral tradition, memorial reworkings or transformations such as these met with no resistance because "no fixed narrative or king list held imagination in check" (Redford, 1992, p. 419).

In Egypt, the experience of the Hyksos invasion and expulsion entered the official king list tradition and was therefore safe from too radical alterations, especially on the chronological level. But the king list tradition was bare of any semantic specification. These documents listed only the names and regnal years, but no evaluation of the kings. My thesis is (and again I find myself in complete agreement with Redford) that the Hyksos tradition received its semantic coloring, its character as a predominantly religious conflict, only after the Amarna age, or, to be more precise, after the extinction of the contemporary generation when the Amarna reminiscences tended to get conflated with the Hyksos tradition. Only now do the Hyksos begin to play the role of adherers to an alien and antagonistic religion. The Amarna experience shaped the Hyksos tradition and created the semantic frame of the "religious enemy" which was filled afterwards by the Assyrians, the Perses, the Greeks, and finally the Jews.

My question, to resume, is not "what really happened" but what became of the recollections that must have existed, in the form of individual remembrances and collective traditions, both in Canaan of the Hyksos' sojourn in Egypt and in Egypt of the Amarna revolution. In my opinion, it is much easier to explain the survival of these memories until the Hellenistic period than their complete disappearance. Herodotus and demotic literature abound with tales, anecdotes, and fables that must have lived on in oral tradition for centuries and even a millennium. (For the case of fables, see Brunner-Traut, 1984.)

The image of the Jew as the religious enemy par excellence—the atheist, iconoclast, sacrilegious criminal, and so forth—turns out to be not a fact of experience but one of memory, that is, of *heavily distorted memory,* the product of cultural projection. The Egyptian encounter with the Jews already took place within the prefabricated semantic frame of the sacrilegious Asiatic as the religious enemy. Manetho still kept things apart. He did not write about Jews but about Egyptian lepers. The equation Osarsiph-Moses, which comes rather surprisingly at the end of his account, looks very much like a later gloss and is commonly treated as such in the literature. It was therefore only Josefus Flavius who read the story as an account of the exodus of the Jews from Egypt.

Tacitus (see Heinen, 1992) transmitted this pseudo-historical tradition to the occident, and his authority as historian imparted the dignity of authentic historical research to this product of imagination, projection, and distorted memory.

References

Anderson, Benedict. 1983. *Imagined Communities: Reflections on the Origins and Spread of Nationalism.* London: Verso.

Assmann, Jan. 1991. "Das ägyptische Prozessionsfest," in J. Assmann and T. Sundermeier (eds.), *Das Fest und das Heilige,* Gütersloh: Gütersloher Verlagshaus.

Assmann, Jan. 1984. *Ägypten: Theologie und Frömmigkeit einer frühen Hochkultur.* Stuttgart: Kohlhammer.

Baczko, Bronislaw. 1984. *Les imaginaires sociaux, mémoires et espoirs collectifs.* Paris: Payot.

Brunner-Traut, Emma. 1984. *Altägyptische Tiergeschichte und Fabel. Gestalt und Strahlkraft.* Darmstadt: Wissenschaftliche Buchgesellschaft.

Castoriadis, Cornelius. 1975. *L'institution imaginaire de la société.* Paris: Editions du seuil.

Eco, U. 1987. "Ars Oblivionalis." *Kos* 30: 40–53. Engl. "An ars oblivionalis? Forget it!" *PMLA* 103: 254–261.

Freud, Sigmund. 1939/1964. *Der Mann Moses und die monotheistische Religion,* in *Gesammelte Werke XVI.* Frankfurt: Suhrkamp.

Funkenstein, Amos. 1993. *Perceptions of Jewish History.* Berkeley: University of California Press.

Gager, John G. 1983. *The Origins of Anti-Semitism.* New York: Oxford University Press.

Gardiner, Alan H. 1938. *Late Egyptian Stories.* Bibliotheca Aegyptiaca I. Brussels: Fondation Reine Elisabeth.

Goedicke, Hans. 1986. *The Quarrel of Apophis and Seqenenre.* San Antonio: Van Siclen Books.

Halbwachs, Maurice. 1925. *Les cadres sociaux de la mémoire.* Paris.

Halbwachs, Maurice. 1950. *La mémoire collective.* Paris: Presses Universitaires de France.

Heinen, H. 1992. "Ägyptische Grundlagen des antiken Antijudaismus. Zum Judenexkurs des Tacitus, Historien V 2–13." *Trierer Theologische Zeitschrift* 101(2): 124–149.

Hobsbawm, Eric, and Terence Ranger, eds. 1983. *The Invention of Tradition.* Cambridge: Cambridge University Press.

Hornung, E. 1992. "The Rediscovery of Akhenaten and His Place in Religion." *Journal of the American Research Center in Egypt* 29: 43–49.

Kasher, Angela. 1985. *The Jews in Hellenistic and Roman Egypt: The Struggle for Equal Rights.* Tübingen: Mohr.

Meyer, Eduard. 1904. *Ägyptische Chronologie.* Berlin: Abhandlungen der Preussischen Akademie der Wissenschaften.

Redford, Donald B. 1970. "The Hyksos Invasion in History and Tradition." *Orientalia* 39: 1–51.

Redford, Donald B. 1986. *Pharaonic King Lists, Annals and Day-Books: A Contribution to the Study of the Egyptian Sense of History.* Mississauga: Benben Publications.

Redford, Donald B. 1992. *Egypt, Canaan, and Israel in Ancient Times.* Princeton: Princeton University Press.

Schott, R. 1968. "Das Geschichtsbewußtsein schriftloser Völker." *Archiv für Begriffsgeschichte* 12: 184.

Stern, Menachem. 1974–1984. *Greek and Latin Authors on Jews and Judaism,* 3 vols. Jerusalem: Magnes Press.

Waddell, G., ed. 1940. *Manetho: History of Egypt and Other Works.* Cambridge, Mass.: Loeb Classical Library.

Walton, F. R., ed. 1967. *Diodorus Siculus, Vol. XII.* Cambridge, Mass.: Loeb Classical Library.

Yerushalmi, Yosef Hayim. 1992. *Freuds Moses: Endliches und Unendliches Judentum.* Berlin: Wagenbach.

Yoyotte, J. 1963. "L'Égypte ancienne et les origines de l'antijudaisme." *RHR* 163: 133–143.

Concluding Reflections

Notes on the Cerebral Topography of Memory and Memory Distortion: A Neurologist's Perspective

15

Marek-Marsel Mesulam

Trying to unravel the relationship between brain structure and memory has been a traditional goal of neurologists, who frequently get to see patients with memory impairment. The importance of memory to all aspects of mental activity might initially lead to the assumption that all parts of the brain should play an equally crucial role in sustaining this function. This expectation appears quite reasonable when considering basic components of memory such as long-term potentiation, habituation, sensitization, and perhaps simple conditioning. Many levels of the nervous system, ranging from sensory receptors in the skin to neurons of the cerebral cortex, tend to display such modifications of activity in response to stimulation. This propensity for change (or plasticity) is an innate property of many nerve cells and accounts for much of the "memory" and "learning" displayed by relatively simple organisms. Elegant developments, such as those outlined by Abel and colleagues in Chapter 11 of this volume, have helped to unravel the cellular and molecular mechanisms associated with these aspects of memory. When viewed from the vantage point of these basic mechanisms, memory is a truly non-localizable function that permeates every corner of the brain.

If we move beyond these fundamentals and consider the conscious recall of past experience, the cerebral topography of memory assumes a surprisingly different appearance. Numerous clinical reports in the neurological literature have shown that extensive damage to the most advanced parts of the human brain such as the frontal and parietal lobes do not interfere with the conscious recall of experience. On the other hand, relatively small amounts of damage restricted to structures such as the hypothalamus, hippocampus, thalamus, and amygdala can cause severe memory disturbances known as amnestic states (Signoret, 1985).

An amnestic individual appears to be fully conscious, coherent, and intelligent, but is unable to remember the content of a conversation or the details of a crucial event that was experienced as recently as a few minutes earlier. The fact that damage to many different cerebral structures can cause amnesia might give the impression that there is no topographic selectivity to the parts of the brain associated with memory. One of the major advances in this field, however, and one that lies at the core of Squire's and McGaugh's contributions to this volume (Chapters 7 and 9), is the realization that there is a great deal of regional specificity, and that persistent amnestic states occur only if the disease process involves a limited set of widely distributed but precisely interconnected areas of the brain which collectively make up a large-scale neural network known as the limbic system (Mesulam, 1990).

A second equally major advance in this field has been the realization that memory is not a unitary process and that it can be divided into at least two subtypes (Schacter et al., 1993): *explicit* memory refers to the intentional, declarative, and conscious recollection of recently experienced events, whereas the presence of *implicit* memory is inferred when exposure to a stimulus or task influences subsequent performance in a setting (such as priming, skill learning, or autonomic conditioning) where the subject may have no conscious recollection of the original stimulus or learning experience. Damage to the limbic system impairs explicit memory but may leave implicit memory processes quite intact. For example, an individual who is amnestic as a consequence of damage to the limbic system may show nearly perfect acquisition of a complex motor skill although he may have no conscious recollection of the sessions in which he learned the task (Milner et al., 1968).

The pivotal relationship between the limbic system and explicit memory was discovered in patients with brain damage. In 1900, Bekhterev described a patient with severe memory impairment who was shown on autopsy to have bilateral brain damage which included components of the limbic system such as the hippocampus and adjacent structures of the temporal lobe (Bekhterev, 1900). A similar patient was described by Glees and Griffith in 1952, but the implications of these case reports for the neurobiology of memory were not fully appreciated until the 1957 paper by Scoville and Milner (Glees and Griffith, 1952; Scoville and Milner, 1957). In this milestone report, Scoville and Milner described the case of H.M., a motor winder who started to have seizures at the age of 10 and who suffered intractable epilepsy for nearly 20 years, at which time he was treated with a neurosurgical procedure involving the bilateral removal of the hippocampus, amygdala, and other limbic structures in the medial parts of the anterior temporal lobe.

This type of surgery had been performed before and did help to control H.M.'s seizures. However, it was soon discovered that the surgical procedure had also led to a severe loss of memory. Prior to surgery, H.M. had relatively normal memory function and an IQ of 112. After surgery, he was unable to remember new facts or experiences, no matter how important. When his family moved a few months after surgery, he could not remember the new address and continued to go to the old house. H.M. has been retested on multiple occasions. Forty years after surgery, his amnesia remains just as severe and he is unable to show meaningful conscious recall of new facts or experiences. In comparison to the memory deficit, other areas of mental function, including his above-average IQ, appear unaffected. H.M. can also acquire new motor skills such as those required for mirror drawing, although he is unable to recall the experience that led to the acquisition of the skill (Milner et al., 1968; Scoville and Milner, 1957). The meticulous clinical investigation of H.M. has led to three major insights in the area of memory research: (1) the integrity of the limbic system is crucial for the conscious recall of recent experience; (2) memory function can be dissociated from other aspects of mental activity; (3) implicit and explicit memory processes have different representations in the brain.

Numerous publications which appeared after the Scoville and Milner paper supported the view that damage to limbic structures in the temporal lobe, especially the hippocampus, could lead to severe and selective deficits of conscious recall. Additional case reports on patients who became amnestic following damage to parts of the brain outside of the temporal lobes subsequently helped to replace the relatively strict localizationist linkage between memory and the hippocampus by a network approach according to which the regions critical for the conscious recall of recent experiences took the form of an interconnected network of limbic structures, only some of which are located in the temporal lobes (Mesulam, 1990). Since the limbic system is a phylogenetically ancient part of the brain, it may initially appear paradoxical that an advanced and distinctly human faculty such as conscious recall should be associated with such an archaic part of the brain. Perhaps this linkage reflects the fact that the progenitor function evolved to register facts related to the discovery of food and the avoidance of danger.

The precise role of the limbic system in memory and learning is not fully understood. According to a recently outlined Selectively Distributed Processing model of brain function (Mesulam, in press; Seeck et al., in press), the limbic system is unlikely to be the site where memories are banked. The sensory information related to past experience appears to be stored in widely distributed form throughout association cortex. This distributed encoding displays a topography of its own so that the visual fragments of an experience are stored predominantly in visual association cortex, the auditory fragments in auditory association cortex, and so on. These sensory association areas, which are also among the most highly advanced parts of the human brain, are likely to provide the most immediate repositories of past experience. The limbic system appears to play its critical role by containing a road map or address book for binding the diverse fragments of individual events into coherent experiences. If a sufficient volume of the limbic system is destroyed, this model predicts that fragments of experience encoded in association cortex would remain intact and continue to sustain implicit memory. However, they would no longer be bound into coherent experiences that can support explicit recall. This Selectively Distributed Processing model of memory provides a neurological basis for the Parallel Distributed Processing model discussed by McClelland in this volume (Chapter 2).

Considering the immense complexity of neural circuitry in the brain, the expectation that recall should be veridical appears unrealistic. The brain does not function as a camcorder to capture replicas of individual events and store them at unique locations. According to Heraclitus, "you cannot step twice into the same river, for fresh waters are ever flowing in upon you." The process of memory evokes an analogous imagery. The recall of an experience results from specific temporal and spatial activity patterns across groups of neurons. Each neuron is likely to belong to a very large number of such groups and to be engaged by large numbers of new experiences. Each new experience is written on top of existing experiences. Consequently, each new memory is likely to be altered by previous memories and to alter existing memories. The distributed storage of memory also enables the same experience to be recalled in many different combinatorial forms and as a result of many different associative approaches.

While this dynamic organization enriches the process of recall, it also makes it vulnerable to distortion. The contributions by Loftus and Ceci to this volume (Chapters 1 and 3) provide dramatic and provocative illustrations of this vulnerability. Memory is both fragile and resilient. Although consciously experienced events may never completely disappear from memory, they are rarely, if ever, reproduced with complete fidelity. All acts of recall are also acts of imagination, retrospective reinterpretations, mini-confabulations. The tendency for distortion is not a consequence of a deficiency in brain function but a reflection of adaptive evolution. Rewards are not given for veridical reproduction but for the adaptive value of what is recalled. History books and courtrooms are full of vivid examples of this principle, a principle that is also likely to have guided the evolution of the human brain into its present form. It could even be argued that a superior talent for veridical recall could constitute a sign of brain disease. In some types of autism, for example, otherwise mentally retarded individuals, also known as "idiot savants," are capable of remarkable feats of accurate recall. These individuals cannot reorganize facts creatively, and their phenomenal memory ability is of little benefit (and is often an impediment) in the pursuit of life achievements.

Although memory processes are naturally prone to distortion, adaptive conduct requires that the resultant re-creations remain within the bounds of the reality principle. Occasionally, under severe emotional stress or after damage to certain parts of the brain such as the frontal lobes (see Moscovitch's discussion in Chapter 8 of this volume), this boundary is crossed and the re-creation of reality, including the filling-in of missing detail about the source of specific events, takes the form of implausible confabulations.

The frontal lobes are among the most highly developed parts of the human brain. The long list of complex functions attributed to the frontal lobes includes the monitoring of contextual plausibility (Mesulam, 1986). Neural networks centered around the frontal lobes could introduce context-dependent boundaries to the distortion (or noise) inherent in memory recall. Damage to certain parts of the frontal lobes could promote confabulatory tendencies by lifting these constraints. The frontal lobes tend to mature relatively late, and this may explain why children are particularly prone to confabulation.

A most dramatic form of confabulation is known as the Capgras syndrome. Patients with this syndrome have the delusional belief that family members and friends have been replaced by impostors. No evidence to the contrary is sufficient to alter this belief, and the patient confabulates extensively in order to rationalize his delusional distortion of reality. The single most frequent type of neurological setting associated with the Capgras syndrome is one where there is a partial (or recovering) limbic lesion together with superimposed damage to the frontal lobes, especially in the right side of the brain (Mesulam, 1988). The combined effects of a marginally functioning limbic system and damage to the frontal lobes appear to provide a setting particularly favorable to confabulatory tendencies.

The contributions to this volume describe some of the advances that have occurred in understanding the biological and psychological mechanisms of memory and its vulnerability to distortion. From the vantage point of the neurologist, it is becoming increasingly clear that the brain mechanisms associated with conscious recall display a rational topography. Only a very small number of brain areas are critical for conscious recall. These areas belong to a distributed neural network known as the limbic system. The core machinery for conscious recall is therefore neither diffuse nor modular but selectively distributed in the form of an interconnected network. At the psychological plane of observation, a major function that can be attributed to this core machinery is to integrate the distributed fragments of events into coherent experiences. The act of conscious recall, including the reconstruction of the relevant experiential and temporal parameters, results from interactions between components of the limbic system and components of association cortex. The architectural and computational complexity of this organization is responsible for the remarkable flexibility and inventiveness of human memory. The vulnerability to distortion appears to be a price, often modest, that has to be paid for these attributes.

This volume, and the conference upon which it is based, support the growing belief that explorations in the general areas of mind/brain/behavior are ripe for meaningful multidisciplinary approaches. The allied fields of neuroscience, neurology, psychiatry, neuroimaging, neuropsychology, and cognitive neuroscience are enjoying unprecedented growth. Although this progress has led to a deluge of new facts, relatively few comprehensive theories have emerged. Multidisciplinary approaches will be crucial for generating theories that can bridge the gap between biology and behavior. It is to be hoped that such unified theories will not confine themselves to a mere vindication of reductionism but will also make a serious attempt to add psychological, social, and humanistic relevance to the rapidly evolving biological cartography of mental function.

References

Bekhterev, V. M. 1900. "Demonstration eines Gehirns mit Zerstörung der vorderen und inneren Theile der Hirnrinde beider Schläfenlappen." *Neurologie Zentralblatt,* 19: 990–991.

Glees, P., and Griffith, H. B. 1952. "Bilateral destruction of the hippocampus (cornu Ammonis) in a case of dementia." *Mschr. Psychiat. Neurol.,* 123: 193–204.

Mesulam, M.-M. 1988. "Neural substrates of behavior; The effects of brain lesions upon mental state." In A. M. Nicoli Jr. (Ed.), *The New Harvard Guide to Psychiatry.* Cambridge, Mass.: Harvard University Press, pp. 91–128.

Mesulam, M.-M. In press. "Neurocognitive networks and selectively distributed processing." *Revue Neurologique.*

Mesulam, M.-M. 1986. "Frontal cortex and behavior." *Annals of Neurology,* 19(4): 320–325.

Mesulam, M.-M. 1990. "Large-scale neurocognitive networks and distributed processing for attention, language, and memory." *Annals of Neurology,* 28(5): 597–613.

Milner, B., Corkin, S., and Teuber, H. L. 1968. "Further analysis of the hippocampal amnesic syndrome: 14-year follow-up study of HM." *Neuropsychologia,* 6: 215–234.

Schacter, D., Chiu, C.-Y. P., and Ochsner, K. N. 1993. "Implicit memory: A selective review." *Annual Review of Neuroscience,* 16: 159–182.

Scoville, W. B., and Milner, B. 1957. "Loss of recent memory after bilateral hippocampal lesions." *Journal of Neurology, Neurosurgery and Psychiatry,* 20: 11–21.

Seeck, M., Schomer, D., Mainwaring, N., Ives, J., Dubuisson, D., Blume, H., Cosgrove, R., Ransil, B. J., and Mesulam, M.-M. In press. "Selectively distributed processing of visual object recognition in the temporal and frontal lobes of the human brain." *Annals of Neurology.*

Signoret, J.-L. 1985. Memory and amnesias. In M.-M. Mesulam (Ed.), *Principles of Behavioral Neurology.* Philadelphia: F. A. Davis, pp. 169–192.

Memory Distortion and Anamnesis: A View from the Human Sciences

16

Lawrence E. Sullivan

To bridge disciplines and establish links across levels of knowledge in the university today, Harvard has begun the Mind, Brain, and Behavior Initiative. This effort gathers neurobiologists, psychologists, historians, sociologists, economists, theologians, legal studies experts, and others. Interfaculty initiatives require focus topics that hold the attention of scholars from many specialties and offer opportunity for genuine engagement with one another's disciplinary perceptions and questions. Memory appears to be one such fruitful topic. Memory can be discussed at the level of biological mechanisms, at the level of cognitive systems, and also on the plane of history or ethnography.

Choosing memory distortion as a particular aspect of the larger issue of memory lends interdisciplinary considerations a sharper edge and an air of urgency. Memory distortion carries negative consequences for individuals and communities in such disturbing forms as personal disorientation, fractured identities, broken relations, litigious action, propagandist rewriting of the historical record, and war-time demagoguery. Memory distortion, it would seem, places human beings at risk of losing touch with their grounding sense of reality. Societies and individuals struggle to avoid these negative consequences and to preserve their grounding sense of reality. As a part of that struggle, then, we would do well to understand memory distortion and to do so with all the resources available from multiple disciplines.

Although a section of this volume is reserved for direct consideration of sociocultural cases, it is good to remember that science is immersed in the sociocultural world at all points in its proceedings and never set apart from it. Memory scientists and their remembering subjects are social actors, one and all. The scientific setting itself, with its clinics, labs, and research processes, occupies an important place in contemporary society. Scientific questions, hypotheses, procedures, and accompanying technology are part and parcel of a fascinating sociocultural history. In fact, the values that attach themselves to science are its social endowment; cultural estimations of science are among its prime motivations, rewards, and critiques. We need not leave the sociocultural world to discuss the biological mechanisms of memory. Indeed, we cannot leave the cultural world to do so, for the terms, data, and equipment that allow us to talk scientifically about memory are the product of culture in specific social locations and historical times.

Cultural Preoccupation: Resisting Memory Distortion and the Forces of Oblivion

The very issues of memory, its central importance to society, and its ramifying connections to concepts like "mind" or "historical behavior" have long been explored in diverse cultures. Some would contend that society is itself a form of memory (Connerton, 1989). Memory distortion is entangled in a knot of issues which we inherit from previous generations of thinkers. We must work with that inheritance in a self-conscious manner if we hope to make new contributions to the human discussion. Even in the compressed space of this chapter, it is helpful to sketch how steadfast and central has been the preoccupation with memory distortion and memory accuracy in myriad societies. Words like "memory," "amnesia," and "anamnesia" enjoy lengthy cultural histories full of subtle distinctions and complex theories. As a historian of religions I am particularly struck by the use of these rich terms in contemporary memory studies because they are also central ones in theories of revelation, salvation, and liturgical practice—from Plato to Roman Catholicism, and in Islam as well as in Judaism.

In the Platonic tradition, which is already a reworking of many diverse evaluations of personal memory and mythic memory in ancient Greece, truth-seeking required recollecting the world of primordial forms which the soul had contemplated in between this and its previous earthly existence. Contemplative knowledge was pure and perfect, but the reincarnated soul drank from the spring of Lethe and forgot the knowledge it had obtained from direct contemplation of the Ideas. Learning is, then, recollection and philosophy, the proper Platonic instrument for bringing to light the accurate anamnesis of the structures of the real, the archaic forms, the transpersonal and eternal truths. Memory, its distortion and its accuracy, remains at the heart of the Western philosophical tradition, from its origin, through the Gnostics and such thinkers as Augustine and Gioacchino de Fiori, to Bergson and Benjamin.

In Roman Catholicism, anamnesis refers to liturgical action which recalls, in an efficacious manner, the saving actions of Jesus. Through liturgical re-

membrance, memory distortion and the oblivion of forgetfulness are overcome, and the intentional consciousness of ritual participants is brought into
the presence of powerful events that may have preceded their own personal
existence (such as the creation of the world, the sojourn of Moses in the
desert, or the death of Christ). Ritual anamnesis makes the ritual participant
an effective and self-aware part of the memorial of remembered events. This
general, sacramental orientation of Catholicism to memory finds specific
application in a wide range of diverse memory-inducing practices, such as
the *Spiritual Exercises* of Ignatius of Loyola, the sixteenth-century founder
of the Jesuits. Inciting exorbitant memory through exercises of imagination,
and pruning memory distortions through strict disciplines of spiritual direction, Ignatius's *Exercises,* which are still widely practiced today, culminate
in the famous donation of memory to the creator. Ignatius's theory of memory (based on the alchemical techniques of "composition of place" in the
imagination) has roots in the *ars memoriae* of Greek sources concerning
Simonides and classical Latin rhetoricians as well as the Renaissance occult
magicians who rediscovered the art and passed it along to budding Enlightenment sciences (Yates, 1966; Couliano, 1987). In *The Memory Palace of
Matteo Ricci,* the Yale historian Jonathan Spence detailed the relationship
of Jesuit memory theories and practices to mystical occultists, on the one
side, and modern sciences, on the other (Spence, 1984).

Memory is so central to Islam that it may be said that "the duty of human
beings is simply to 'remember' *(dhikr)*" (Chittick, 1994, p. 52). Having remembered, humans find the original disposition with which they were created, and which allows them to understand things as they truly are. Like
the sun, the original disposition can become clouded by the distortions of
memory in the human environment but is found bright and shining when
the clouds disperse through accurate memory. The function of the prophet
is "to remind *(dhikr)*" people of what they already know but have forgotten
or have distorted through oblivion or inaccurate recall. According to the
view of the Islamic thinker Ibn al-'Arabi, the remembering soul becomes
transmuted and suffused with spiritual light, which is consubstantial with
the primordial faith of Abraham, which in its turn was a clear reflective
awareness of the luminous spirit breathed into the dark body-clay of the
first human being by the creator.

Memory without distortion is also a central concern in Judaism, where
there exist halakhic obligations to remember key events that an individual
may never have known through immediate experience. Yosef Yerushalmi
observes that, in Judaism, "the injunction to remember [is] felt as a religious
imperative to an entire people . . . The command to remember is absolute"
(Yerushalmi, 1982, pp. 9–10); this is fulfilled through the interplay of ritual
and recital which occurs at festivals. Moshe Halevi Spero has pointed out
the ritual character of memory, of observing the *mitsvot* involving *zekhirah*

(Spero, 1981). Various *zakhor* imperatives require the individual to envision, for example, that he himself left Egypt in the Exodus. The command to remember key events is often obeyed in institutionalized feasts and festivals. Sukkot and Pesach recall the Exodus from Egypt (as may the daily recitation of the *Shema*). God's ongoing battle with Amalek is remembered in the readings on the Sabbath before Purim and in the Torah reading for the morning of Purim. The remembrance of the binding of Isaac occurs in the Torah readings for Rosh Hashanah as well as in the *tahanunim* prayers recited on Mondays and Thursdays. In the same way other obligatory and devotional remembrances are lived out in ritual practice. How such feats of memory can be accomplished without distortion has been a longstanding concern in Jewish practice and theory. The concern has generated an epistemological and philosophical literature on the relationship of memory to historical knowledge, on the one hand, and, on the other hand, the relationship of ritual action to the action experienced in history (Yerushalmi, 1982, pp. 42–52, 93–95). To Rabbi Joseph B. Soloveitchik, observant memory gives the experience of history an ontical quality:

> Experiential memory . . . recalls experiences by evoking the feelings of the past event . . . whatever was horrible and frightening should be remembered as horrible and frightening, no matter how much time has elapsed since the event transpired . . . In short, when remembering the past, the Jew relives the event as if it were a present reality. (Soloveitchik, 1974, pp. 55–56; cited in Spero, 1981, p. 63)

Soloveitchik held that the ontical quality of time engendered by ritual remembering—by the fulfillment of *zakhor*—transforms the Jewish experience of existence in time. Through such observances of memory the distortions of a purely quantitative experience of time are overcome. An exhaustively quantitative time-framework creates a distorting "archaeological consciousness of periods" that never fully integrates past events into one's own existence. But the qualitative consciousness of time induced by regular ritual remembering at the festivals merges the past, present, and future into a single "historic stream of Jewish spirit" (Soloveitchik, 1966, p. 21; cited in Spero, 1981, p. 63). "We not only tell stories describing events; we tell stories precipitating the re-experiences of events which transpired millennia ago" (Soloveitchik, 1978, p. 24; cited in Spero, 1981, p. 73). "Every festival is a historical dynamo regenerating and reproducing the past into a living form of our collective spirit. It is a re-living of the whole of history from its very beginning" (Adlerblum, 1960, p. 55).

Overcoming forgetfulness and distortion through anamnesis is not only central to philosophies of the West and the Abrahamic faiths. Terms cognate and analogous to "anamnesis" may be found in many of the world's religions, each with its distinctive evaluation (Eliade, 1963). Through bodily exercises, elaborate meditations, and alchemical practices, Taoists seek to remember elaborate inner landscapes and, ultimately, the matrix from which their life (and all life) springs (Shipper, 1980; Girardot, 1983). In West African societies, memory distortion, made evident through misfortune, is sorted out in complex divinatory rites for entire social groups so that communities may understand more clearly the histories that have produced them. These are social histories of the community as a whole as well as the spiritual histories (often lengthy genealogical trajectories) of the many elements of the soul which pre-exist their assembly within a living individual (Pelton, 1979). A pivotal moment in the initiation of many Australian aboriginal societies is an experience of genuine anamnesis, recognizing one's identification with ancestors who have walked about the landscape in the great dream time and who have left signs of their passing which are consubstantial with the initiand. Such benchmark experiences of remembering—quests through geographic space and historical time transformed, through acts of anamnesis, into journeys of self-discovery—become fundamental to one's identity and beacons of certitude in the ocean of free-form experiences and memory distortions which flood day-to-day life. For Samkhya-Yoga as well as for Vedanta traditions of South Asia, the wisdom that is a goal of life and the resultant deliverance *(mukti)* from the slavery of ignorance come when the self *(atman, purusha)* recovers its memory and becomes conscious of the identity that was truly its own all along. Short of such deliverance, achieved in asceticism and meditation but also in ritual activities such as dance and in secret signs or mystical language, one sleeps in an ignorance spawned by memory distortion and forgetfulness of all the determining influences that have preceded and shaped one's existence. Sánkara, the eighth century Indian philosopher, commenting on the *Chandogya Upanishad,* remarked that such memory distortions were like a monstrous net or like the blindfold of illusion that thieves set over a victim before carting him away. He may feel lost and wandering, but, through anamnesis, the victim discovers that his true being is within him all along and is thereby freed to discover that what Being is, is the very same thing that he too is. In the Buddhist traditions of Southeast and East Asia, it is pointed out that the Buddha remembered all his former lives and was able, in this omniscient manner, to extinguish the desires that engendered the distortions of each one of them, thus bringing the cycle of rebirths to a close, abolishing the human condition of distorted memory and achieving Nirvana.

In our struggle to understand memory and memory distortion, it is amazing how little need is felt for recourse to the manifold experiences of humans in other cultures and times. And yet, how else but through some extended comparison will we grasp what is distinctive about our own questions, concepts, and tentative answers? That is, how will we get a defining sense of our own struggle to understand memory, unless we line up our attempts as one among the variants in a series of human quests to fathom memory?

One of the challenges to memory studies in the contemporary scene is how to examine more seriously the real-time experiences of memory, as exercised in cultures throughout history, within the artificially narrowed confines of the experimental sciences. There are at least two major sides to the problem: language and practice. "Memory," "amnesia," "anamnesis" and other technical terms in the many languages in which people work out their concerns are words shaped by the particular history of their use. They carry with them not only their narrow definitions—the activities that the words denote—but the wider world of connotations that have encrusted like barnacles on them as they glided through the course of time. The problem here is not simply lexical, as in the word-for-word translation of a technical term for memory distortion from some Melanesian language into English. The language problem here is cosmological: conveying adequately the meaning of the world in which such words make sense to those acting and speaking within a significantly different worldview.

As regards the second side of the problem, the aspect of practice, we must observe that, throughout history, remembering in such a way as to minimize memory distortion has rarely been a cerebral exercise only. More commonly, remembering is an elaborate act central to an entire system of ritualized bodily practices, ranging from quiet meditations, to arduous initiations, to dramatic public spectacles (Connerton, 1989). Generally, we do not have a long-practiced ritual experience lying at the basis of our knowledge about memory and find the existence of such systems difficult to evaluate. Perhaps because they do not lend themselves to existing experimental designs or perhaps for other reasons, the systems of practice most involved with cultural theories of memory have not been the subject of much serious memory research. An additional obstacle is the lack of self-conscious awareness, on the part of the experimenter, of the ritual-like character of the experimental setting, a parallelism that could be a source of sympathetic and yet scientific interest in other ritual settings involved with understanding memory.

Tracing Models and Their Histories: On Not Forgetting Sociocultural Origins and Contexts

For all its ignoring of culture and history, the study of the brain seems rife with terms taken from other cultural worldviews and periods. Those source-realms have now fallen into relative oblivion—perhaps an example of source amnesia within memory studies. Some examples may help. The hippocampus is a figure from Greek mythology and refers to the adventurous seahorse with two forelegs and a curved tail. *Amygdala* means "almond." But it is the almond as it is known through mythology and folklore, in the Mediterranean and more widely in Indo-European culture. Here the almond is the emblem of fertility and the source also of hidden but lethal power. In the history of art, the almond appears as a frame for revelations. *Synapse* is a technical term borrowed from Greek architecture. It describes a "connection" in space where two passageways join and the ceiling work is fitted so that there are no columns. Thus, "apt" means "fitting."

Many of the terms important to our memory studies have a history outside of them: thalamus, limbic, cybernetic, mechanism, parallel processing, neocortex, strategy, knock-out, system, and so on. These images and metaphors are not negligible. They organize information and pattern our thought in ways that are both enabling and constraining. Such images come from the sociocultural world and its history. The world of memory studies, through its borrowed vocabularies, is something of a cauldron of cultures and histories without really being cognizant of the fact—a symptom of its source amnesia. But the loan-words taken from history or mythology often serve only the most meager purpose: describing gross anatomy. Key organs suggest shapes vaguely reminiscent of the seahorse and the almond, for example. Such vague and static metaphors tell us little about the urgent points we wish to know more about today. We want to know about function and process, about the dynamics of systems and the interactions among levels. Finding new concepts and models of interactivity, dynamism, system, and levels of function may be precisely the area in which the coherent ideas of other cultural systems may be most helpful. But at this level of sophistication and suggestibility, more than a passing acquaintance with gross features is required. Before we delve into Islamic or Buddhist history, the dynamic patterns built into the cultural context of the very images we often extract from our own contexts, without due consideration, may help to make a point. There is a need to paint in the cultural background and history of stimulating concepts and models.

The term *parallel distributive processing* is an interesting example. It is not an ancient Greek term, although it does come from the science of computational analysis, which has an ancient history. The term gains its contemporary power of explanation, however, from the world of modern computers. Parallel distributive processing refers to the way in which long columns of numbers with multiple integers can be added in a parallel way rather than serially, waiting for each column to total before distributing an additional sum to the next column.

The image of parallel distributive processing, which is so energizing an image for at least one school of memory studies, should not be taken as a natural given, self-evident apart from the peculiar circumstances of its arising. Parallel distributive processing actually sinks one of its roots in the mystical experience of a contemporary mathematician who discovered the equation for the parallel processing of long series of numbers with multiple integers. This is Orest Bedrij, a Ukrainian émigré who worked out fundamental mathematical equations patented by IBM. Bedrij subsequently became IBM's technical director at the California Institute of Technology, Jet Propulsion Laboratory and was responsible for the development and integration of a computer complex that controlled the first soft landing on the moon (Bedrij, 1988; Bedrij, 1978). To discover the equations for parallel processing, Bedrij prayed and fasted intensely for a long period of time, as was his wont in discovering new formulas. He ceased any attempt at deliberate calculation and sat motionless facing a blank wall where the equations eventually appeared. Theories of memory that might draw their inspiration from the image of parallel distributive processing may do well to take into consideration the entire sociocultural context that led to the construction of the term and its significance. By tracing the entire process through its sociocultural world—Bedrij's theology, cosmology, and prayer practices—one uncovers the full and true dimensions of the interactive processes of mind, brain, and behavior that gave rise to the image and its explanatory power.

The full biographical and cultural tracing of Western-based "domestic-made models" (such as transformational grammar, or constructivist performance), which have already proven generative for the memory sciences, is only one side of the exploration of the sociocultural world. The other side of the effort is to hold up to view new, suggestive models from cultures less well known to practicing memory scientists. With time and sufficient familiarity, these cultural paradigms of interactivity and cultural theories of memory may provoke organizing metaphors and stimulate new models for understanding the dynamic interactions that undergird accurate memory. Borana time-reckoning and memory systems, as outlined in Asmaron Legesse's fine book *Gada: Three Approaches to the Study of African Society* (Legesse, 1973), and Ifa divination, as analyzed in William Bascom's *Sixteen Cowries: Yoruba Divination from Africa to the New World* (Bascom, 1980), stand out as strong candidates for exploration. Here are highly complicated, dynamic systems that are, at one and the same time, social performances, aesthetic expressions, information-retrieval systems, and mnemonic devices for encoding cultural and personal history. Iconic and performative, they are not centered over verbal declarations. Though they aim to be comprehensive memory repositories, they appear to be open systems, built around stochastic strategies. The same might be said of the *quipu* system (a ritual and textile-based mnemic system) of the Incas, as analyzed in a work forthcoming from Gary Urton. These cultural systems can offer richer and more complicated analogies than the unidimensional metaphors, like "synapse," which we may borrow from Greek architecture. Close examination of such dynamic cultural systems may help us imagine how every new piece of information alters memories and is altered by them and how every recall is in some way a reconstruction. It should be emphasized that reliable knowledge about such systems in non-literate societies is new (though it is often mistakenly presented in the framework of a "primitive" society), and its value in stimulating new lines of contemporary thought has yet to be appreciated.

The encouragement that Edwin Land gave to the interaction among disciplines applies also to the exchange of cultural models: "The transfer of concepts as models from one field to another requires intimacy, informality, and friendliness because the transfer usually is not a conscious process. Models for physics may come from music, for chemistry from physics, for art from cosmology . . . The great historic periods of spectacular human advance, within time spans of relatively few generations, may have been periods in which society made possible the concentrated interplay of the separate contributions of creative individuals" (Land, 1979).

The exploration of models arising in the manifold cultures of the world by the Western sciences is underdeveloped in all the sciences (Nandy, 1990). But the interplay, where it has occurred and been chronicled, is promising. One can think not only of the historical cases of Fibonacci of Pisa, who introduced Hindu and Arab mathematics into the West in the thirteenth century, and the Academy of Alphonso X in Castile and that of Marsilio Ficino in Renaissance Italy. Antonio LaFuente and his colleagues in Madrid have chronicled the influence of sciences indigenous to New World societies on Europe, especially during the Bourbon reign (LaFuente, 1992). More recently, scientists have drawn inspiration and organizing models from cultural systems outside the West, such as the Danish physicist Neils Bohr, fascinated by Taoism. Of course, occult models have also been considered exotic to mainline science. The ways in which Enlightenment scientists have drawn upon occult and magical paradigms to think "outside the box" and spur on their scientific imaginations are now better documented in the lives of Newton, Boyle, Ashmole, and Fludd. These men were all serious alchemists and considered their scientific discoveries related to their occult exercises. Ioan Couliano has traced the historical precedents (in mystical literature and practice) and comparative models of Einstein's notion of the fourth dimension in *Out of This World* (Couliano, 1992). Nikola Tesla himself, one of the great inventors of the modern period, whose discoveries undergird contemporary Magnetic Resonance Imagery technology that probes the brain, styled himself as a Serbo-Croatian magician and mystic (Hunt and Draper, 1964).

The Hidden Model of Tragedy: Connections between Memory, Misfortune, and Writing

Striking in the development of memory studies and the understanding of memory distortion is the role of trauma, misfortune, and accident. In some instances, trauma marks memorable events; in others, trauma makes more difficult the recovery of the memory. Through pathology and the study of patients who present with disorders, trauma and misfortune also figure importantly in the processes wherein researchers gain further knowledge about memory. The question arises whether failure and mishap can be staged in order to encourage accurate memory. Examining the effect of rehearsed or staged accidents on memory, as some of the researchers in this volume have done, raises the question of how religions and other ritualized activities (courtroom dramas, athletics, theatrical productions) sustain high arousal, which is conducive to good recall, even when gestures are enacted, re-enacted, and routinized. After all, memories of events do not unfold in a dry way but can be transfused with affect and even with the physiological responses original to the experience. What does it mean to enact and re-enact a crisis, in terms of the impression made on memory? Paul Connerton might claim that memory, in such ceremonialized presentations, becomes incorporated into the body. In this respect, it is worth noting how frequently religious rituals center on traumatic events or commemorate them: sacrifices, decisive battles or contests, the departures of the gods, the closing of the mythic age, the crisis of sickness or death. Divinatory rites, which often provoke elaborate exercises of collective memory as community members search their memories for behaviors relevant to problems being diagnosed, are occasioned by misfortune. Regarding rituals in general, investigators have pointed out that emotions and physiological states are often essential elements and not simply accidental by-products of ritual. Irving Goldman, for example, reported that the Cubeo people of Southern Colombia have been known to call off their important commemorative rituals in mid-stride when the appropriate emotional tone had not been achieved or when the re-presentation of past events was distorted or absent (Goldman, 1963).

Another striking aspect of recent research on memory is its dependence on words, declarations, and even writing. The subject is asked to speak, write, or identify written words; the researcher records what is said so that the written record may serve as a future benchmark for later comparison. In written culture, grounded historically on the sacrality of scripture as embodied in the unique canons of the monotheisms, we learn to think that memory can be brought before the tribunal of history, especially written history. Particularly since the time of the Protestant Reformation and its emphasis on the authority of lay literacy, we prize a notion of accuracy which holds memory accountable to written record (Frei, 1974). Even in cultures and times where written records were absent, the new standards based on literacy now prevail to judge them: the oral traditions may be seen as unreliable compared to the accuracy that a written record of events *might* have provided. Our concepts of the accuracy and "truth" of memory may be out of tune with the way most human beings have evaluated the accuracy and power of memory. Inca and Polynesian societies can remind us that complex states, built on finely calibrated collective memories, can function without recourse to the notions of accuracy inherent in our current studies and ultimately predicated on certain standards of literacy and the political economy of printing in the modern West. Ought we to deem the variants of their central accounts instances of "memory distortion"? Probably not. Rather, awareness of the fluidity of collective memory, evident in such cultural cases, should raise challenging questions to us concerning the narrow frame of assumptions about accuracy which undergird our current studies of memory distortion.

Ironically, we have written records of prodigious feats of memory in non-literate societies through the study, for example, of epic poetry recited by illiterate bards (Lord, 1960). Stunning testimonies to the accuracy of memory in non-literate societies have also been examined by the French paleontologist André Leroi-Gourhan and by the Italian rock art and petroglyph specialist Emanuel Anati. These are the prehistoric paintings found in cavernous networks in France and Spain (for example, in Lascaux, Dordogne, and Altamira). Statistical analysis has led researchers to hypothesize the existence of a finite number of fixed patterns in the complex painted structures that stretch, sometimes for miles, in the dark tunnels beneath the ground. These lengthy tunnels reveal themselves to be single works of art, with arrangements of abstract motifs set in symmetries from one end of the network to the other, and converging on a single chamber in the center. What is most amazing is that the artistic motifs, their carefully orchestrated and complex arrangements, and their overall organizational structure—all of which are quite elegant but also quite arbitrary—were remembered and transmitted over the course of thousands of years (Leroi-Gourhan, 1964). Explanations of how all this was remembered and passed along in a non-literate society veer onto much of the same theoretical ground traversed in our conference discussions of memory: constructivism, narrative structure, emplotment, deep structures, transformational grammar, and performance theory.

In non-literate societies, accuracy of memory seems assured and assessed not through writing, of course, but through a number of performative exercises: commemorative ceremonies, oaths, sacrifices, covenants, ordeals, divinations, or magical practices. From time to time, even Western literati have reappropriated these performative techniques of the art of accurate memory. My concern at this juncture is not so much to discover overt practices of the art of memory among modern researchers, but to ask whether there are other, less acknowledged assumptions concerning memory which might underlie the practices of the contemporary experimental setting.

Truth and Time in the Experimental Setting and Memory as Microcosm

Two less acknowledged assumptions seem embedded in the omnipresent notions of "replicability" and "adaptation." Both terms conjure images and constructs of memory that structure the experimental setting. The notion of replicability inserts into each instance of an experiment the implied recollectible history, past and present, peculiar to that specific series of similar experiments. Replicability inserts a notion of immutability and changelessness. "Adaptation," on the other hand, invokes the immense, remote, and speculative history of evolution, of mutability, and change as an explanation for static features that emerge in the experimental setting. Ironically, the changing history of a species accounts for the fixed features found in the current specimen. Evolutionary history is an especially spectral history "remembered" even though the researcher did not experience the events directly.

Memory distortion may be found, then, on an unexpected level—within the framing structure of experimental design itself. Founded as it is on the temporal constructs of "replicability" and "adaptation," the experimental setting may be overdetermined and have difficulties adapting to the study of memory as it is experienced in real-time cultural settings. The ability to control conditions in experimental situations is of great value. At the same time, it must be said that the experimental setting, by definition, narrows, resets, and redefines "memory" in ways that remove it from the uncontrolled associations with which memory is entangled in life outside the experimental setting. Removing the study of "memory" from the large number of cultural contexts in which it flourishes has its cost. Goethe once objected to Newton that the latter's studies of "light" did not deal much with light at all, only the spectral phenomena which Newton had forced through a prism. In order to understand light, Goethe insisted, one would have to step outside into the sunlight. So, too, our experimental studies of memory restrict the setting and perhaps even distort the meaning of the term "memory." Armed with whatever hypotheses and suggestions experimental data may furnish, we would do well to step back into the real-time cultural and historical world of societies who remember and who also have articulate theories about memory in order to customize experimental designs appropriate to the ethnographic and historical level of experience. Would it not be possible to design studies comparing the memory capacities and deficiencies of long-term meditators, specialists in ritual remembering, confabulators, and those who practice no such usages? It is important that our tighter definitions of memory and our unspoken assumptions about the relations between time, change, replicability, and truth not trivialize longstanding concepts of memory at work in historical cultures.

Through memory and the distinctive forms of human learning that memory enables, the brain helps to constitute the human individual as a self-conscious microcosm. That is, the features of the larger, macrocosmic world become known and, above all, remembered in such a way as to form a coherent world of effective images within the mind. Arranging, exploring, and manipulating the resultant system of correspondences that obtains between macro- and microcosm constitute a project of learning and memory that is both individual and collective in scope. Through memory, the history of the wider world takes up lodgings within and among individuals as an ordered, imaginal world *en miniature,* with its attendant dynamic cognitive structures, symbolic orders, and biological mechanisms. The imaginal world of memory seems constantly under renovation and, therefore, must be constantly at risk of distortion. New bits of information alter older memories and are altered by them. Not all memories are lived (some are read or taught or suggested); not all lived experiences are remembered. Our contemporary *mundus imaginalis*, formed so emphatically by the sciences, is composed of much more than current and personal associations (such as the knowledge of family members, favorite songs, or neighboring streets) or longer spans of human history (such as American history or the principles of mathematics as they are handed on from Euclid and Newton to Maxwell and Minkowski). In a way that marks modern memory with a special character, the natural sciences have also shoe-horned into human memory the representations of the remotely distant material processes that precede the existence of our human species, such as the formation of the universe and its chemical transactions, or the evolutionary development of the brain itself. The sciences represent spectacular and fantastic exercises of memory, recovering knowledge of events at which humans were not even present in the first place (the evolution of the brain, the creation of heavy elements in supernova explosions, and so on). Memory, through the system of correspondences it creates between macrocosm and microcosm, becomes the way in which human intention interiorizes the material world and insinuates itself into it at the same time. Through memory, for example, the astronomic and geological sciences become the ways in which the dramas of the material universe, which pre-exist human species, are drawn into the orbit of human understanding, intention, and will. Through the memory capacities and processes transacted by the brain, which is itself the outcome of a history of sociocultural interactions, the material universe—the elementary chemical formation of matter and other self-organizing material systems that came into being without human intention—is drawn into the purposes and accidents of the sociocultural world.

Since they live by their bold and fantastic hypotheses, however, the sciences and the microcosm informed by them in the mind also push constantly toward the edge of memory distortion, hoping that such supportive notions as "replicability" and "adaptation" will keep them from falling over that edge. As knowledge of past events expands and becomes finer-grained, human memory condenses the significant events of time into ever more economical and multivalent representations. In this way, the process of memory, as it appears to operate in the historical and natural sciences, betrays its relationship to the process of symbolization and its kinship to the sense-making process of cosmology.

Thus, memory attunes the individual to the world, drawing ever more of the outer world into relevant interaction with the inner world reflected in the mind. In accurate memory, inner microcosm maps outer macrocosm (mapping being a work of intelligent reflection, reduction, and sense-making and not a merely passive mirroring). Memory distortion, on the other hand, disrupts or fails to support the reflective, intelligent, and creative relation-ship between the world and the effective images we form of it in memory.

Of course, the talk of "inner" and "outer" worlds is suspicious, since social actors, including their brains and minds, are a significant part of the outer world. Moreover, the physical and social aspects of the world serve as the priming elements and cues which set up and trigger recall. The "outer world" must therefore be seen as an integral part of the "inner" process of memory and not just external to it. Our understanding of memory would not be well served if memory were etherealized and disembodied. By the same token, the imaginal world should not be dematerialized.

Because that material outer world, perceived through the senses, is at the same time a symbolic one, memory need not always distort but can, in an im-portant sense, accurately and effectively represent recollections even as mem-ory carries its multivalent (and sometimes ambiguous) charges of meaning and cross-reference. The game-board world created by, and constantly shift-ing in, the imagination is held in the mind through memory. This keeping-in-mind, effected by memory, allows for the manipulation and transforma-tion of the outer macrocosm in such expressions as the applied sciences, drama, learning, and rhetorical persuasion. From the point of view of the human sciences the question is: by what cultural and historical lights and by what evaluative, critical process might the mind, on either the individual or the collective level, correct itself to overcome memory distortions that may emerge while the sciences, especially the sciences of the brain and of memory, generate new knowledge and act upon it?

References

Adlerblum, Nima H. 1960. "The Collective Jewish Spirit: An Interpretation of Jew-ish Philosophy." *Tradition* 3:1 (Fall): 44–59.

Babb, Lawrence A. 1982. "Amnesia and Remembrance in a Hindu Theory of His-tory." *Asian Folklore Studies* 41 (1): 49–66.

Bascom, William. 1980. *Sixteen Cowries: Yoruba Divination from Africa to the New World*. Bloomington: Indiana University Press.

Bedrij, Orest. 1977. *One*. San Francisco: Strawberry Hill Press.

Bedrij, Orest. 1988. *You: The Essence of Science and the Spirit of Living*. Warwick, N.Y.: Amity House Press.

Chittick, William C. 1994. *Imaginal Worlds: Ibn al-'Arabi and the Problem of Reli-gious Diversity*. Albany, N.Y.: State University of New York Press.

Connerton, Paul. 1989. *How Societies Remember*. Cambridge: Cambridge Univer-sity Press.

Couliano, Ioan. 1987. *Eros and Magic in the Renaissance*. Translated by Margaret Cook. Chicago: University of Chicago Press.

Couliano, Ioan. 1991. *Out of This World: A History of Otherworldly Journeys from Gilgamesh to Albert Einstein.* Boston: Shambala.

DeConcini, Barbara. 1990. *Narrative Remembering.* Lanham, Md.: University Press of America.

Dupré, Louis. 1975. "Alienation and Redemption Through Time and Memory: An Essay on Religious Time Consciousness." *Journal of the American Academy of Religion* 43 (December): 671–679.

Eliade, Mircea. 1963. "Mythologies of Memory and Forgetting." *History of Religions* 2:2 (Winter): 329–344.

Frei, Hans. 1974. *The Eclipse of Biblical Narrative: A Study in Eighteenth and Nineteenth Century Hermeneutics.* New Haven: Yale University Press.

Girardot, Norman J. 1983. *Myth and Meaning in Early Taoism: The Theme of Chaos (hun-tun).* Los Angeles: University of California Press.

Goldman, Irving. 1963. *The Cubeo Indians of the Northwest Amazon.* Urbana, Ill.: University of Illinois Press.

Hunt, Inez and Wanetta W. Draper. 1964. *Lightning in His Hand: The Life Story of Nikola Tesla.* Denver: Sage Books.

LaFuente, Antonio, and J. Sala Catala, eds. 1992. *Ciencia Colonial En America.* Madrid: Alianza.

Land, Edwin. 1979. Address inaugurating the American Academy of Arts and Sciences. April 2, 1979.

Legesse, Asmaron. 1973. *Gada: Three Approaches to the Study of African Society.* New York: Free Press.

Leroi-Gourhan, André. 1964. *Les religions de la préhistoire (Paleolithique).* Paris: Presses Universitaires de France.

Lord, Albert. 1960. *The Singer of Tales.* Cambridge, Mass.: Harvard University Press.

Nandy, Ashis. 1980. *Alternative Sciences: Creativity and Authenticity in Two Indian Scientists.* New Delhi: Allied.

Pelton, Robert D. 1979. *The Trickster in West Africa: A Study of Mythic Irony and Sacred Delight.* Los Angeles: University of California Press.

Schipper, Kristofer. 1980. *Le corps taoiste: corps physique, corps social.* Paris: Presses universitaires de Paris.

Smith, Jonathan Z. 1987. *To Take Place: Toward Theory in Ritual.* Chicago: University of Chicago Press.

Soloveitchik, Joseph B. 1978. "Sacred and Profane: *Kodesh* and *Chol* in World Perspectives," *Gesher* 3(1): 5–29.

Soloveitchik, Joseph Dov. 1994. *Shiurei Harav: A Conspectus of the Public Lectures of Joseph B. Soloveitchik,* ed. Joseph Epstein. Hoboken: Ktav.

Spence, Jonathan D. 1984. *The Memory Palace of Matteo Ricci.* New York: Elizabeth Sifton Books, Viking Penguin, Inc.

Spero, Moshe Halevi. 1981. "Remembering and Historical Awareness. Part II: Psychological Aspects of a Halakhic State of Mind." *Tradition: A Journal of Orthodox Thought* 19:1 (Spring): 59–75.

Yates, Frances A. 1966. *The Art of Memory.* Chicago: University of Chicago Press.

Yerushalmi, Yosef Hayim. 1982. *Zakhor: Jewish History and Jewish Memory.* Seattle: University of Washington Press.

Contributors
Index

Contributors

TED ABEL, Columbia University, Center for Neurobiology and Behavior, New York, N.Y.

CRISTINA ALBERINI, Columbia University, Center for Neurobiology and Behavior, New York, N.Y.

KIM E. ARMSTRONG, Beckman Institute, University of Illinois, Department of Psychology, Urbana, Ill.

JAN ASSMANN, Ägyptologisches Institut, Heidelberg, Germany

STEPHEN J. CECI, Cornell University, Human Development and Family Studies, Ithaca, N.Y.

DENNIS S. CHARNEY, Yale University, Department of Psychiatry at West Haven Veterans Affairs Medical Center, West Haven, Conn.

THOMAS A. COMERY, Beckman Institute, University of Illinois, Neuroscience Program, Urbana, Ill.

JOSEPH T. COYLE, Harvard University Medical School and McLean Hospital, Consolidated Department of Psychiatry, Belmont, Mass.

RICHARD DASHIELL, University of Washington, Department of Psychology, Seattle, Wash.

JULIE FELDMAN, University of Washington, Department of Psychology, Seattle, Wash.

GERALD D. FISCHBACH, Harvard Medical School, Department of Neurobiology, Boston, Mass.

MIRELLA GHIRARDI, Columbia University, Center for Neurobiology and Behavior, New York, N.Y.

WILLIAM T. GREENOUGH, Beckman Institute, University of Illinois, Department of Psychology, Urbana, Ill.

YAN-YOU HUANG, Columbia University, Center for Neurobiology and Behavior, New York, N.Y.

AARON G. HUMPHREYS, Beckman Institute, University of Illinois, Neuroscience Program, Urbana, Ill.

THERESA A. JONES, Beckman Institute, University of Illinois, Department of Psychology, Urbana, Ill.

MICHAEL KAMMEN, Cornell University, Department of History, Ithaca, N.Y.

ERIC R. KANDEL, Columbia University, Center for Neurobiology and Behavior, New York, N.Y.

JEFF A. KLEIM, Beckman Institute, University of Illinois, Department of Psychology, Urbana, Ill.

JOHN H. KRYSTAL, Yale University, Department of Psychiatry at West Haven Veterans Affairs Medical Center, West Haven, Conn.

ELIZABETH F. LOFTUS, University of Washington, Department of Psychology, Seattle, Wash.

JAMES L. MCCLELLAND, Carnegie-Mellon University, Department of Psychology, Pittsburgh, Pa.

JAMES L. MCGAUGH, University of California, Center for the Neurobiology of Learning and Memory, Department of Psychology, Irvine, Calif.

MAREK-MARSEL MESULAM, Northwestern University Medical School, Behavioral and Cognitive Neurology and the Alzheimer Program, Departments of Neurology and Psychiatry, Chicago, Ill.

SUSAN MINEKA, Northwestern University, Department of Psychology, Evanston, Ill.

MORRIS MOSCOVITCH, Erindale College, Department of Psychology, Ontario, Canada

PETER NGUYEN, Columbia University, Center for Neurobiology and Behavior, New York, N.Y.

KATHLEEN NUGENT, Northwestern University, Department of Psychology, Evanston, Ill.

DANIEL L. SCHACTER, Harvard University, Department of Psychology, Cambridge, Mass.

MICHAEL SCHUDSON, University of California at San Diego, Department of Sociology, LaJolla, Calif.

STEVEN M. SOUTHWICK, Yale University, Department of Psychiatry at West Haven Veterans Affairs Medical Center, West Haven, Conn.

DAVID SPIEGEL, Stanford University–School of Medicine, Department of Psychiatry and Behavioral Sciences, Stanford, Calif.

LARRY R. SQUIRE, Department of Veterans Affairs and University of California at San Diego, Department of Psychiatry and Neurosciences, San Diego, Calif.

LAWRENCE E. SULLIVAN, Harvard University, Center for the Study of World Religions, Cambridge, Mass.

RODNEY A. SWAIN, Beckman Institute, University of Illinois, Department of Psychology, Urbana, Ill.

Index

Abreaction, 163
Absorption, 130
ACTH, 257
Actinomycin D, 314
Activation of mental representations, 186
Activity, vascular response to, 277
Adaptability, 220
Adaptation, 396–397, 398
Adenosine 3′,5′-cyclic monophosphate, 303–306, 314–315
Adenylyl cyclase, 303, 306, 314
Adrenaline, 318
Adrenergic system, 258–260, 264–265
Age of Jackson, 332
Agoraphobia, 182, 183
Akhenaten, 366–375
Alcohol, effects of chronic exposure on dendritic morphology, 280–281
Alcott, Bronson, 342
Alexithymia, 158
All the President's Men (Woodward and Bernstein), 356–357
American foreign policy, 335–336
American history, distortion of, 329–345
American presidents: distortion of collective memory of, 336–337; abuse of powers of office by, 349–350
Amnesia: defined, 133; drug-induced, for treating PTSD, 162; impaired explicit memory with, 177–178; neuroanatomical studies of, 200–202; preserved memory functions in, 203–206; impaired recogni-

tion memory in, 209–210; source memory studies of, 216–218; regarding racial issues, 334–335; structural, 366; brain structures involved in, 379–380; after surgical removal of limbic system, 380–381. *See also* Confabulation; Dissociative amnesia; Functional amnesia; Hypnotic amnesia; Infantile amnesia; Korsakoff's syndrome; Retrograde amnesia; Source amnesia
Amphetamine, 257, 263
Amputation, effect on representation area, 286–287
Amygdala: role in emotion-related memory, 26, 259–264; role in fear conditioning, 151, 153; role in behavioral sensitization, 154; memory functions of, 207; synaptic plasticity after training, 262–263; hormonal effects on memory storage in, 318; etymology of term, 391, 392
Amytal, 162
Anamnesis, role in world's religions, 386–400
Anisomycin, 314
Anosognosia, 229, 230, 231, 319
Anterior communicating artery, 227, 230–231, 241
Antianxiety drugs, 162
Antidepressants, 164–165
Antijudaism in Ancient Egypt, 365–376
Anxiety, 173–189; Beck's schemata model for, 175; attentional bias in, 176–177;